GROUND

BOOKS BY NATUREZA GABRIEL

praise for *Restorative Practices of Wellbeing*

"A remarkable book."
—Dr. Stephen Porges, Developer of the Polyvagal Theory

"An excellent guide to wellbeing and wholeness that is greatly needed today ..."
—Ilarion Merculieff, President of Global Center for Indigenous Leadership and Lifeways

"A treasured cookbook for the spirit."
— Roshi Fleet Maull

praise for *Keywords: A Field Guide to the Missing Words*

"An extraordinary way-finding to what is missing, what has been cut out of the heart of humanity and which can be fully restored by our attention ... Gabriel is making our way of being holy again by the quality of attention he brings to the words that are missing, re-storing and re-connecting us with the ineffable so we can re-member ourselves into our ancestral future."
— Peter Tavernise

praise for *The Neurobiology of Connection*

"Truly a masterwork, this is a rare combination of scientific insight, spiritual wisdom, and practical tools for daily life. Beautifully written, it's warm and inviting, like a clear path through green forest groves. Poetic, personal, comprehensive, and endlessly useful, in these pages you're in the company of a brilliant and warm-hearted guide to lasting well-being, love, and inner peace."
— Rick Hanson, PhD, author of *Buddha's Brain: The Practical Neuroscience of Happiness, Love, and Wisdom*

"A marvelous text, full of brilliant trans-disciplinary insights!"
— Darcia Narvaez, PhD, Developer of the Evolved Nest

> "You shall claim your rightful inheritance through the soles of your feet..."
>
> – J. Ariel Guy, quoting a passage from the Talmud that we have not since been able to find

GROUND

NATUREZA GABRIEL

© 2025 Jaguar Imprints & Hearth Science, Inc.

v. 11112025

All rights reserved. No part of this publication may be reproduced, stored in a retrieval system or transmited in any form or by any means, electronic, mechanical, photocopying, recording or otherwise without the prior permision of the publisher or in accordance with the provisions of the Copyright, Designs and Patents Act 1988 or under the terms of any license permitting limited copying issued by the Copyright Licensing Agency.

Published by
Jaguar Imprints
PO Box 567
Nicasio, CA 94946

THIS IS NOT A BOOK.
THIS IS AN INITIATION.
PREPARE ACCORDINGLY.

GROUND

HOW MODERNITY DISCONNECTED FROM THE EARTH, WHY IT MATTERS, & HOW TO FIX IT

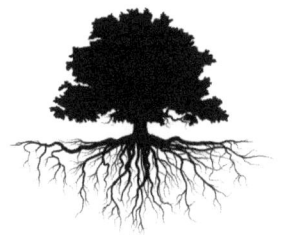

NATUREZA GABRIEL
DEVELOPER OF AUTONOMICS

CONTENTS

Fractal	xv

Setting the Stage

01- Introduction	1
02- Ladder	5
03- Blind Leading the Blind	12
04- Necrotic Neuroscience	17
05- Grounding System	24

Civilization

06- Yoga Class	30
07- War	35
08- Death's Head	41
09- Digging out the Taproot of Supremacy	45
10- Heirarchy	52
11- Tragic Exiles	58
12- Original Exile	63
13- Cain & Abel	71
14- Deepest Belly of Forsaken	79
15- An Intrusive God	92

16- Always Digging Out	94
17- Prohibition on Lamentation	102
18- The Nike of Samothrace	112
19- Inverting the Logic of Enclosure	120
20- Wrong Angles	134
21- At the Origin of Consciousness, A Crime Scene	153
22- Gate of Union	162
23- Toiling in a Mine	171

Lineage

24- Archeology of Shadows	178
25- Descent	182
26- Localized Shutdown	190
27- Fishmonger	195
28- Father of Fathers	199
29- Feet Not Touching the Ground	205
30- Clear Seeing	208
31- How the Wound is Passed	212
32- Variants of Shutdown	218
33- Everyday Powerlessness	228
34- Archeology Again	233
35- I Cannot Bear It	239
36- Sweep it Under the Rug	248
37- Dream the Deepest Shutdown	252
38- Line the Ancestors Up	260
39- Sometimes God is a Blade	270

Physiology

40- The Grounding System	279
41- Diseases of the Grounding System	282

42- Eat More Dirt	292
43- Trinity	298
44- Refined Sugar	304
45- The Body is the Sacrifice Site	309
46- Permeability	319
47- Open to Something that Hurts Us	322

Activism

48- Audacity	333
49- Ancestral Fireplace	337
50- Observations Derivative Thereto	341
51- Furthermore	345
52- Breathe	349
53- Allowing	352
54- Full Spiral	377

Resources

Grounding Practices	385
Illnesses	392
Autonomic Mandala	394
An Interview with Natureza Gabriel	396
About the Author	405

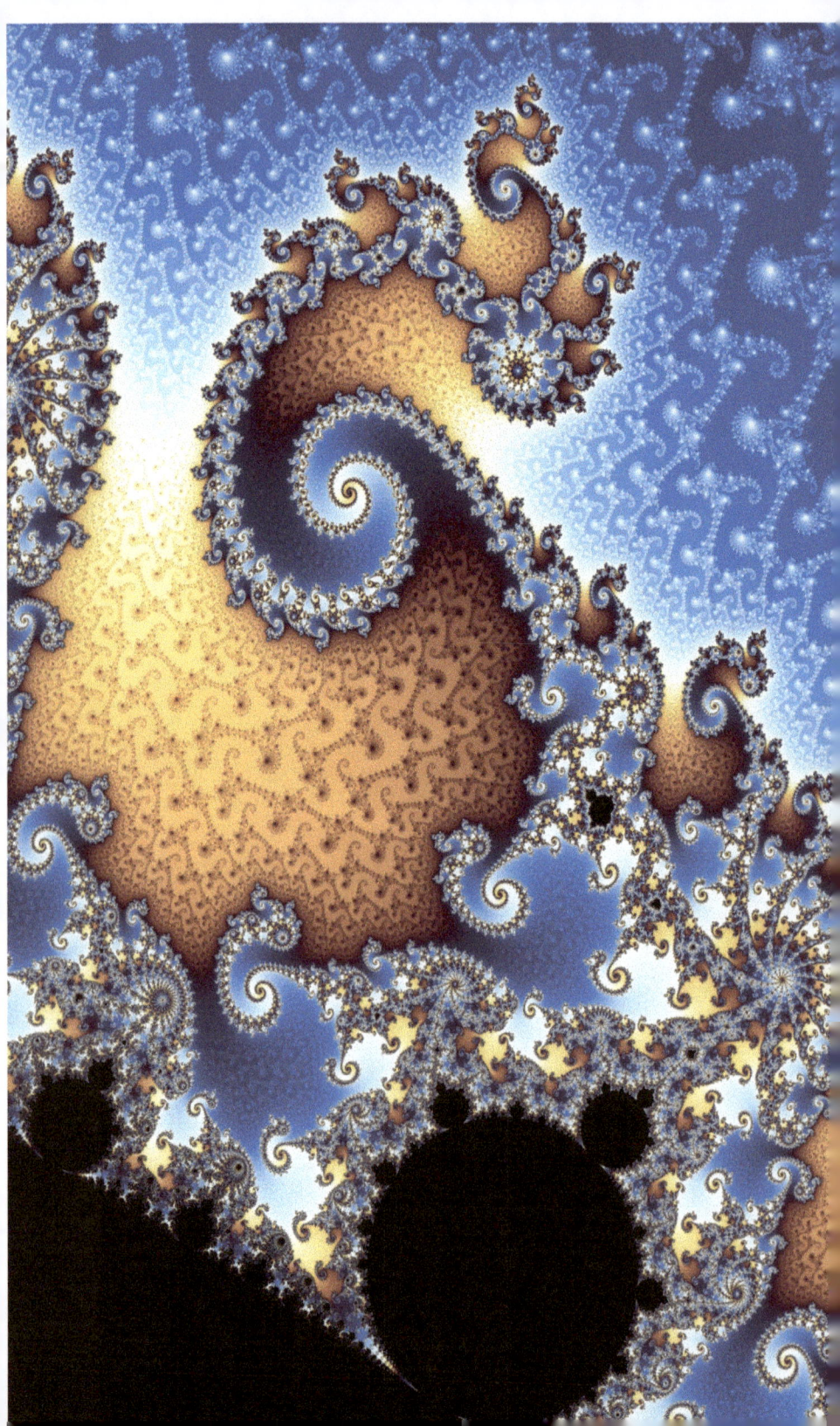

Fractal

This is the second book in the Autonomics Trilogy, which began with *The Neurobiology of Connection*. My objective in the trilogy is to treat, as deeply as possible, and with as much poetry as science, on the three primary autonomic neurological systems that comprise the mammalian ANS. I have been accused of writing about culture as much as I am writing about neurology, and you can decide whether this accusation has merit. I am concerned with *meaning* and how all of this matters deeply to our lives. I do not wish to separate how the neurology works from the societal, cultural, and civilizational contexts in which it is operating, because they fundamentally inform one another, for better and worse.

Writing for me is as much a process of exploration as of exposition– I write both to learn what I know, and to share it. I experience the act of writing as a way-of-knowing, and at the outset of this second book I'd like to let you know that although *GROUND* is part of this trilogy, and while the name is largely a reference to the GROUNDING SYSTEM, our oldest sub-diaphragmatic autonomic neurology, the method, articulation, and meaning-making of this book is different than the previous one. Perhaps this is because I am attempting, in this series, to let the respective neural architectures themselves author the book.

In *The Neurobiology of Connection*, it was my own connection system speaking with you. This elocution– of the face, heart, and hands– had a certain timbre, a certain cadence, and ways of unveiling itself that felt fundamentally conversational. As though we were having coffee together, or telling stories around a campfire, that book spoke itself known. Now, it is my grounding system authoring. And this ancient unmyelinated system, with its chthonic neurology whose throne is the deep belly, whose intelligence is the hara, its ability to present through whispers arising across the soles of the feet, the earth itself speaking upwards into my body, has birthed an entirely different logic.

The story that wants to be told here is a story of our uprooting from the earth, and this is a civilization-long story that begins about twelve thousand years ago. The story that wants to tell itself through my hands, through fingers typing, makes its way to me up out of the earth, in a pattern of her fundamental rhythms, and in gestalt. Holisms recursive.

When we have a gut feeling, it is not precise the way that a facial expression is. In the domain of the connection system, we are dealing with the slightest head nod, a quick gaze, crinkles around smiling eyes. Yet the deep belly speaks, at least to me, through a different kind of knowing. It speaks synechdocally: a part standing in for the whole. A full figure; something talismanic.

And it is this knowing that I have permitted to govern the architecture of the book. It will require that I tell three different layers of story. One about our civilization, which will take the form of a series of essays. One about my family of origin, that would probably be genred as memoir. And one about the nature of the sovereign body, and what happens when it is denatured by domination, that is a proper autonomic story.

On the page previous is a close-up of part of the Mandelbrot Set, the visual display of an iterative equation that creates an image commonly known as a fractal. Fractals are self-similar at varying levels of scale. Which is to say that you can see the recursion of patterns at small and large sizes. You can zoom in on the image infinitely, and it will continue to repeat its pattern language. Fractality is one of the fundamental design languages of nature. Benoit Mandelbrot is credited with discovering fractals, but it would be more accurate to say that he translated them into mathematical language. Nature has been designing this way since always. Life is fractal. Light is fractal. Fractality is a meta-pattern for experience.

This book has arrived as a fractal. It is recursive at several levels of scale, and will explore a set of meta-patterns that operate from the level of civilization, to the level of the family, to the individual life, all the way down to cellular and molecular levels.

Because the story I need to tell here is self-similar at varying levels of scale, there may be times when I need to jump from one scale to another and then back. Studying the pattern may help you become more comfortable with this narrative motion pattern, which is not linear, and therefore possibly not the narrative pattern you have been acculturated to expect. Yet your right brain already knows how to do this. If you make art, or music, go tracking, or enter a flowstate, you are doing it anyway. Like I said, it is how Nature designs.

And so, an inquiry into the Grounding System, through three related fractal inquiries: what happened to our grounding systems collectively as we, civilizationally, deviated from the deep ancestral baseline in safety and connection. What happened in my own family over the past several generations that conditioned the autonomic environment in which I grew up, and ultimately escaped from, and finally a proper inquiry into the physiology of these systems themselves.

I provide this brief interlude as orientation, particularly as some of the early readers of this text familiar with my writings on autonomic physiology were not quite sure what to make of the discourse on civilization or the memoir. Oriented thusly to impending disorientation we begin.

-*Natureza* Gabriel

01-Introduction

I begin with the ritual of making myself a cup of tea. Water in a kettle. Bluelick of flame. Sachet in earthenware cup.

It was 1:53 am by my clock when I rose, early in the morning, very. But I didn't open my eyes until I had lain for some time in bed, assessing my body, determining I was truly awake. I stopped setting an alarm years ago. These days, my sole metric for arising is the body clock. Outside, it is a sunday January in early 2025, long before dawn. I can hear the wind rustling the bushes, raking its fingers through the scraggly heads of palm trees.

The moon is nearly full, something I ascertain visually descending the stairs- the rear quadrant of our backyard is silvered by her light. Stepping out a luminous stillness pervades.

Before I drink, sitting at the breakfast table where I write, I inhale the steaming cup. Currents of rising air are visible on its surface, and it smells of woodsmoke, tar, and soil. The name for this tea, *Lapsang Souchong*- pine wood small sort- refers to the pine wood it is smoked over, and the fact that these are the smaller leaves of the plant, the fourth and fifth picking. The originating legend of the tea is that it was created in China in 1646 by villagers in the Wuyi mountains of Fujian province who were fleeing Qing soldiers advancing through their area on the Manchu unification campaign. Before they fled, to avoid spoilage of the newly picked leaves, they accelerated their drying over pinewood fires, and then buried the tealeaves in sacks. This explains their characteristic bite of smoke and why they exhale earth. Partially oxidized, the tea was a hit with the Dutch traders who needed some form of preservation to get it back to Europe over several months in the hold of a ship without succumbing to rot. They kept asking for more.

The elemental alchemy of fire, water, plants, and earth yields, on the one hand, this ritual libation in my cup: a ceremony at the inception of this book. On the other hand, five hundred miles south, Los Angeles is on fire. A slightly different alchemy, a reverse alchemy if you will, has seen ignite, over the past four days, the most expensive and culturally devastating wildfires in the history of that city whose founding nightmare certainly involved immolation. Carved from the desert with water borrowed from elsewhere, the city of angels stars in the paradisiacal dream of California.

The dark twin of the silvering of my backyard by moonlight is a photograph I saw yesterday in *The New York Times* of houses reduced to ashen footprints punctuated by eerily intact chimneys, cars wireframed husks of themselves, in the foreground some metal leakage– the car's melted battery?– now formless: a puddled slick of quicksilver.

There is one rule, and one rule only that I have given myself for this book, which is that when I sit down to write I take off my shoes. That each writing session begins with my feet on the ground. My prayer is that the book arrives as an upload from the earth.

I write to understand what I know, and to become more deeply who I am. I write like a blind man feeling his way around a cave, memorializing its contours in the close dark. I write to consolidate memory, to assemble strands of thinking and feeling and sense-making into a tapestry of meaning-making in which I can clothe myself. I am writing *to* you, but I am writing *for* myself, to clothe myself in the deep coherence of earth, her many ancient tongues. To unite my body with her heartbeat.

I need to unite these strands of deep history, and imperial domination, and the long history of displacement in my family, with an understanding of my own neurophysiological process of healing, and an analysis of why the modern world is collectively enacting a suicide narrative. I want a working model of how humanity has become untethered, how our roots have been cut, how we find ourselves as a collective out here floating in outer dark, how the best dreams we can seem to muster are the imaginings of batshit-crazy apocalyptic dickhead billionaire thieves whose feverdreams are of exiting the only biosphere in the known universe in flamboyantly fire-powered models of their imaginary fully-erect cocks.

So that they can go fucking where? To Mars? A war planet of lifeless ochre dust?

I'd like to trace the pathway of how we got so lost, but more importantly I would like to write new neural pathways for how we might get found. I am always and forever writing about how we might get home...that is the deepest compass in my blood.

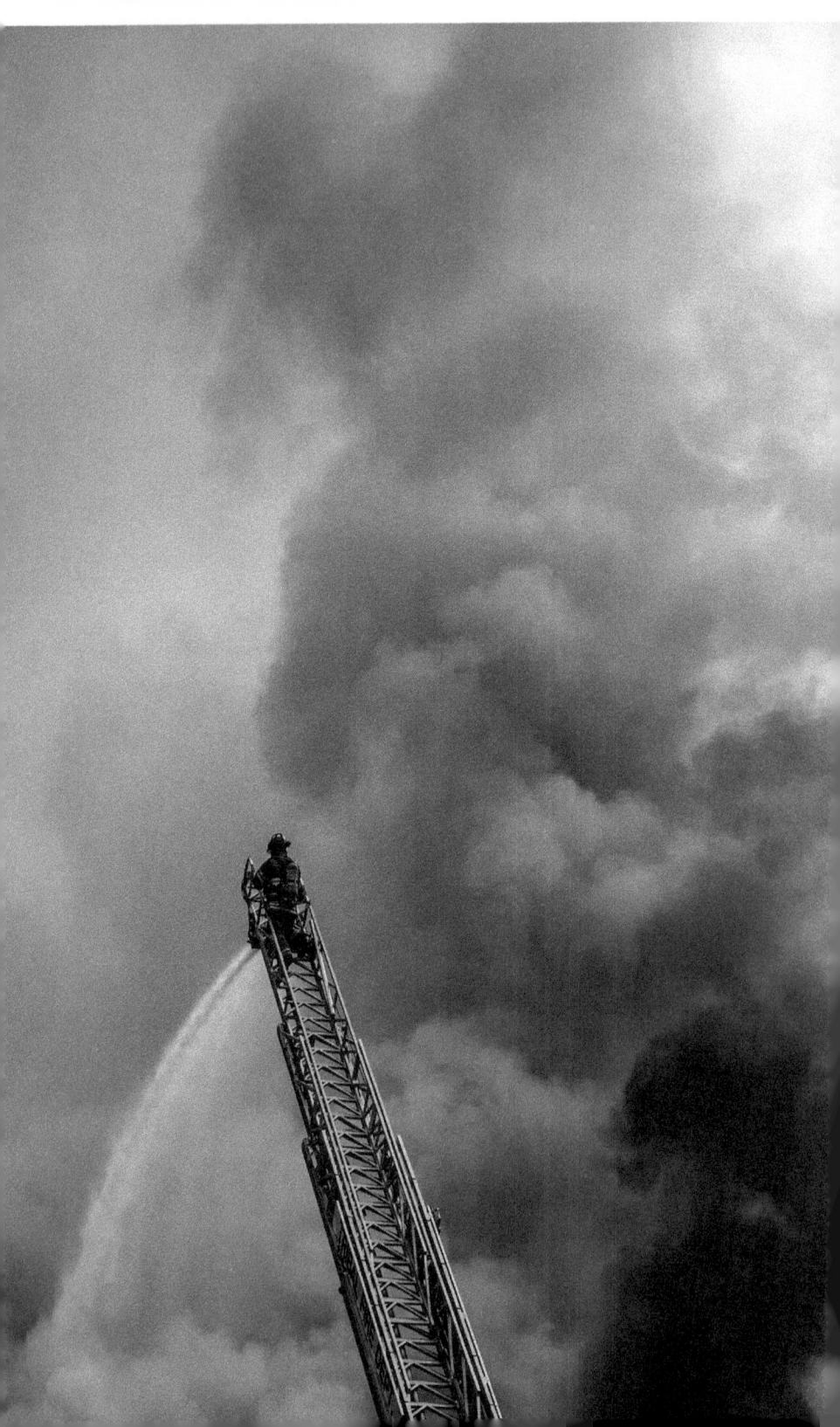

02-The Ladder

My thesis is fairly straightforward: we can examine it together and decide whether or not it has merit. It seems to me that something has happened in our lineage history in the process of becoming 'modern', or more specifically in the process of developing a modern notion of self, that we conceptualize in terms of a uniquely contemporary sense of identity or consciousness of what it means to be 'human', but that seems to me in actuality the neurobiological sequelae of a physiological alteration in the individual and collective normative neurological baseline of humanity as a result of individual, multi-generational, and civilizational trauma: a normalizing of alienation. I am proposing, at the outset of the book, that our modern notion of self – how we experience the intimacy of our private inwardness – is a neurological byproduct of alienation.

Our modern experience of identity is an epiphenomen of alienation.

I've been circling these thoughts for years, spiraling around them like a raptor rising on thermals, but I want to distill the pattern here so we can make good use of it together. The contemporary emanation of this thoughtform was accidentally distilled by Descartes, whose utterance *Je pense, donc je suis* [I think, therefore I am] is among its simplest formulations. Descartes wrote this phrase in the *Discourse on Method* in 1637, 388 years ago. The legacy of this assertion locates identity firmly in thinking, an activity that takes place in the cranial brain. One of its significant corollaries, which follows firmly in its wake, gives rise to the modern neuroscience with which we are familiar. Its broad contours would be as follows: *I think, therefore I am.* The organ in which thinking takes place in words and pictures, therefore, has pride of place in our neurology. This organ is the cranial brain, therefore the brain is the centerpiece of our neurology, because it is where identity resides.

The Cartesian frame is, in my view, the consolidation of a trend that began to accelerate in earnest about 12,000 years ago, but whose *acceleration has accelerated*[1] over the past 500 years exponentially, and is doing so again in this age of artificial intelligence.[2] I would like to argue that 'Je pense, donc je suis' is co-equal and contemporaneous with another related thoughtform, distilled most notably in the papal bull *Inter Caetara*, of 1493, and which gave to the Catholic Kings of Castile and Leon, based on the asserted apostolic authority of the Catholic church, ownership of the earth entire: all latitudes and longitudes outside the then-present dominion of European christian kings. This assertion of absolute *spiritual* authority, which became the subsequent foundation of *legal* authority, and the political expedience that gifted imperial domination rights to Catholic kings, is but the most current and present-world-order-informing example of an imperial logic of domination. What is implicit in this construction, which established both the spiritual and legal basis of colonialism, is the notion of ownership of the earth and its inhabitants.

Relations of ownership are predicated on hierarchy. Hierarchy

---

1 In physics, the acceleration of acceleration is called *jerk* (the third derivative of position with respect to time). A vector quantity, it is often used in engineering and mechanics to describe comfort in transportation, or to analyze the destructive effects of motion of machinery. In this era of endstage capitalism, AI accelerationism, and climate catastrophe we are collectively feeling the jerk as a sense of being thrown about by increasing ambient chaos.

2 For the cultural and evolutionary timelines of this deviation from the ancestral baseline, see the work of Darcia Narvaez, Ph.D., including the concept of the Evolved Nest. See *Neurobiology and the Development of Human Morality*, 2014.

is necessarily organized on a vertical axis. Empires require both an elite and an exploited class. If you are going to privilege one group of people with more of something, you have to extract the surplus you are giving them from someone (or somewhere) else. Imperial mechanics are the extraction of life and labor from a group that is exploited, and its systematic transfer to a group that is elite. A group below becomes the base of labor and life that is extracted to send surplus to a group above. The emperor (in the latin: *auctoritas, augustus, potestas, imperium, potentia, licentia, ius, etc.*) sits atop this hierarchy.

Emperors worship skygods, by definition.

Since Jesus, whose religion became officialized in the Roman Empire in 380 AD when Emperor Theodosius I issued the Edict of Thessalonica, was not a skygod by his own word, the Romans had to turn him into one.

Why does empire require skygods? Because hierarchy is a ladder, and humans are quite literal. In order to be a ladder, the rungs must ascend and descend. At the top of the earthly ladder is the Emperor, whose position and body concretizes the apex. The emperor's claim to authority *(auctoritas)* is that it derives from divine right, mirroring a celestial hierarchy. And because (unfortunately) we create cosmology in our own image, there is thus a corresponding celestial ladder, and at its top a skygod, because held within the sway of the earth's gravitational field, sky is the top.

Empires tilt monotheistic, because the skygod references the Emperor, and there is but one of each. Animistic and polytheistic traditions undercut absolute authority; they confuse the matter of who is in charge. So in Empire there is *THE* skygod.

Jesus, whose profound humility precluded him being an obvious candidate for such elevation, was therefore re-sized by the Romans, re-moved from the earthly plane, and re-located to the Celestial. From his doctrine, which was largely horizontal (he never once referred to himself as the Son of God, but always as the Son of Man) were excised all of the chthonic and earth-based elements, the Nature worship, the elevation of the feminine. Half of the teachings were destroyed so thoroughly there is no official trace remaining, until the religion was tailored to the political requirements of an imperial mind with the precision of a Saville Row suit[3].

Because the earthly ladder has a top and a bottom, and because authority is fixed at the top and systematically denied at the bottom, the corresponding celestial scheme is the same. At the top is the skygod, at the bottom its opposite. If you know anything about Aramaic, the language that Jesus spoke, and anything about how he referred to the Divine, this is already confusing, because one of the many names that he used for the Divinity, in its sovereign Queendom, is 'the One with no Opposite.' The word *alaha* in Aramaic, which shares etymology with the Arabic word *Allah*, and is often translated as 'sacred' literally means 'the One with no Opposite.' The configuration of an antagonist to the Creator, an inverted image, someone at the bottom of the ladder, was again necessitated by imperial mind.[4]

What I would like to focalize here, to bring strongly to your attention, is the correspondence between a theory of self that localizes identity at the top of the ladder (brain-centric), and a theory of social organization (imperial) that localizes authority at the top of the ladder. Both of these constructs are

---

3 Saville Row is the street in London's Mayfair district globally famous for its traditional high-end bespoke tailoring for men.

4 Imperial mind elevates the importance of the demonic, in which Jesus was not particularly interested. The most common word Jesus actually used for evil means 'unripe' in Aramaic. Jesus dealt with evil the way eagles deal with crows: primarily ignoring them, destroying them if they get too close, annoying, or dangerous. Imperial mind, by contrast, requires a fixation, fascination, terror of, and engagement with the demonic, because imperial mind is schizophrenic and needs to examine the negative pole. See for example the Renaissance Italian obsessions with measuring the thickness of the rooftop of Hell, and apocalypse merchant Peter Thiel's fixation on the Antichrist.

premised on verticality. Synonyms for the top of the ladder? *Divine. Heaven. Sky. Father. Head. Goodness. Self. Brain. Identity.* This is not an accident.

There are several questions that I would like you to ask yourself. The first is *How did the earth under our feet become equated with Hell?* Because that is what has happened, it was a sleight of hand, a unique byproduct of the thoughtforms of western civilization, and done on purpose. By way of evidence, I suggest to you the following simple experiment. Talk to someone who was raised in a non-christianized part of Asia, and ask them to complete the following sentence: *Heaven and...*

What they will likely say is *Earth*. I don't need to tell you what a person raised in a western context will say, because you've already said it in your mind, and it was not Earth. So how did this happen? How and why are we so disconnected from the Earth that we have had the psychic necessity to disfigure Our Mother into a hell realm? What dark magic is that?

Given that the Good Earth provides literally everything our bodies require- the air we breathe, the food we eat, the water that we drink, all of the materials that we use, literally everything that we will be in contact with for our entire lives, assuming we don't ascend in Elon's squat rocket-dick to Mars- how is it that we have confused this earthly paradise for hell? Because this confusion in the basement of the modern psyche is part of why we are turning this earthly paradise into hell.

The second question that I would like you to ask yourself is, *What happened to the horizontal axis?* The vertical axis of Empire is perpendicular to the horizontal axis of relating. The vertical axis, concerned with domination and subjugation, has an entirely different set of concerns than the horizontal, which is concerned with kinship and reciprocity.

How have we birthed (stillbirthed) a civilization (so-called) and a sense of self (so-called) where both our forms of social organization and our sense of identity are so firmly entrenched in a domination paradigm? Where the primary metaphors through which we organize self and society are transactional and based on seeking power over, where our metaphors for success are figurations of the thoughtforms of annihilation?[5]

We want to control our bodies, curate their appearances and how we are seen. We want to be photographed in certain light at the angle that gives us the finest jawline. We want to subjugate our insecurities, to crush and kill them and we speak to them in a language of command and control. To destroy our vulnerabilities not embrace them. We want to be rich and we don't care how the coin comes to us. We want to be the boss: firmly in charge. We want to be at the top of the ladder, and because of physics, this means pushing someone or something else down to get ourselves up higher. How and why did this happen? What is the furious engine of all this psychic displacement? What on earth are we so afraid to feel?

---

[5] In some of the milieus I inhabit, if you ask someone to explain a work success, they will talk about 'killing it', 'crushing it', or 'destroying'. Without considering it, we clothe our notions of success in the casual language of war. In the United States, where I reside, federal civic 'celebrations' are demonstrations of annihilation packaged as entertainment and pageantry. A recent military celebration featured the shooting of live ordinance over a California highway that had to be shut down while this was happening, with the not astonishing result that some of it exploded prematurely (imagine! ordinance exploding!) and damaged police vehicles parked on the thoroughfare.

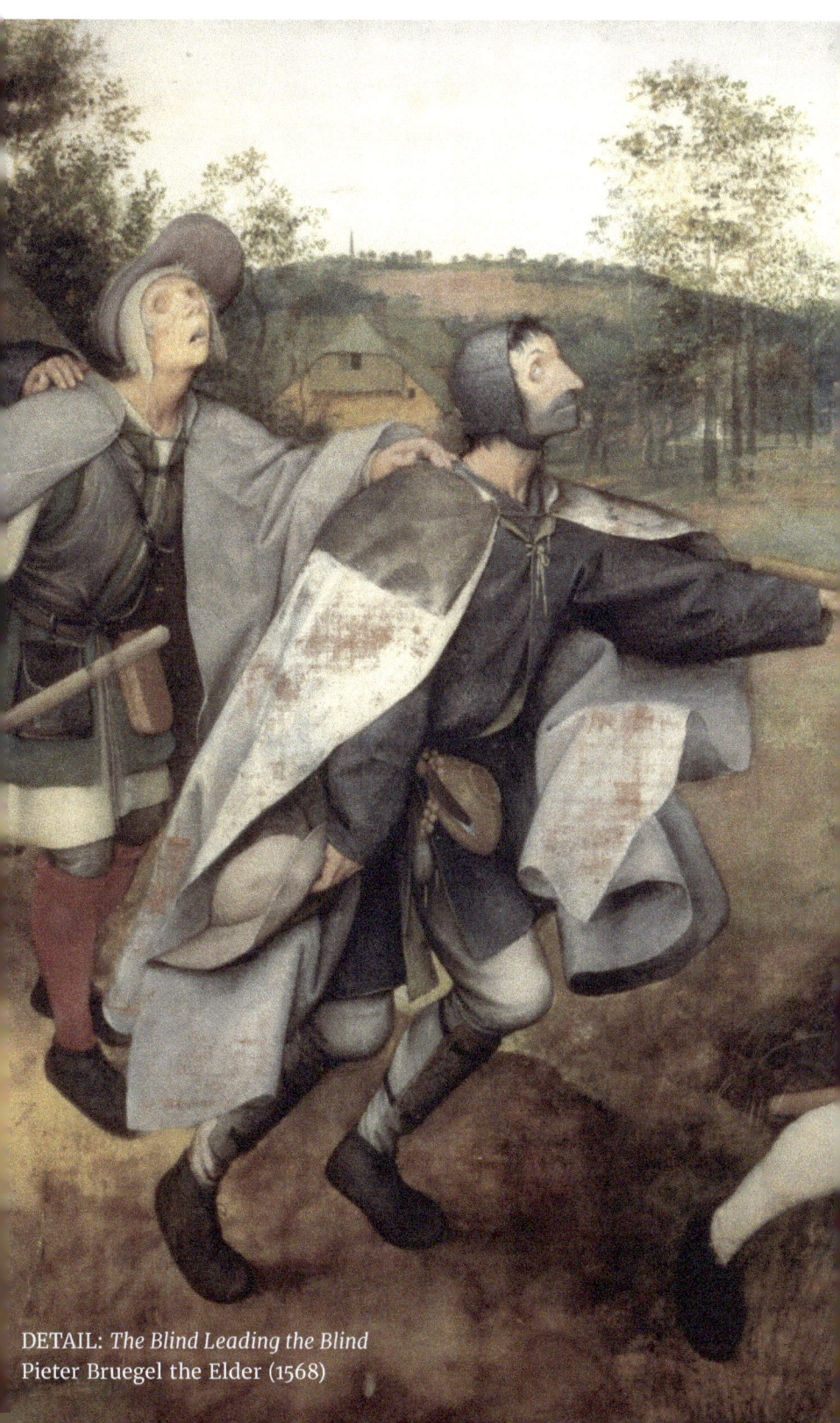

DETAIL: *The Blind Leading the Blind*
Pieter Bruegel the Elder (1568)

03–Blind Leading the blind

Somehow, despite our advanced biochemistry, precision medicine, 3D imaging of the body entire, engineering ability to catch a rocket on a pair of chopsticks, two nanometer transistors, large language models, and a hundred and fifty years of neuroscience, modern medicine and mental health do not understand the Autonomic Nervous System AT ALL. I say this with confidence because the organization I founded has validated a new foundation model of autonomic physiology, *Autonomics*, that successfully contradicts several hundred years of established neuroscience, essentially crashing the discipline like an antique hard-drive.[1]

We have redrawn the functional maps undergirding the autonomic systems and their coordination, going back to fundamental principles of neurogenesis and axon growth, having demonstrated that the physiological models (unlike neuro-anatomical models, which are concerned with neural structure, neuro-physiological models are concerned with how neural systems function *in vivo*) undergirding the mainstream conceptualization of autonomic responses to safety, danger, and lifethreat[2] have been structurally incomplete or flat wrong for the past two hundred years.

---

[1] See the Hearth Science whitepapers, *Towards an Accurate In Vivo Reconceptualizing of Autonomic State, A Typology of Chronic Defensive Autonomic States as Specific Antecedents to Disease Etiology,* and *AUTONOMIC DIAGNOSTICS: Towards Accurate In Vivo Autonomic Measurement.*

[2] The popular shorthand for this is relaxation versus stress responses

Of the many reasons that this is so– one of the most interesting and likely overlooked is that the neurological baseline of modern humans is already deviated from the ancestral baseline of optimal human functioning. Scientists whose own normative sense of identity is informed by a civilization-wide and multi-generational compromise of autonomic function, denying them physiological access to the harmonized functioning of these systems, and unaware that their own systems are functioning sub-optimally, are unlikely to map the complete systems. They are also unaware that they are not mapping the complete systems, because they do not live in the experience of having all of these systems available to them. People who cannot see color should not develop color theory, but this is exactly what has happened in neuroscience. People who have conflated self with thinking have created the neurological maps for how the nervous system works, and they are, like their authors, stuck in the head.[3]

What we have mapped in traditional neurology is the neurology of *traumatized homo sapiens*. We have confused this with the neurology of *homo sapiens*.

People become primarily identified with thinking as a result of trauma. To experience ourselves (our identities) as a flow of words and images is not a metric of being, but rather a metric of alienation. This is not to say that cognition is not a necessary or signature attribute of human consciousness, but rather that the default organization of self-schema inside of the experience of cognition is a neurobiological sequelae of being traumatized. Humans retreat to their thinking when they have lost contact with the pleasurable experience of embodied awareness.

In this book, I would like to tell the deep and ancestral story of how this has happened, why it matters, and what we can do about it. It has occurred both gradually and acceleratingly

---

[3] Unfortunately, these same brain-centric halfmaps have been instantiated in the Large Language Models (LLMs) running AI. We have therefore created hardcoded silicon emanations of our own alienation.

over the past twelve thousand years. The origin stories of western civilization are politically coded explanations for why this has happened, framed in the cosmological *lingua franca* of the day, which was religion when these stories were written, but probably is no longer. The story of the Fall, in Genesis, is a story that is attempting to explain how we fell out of embodied kinship with *All That Is*.

I would like to tell a version of this story that is civilizational, and that examines this phenomenon over the past 12,000 years. Next I would like to tell a version of this story that is generational, examining it over the past hundred or so years in the family I grew up in. It may sound strongly like I am criticizing my family of origin, but the critical lens is not personal. I'm not saying that it was their fault: the fault is broader. But this was the milieu in which I was acculturated, so it is the only familial circumstance I have authority to speak about from direct experience. And then I would like to tell a version of this story that is biographical, examining it over my own lifespan, which is on the fifty year mark at present: half a century.

Throughout these tellings, I would like to tell it neurophysiologically, weaving the strands of the stories above with what we understand about autonomic physiology, which is the focus and *focolare*[4] of my own work for the past thirty years.

I posit the following credentials for narrating this story: like humanity as a lineage, I was born in deep contact with the Living World, grew up deeply attached to Place, and was then exiled from this attachment as a young child (at seven years old). This exile, which I could not put into words until I was an adult as it was too overwhelming and painful to touch or name, profoundly altered my neurophysiology in ways that I did not understand for decades. In seeking to heal myself, to reclaim what I knew I once had but lost, I began a multi-decade study of autonomic physiology, which has resulted after

---

4 hearth; fireplace.

thirty years in the creation of a new foundation model of autonomic physiology that is likely the first accurate map of its *in vivo* functioning of this civilizational epoch.

In attempting to heal I was not helped by my family, despite their love for me, because they were also alienated in the fundamental neurophysiological ways I was trying to address, and therefore could not accurately perceive what had happened. (It is very hard to see something in someone else that you do not perceive in yourself, or help someone cross a river that you have not crossed.)

Neither was I able to seek solace in the wisdom of the culture (American circa 1975-present), nor the civilization in which I found myself growing, because the nation-state and the civilization itself emerged out of the alienation into which I found myself thrust. It was therefore necessary, in my work of healing, to go outside of my family (generational familial milieu), culture (colonial cultural milieu), and civilization (cosmological historical milieu) to find the traces of what I knew must exist as healing technologies. They do, of course, exist.

So although at this point I assert myself one of the world's leading experts in these intersections, this material is not academic for me. I have had to claw my life back. There is very little skin I have that is not in this game. Furthermore, the meta-catastrophe bearing down on everyone inhabiting this terrestrial sphere- a poly-collapse of life-sustaining systems- because of the fact that modern humans do not understand this- impels urgency to the project. So I need you to understand what I am saying.

I am going to show you how we have been cut off at the roots not so that you can languish in agony and die here, dissociate in virtual realities, or give up hope, abandon the planet, and leave for Mars, but so that you can figure out how the fuck to regrow your roots, as if your very life, and life of everyone you know depended on it.

04 - Necrotic Neuroscience

The Autonomic Nervous System (ANS) is the most important biological system that modern people know the least about. A well-informed adult has at least some sense of the immune system, how breathing works, how the heart and the circulatory system function, how digestion metabolizes the nutrients in our food. Yet almost no one outside of specialist circles understands the degree to which the functioning of the ANS governs our moment-to-moment experience of wellbeing, or the degree to which it communicates with every other biological system mentioned above, often governing them. Its study thus far has been confined to a cadre of specialist professionals, and has remained esoteric, although the tide is turning over the past two decades as the first systematic models have described the way that the ANS is implicated in various types of traumatic stress, leading to affirmation and refinement of somatic therapies capable of working more directly with allostatic load retained in the body, which is a good part of what trauma is.

We have understood the role that the ANS plays in stress for at least a hundred years, since the 1920s, but have only functionally differentiated the three component systems whose coordinated (and de-coordinated) actions comprise it since 1994, when Stephen Porges published the Polyvagal Theory. One of Porges' seminal breakthroughs was the differentiation of two vagal systems: one ancient, unmyelinated, and primarily sub-diaphragmatic, subtending the viscera and guts; the other myelinated, above the respiratory diaphragm, and subtending in part the face, voice, heart, and lungs. Porges, using comparative evolutionary neuro-anatomy, and his own embodied experience, was able to formulate an evolutionary scaffolding explanation for how these two systems, which share the neural conduit known as the vagus nerve, both came to exist, while subtending different circuits with differential action on bodily systems.

The story of the origin of Polyvagal Theory, how it corroborated Steve's adolescent experience playing the clarinet (effectively a vagal exercise), and his subsequent detective work to identify the origin and location of the neural circuits responsible is extraordinary, and merits its own telling. It is also part of a much larger lineage history of neuroscience, which our work at Hearth Science has been re-writing for years. The history of neuroscience is a history that was indelibly marked by implicit bias in its origins. The field is officially about a hundred and fifty years old. We could argue effectively it was born with Santiago Ramón y Cajals, whose visionary drawings of neural structure beginning around 1888, after perfecting a silver staining technique that allowed for detailed visualization of neurons, originated the field as a discrete domain of study. Ramón y Cajals, like most educated Europeans of his day, was so deeply under the sway of Cartesian dogma (*I think, therefore I am*) that he did not recognize it was a paradigm within which he was operating. Like many of the paradigms in which we swim, Ramón y Cajals simply assumed that 'I think, therefore I am' is the way that things are.

The organ that does the thinking in words and pictures is the cranial brain. And so, in Ramón y Cajals' neuroscience, and in the discipline ever since, the brain has been the *de facto* center of the study of neurology. This is true to such a degree that most modern western people use the words mind and brain almost interchangably. There has been a trend in neuroscience over the past fifty years, of which Porges is a part, to extend the domain of inquiry deeper and deeper into the brain: to extend inquiry from cortex, to midbrain, to brainstem. Paul Maclean, the American neuroscientist responsible for the Triune Brain model (which has been 'disproven' and is no longer in vogue) was one of the first to recognize that deeper and more ancient neural circuitry provides the physiological foundations upon which more recently evolved structures depend for inputs and tempering. Although this was understood generally in the field prior to his work, the functional significance of this recognition was really not established until Maclean brought it home for us in evolutionary terms. To Maclean we owe the awareness that if the deepest reptilian layers of awareness are responding to threat, cognition, which is largely a cortical process, is not available to us. Porges was able to bring the field's attention strongly to the brainstem, the deepest and oldest 'basement' of the brain, and to differentiate the 'origin' of the two vagal circuits deep within it in the medulla oblongata. In this way he sought to expand the purview of the field to look deeper and deeper into the oldest parts of the brain, with a view to understanding how they influence visceral function, identity, perception, and ultimately behavior. His work strongly directs us to the neural substrates of feeling and his importance in the field cannot be overstated.

While I am eternally grateful to Porges, with whom I worked collaboratively for a number of years, and with whose company my firm had an intellectual property development agreement, I would like to point out that even studying the deepest and oldest structures in the brain remains within the paradigm of the brain-centric. Modern neurology, thus far, has really been the study of the brain and the central nervous system. Autonomic physiology, as we really begin to grasp how it actually works, completely shatters this hold.

Because of the field Porges was in, the lineage context out of which Polyvagal Theory arrives, and the degree to which academic research must be architected on top of prior knowledge edifices to obtain validity, Porges built Polyvagal Theory on top of inherited neuro-anatomical maps. The problem here is rather elementary. If someone sets sail for a new world and comes back with a cartography, and you set out for the same shore a hundred years later, you had better be damn sure that the first set of maps is accurate if you are planning to use them to navigate. If you don't double-check the maps that you inherit, and they turn out to be wrong, all the layers that you've built on top of them are going to be faulty.

In 2019, while collaborating with Porges on the first official visual depictions of Polyvagal Theory, I had two direct intimations that we needed to re-visit and verify the source maps. One involved the celiac ganglia, a neural intersection in the abdomen that coordinates autonomic neurology flowing into the digestive system, the other involved the neural extension of what we call the Connection System, and that Porges before us calls the 'ventral vagal' or Social Engagement physiology. In both cases I had a clear and unambiguous interoceptive experience of my own neurology that clearly contradicted the established maps, and that I was able to reproduce consistently with other people, again in contradiction to the established maps.

It is necessary at this moment to point out another feature of the discipline of neuroscience, which bears on our present conversation. It can be summarized as follows: anatomy and physiology are not the same thing. You can have a map of the entire subway system of New York (anatomy), but if you do not understand in which direction trains are moving at what time, you do not have an understanding of the ways in which the system moves the information it carries (physiology). While a non-trivial number of the refinements that our work has made to neuroscience contradict the established anatomy, most of its foundation arguments with the discipline contradict its established physiology. In plain language, much of neuroscience understands how the nervous system is structured without understanding how it works.

This is in part due, again, to how the knowledge was accreted. Most anatomical studies that gave origin to our detailed anatomical maps were done on cadavers. This necrotic anatomy, conducted beginning during the High Renaissance, has two very serious limitations. First of all, in the same way that trees, when they die, lose their leaves, humans when they die, lose the finest ramifications of neurology (the smallest neural conduits and their associated receptors) which are the sources of afferent (flowing toward the cranial brain) neurology and the terminations of efferent (flowing away from the cranial brain) neurology. Secondly, neurons in corpses are not firing, so you cannot determine in which directions their information is flowing. To understand physiology we have to understand how neural systems are linked, and how information moves through them. While given the complexity of neurological systems, and the numbers of synaptic connections they include, this is almost practically impossible, our current neuroscience has an extremely rudimentary understanding of information flow in neural conduits.

What this meant for me personally, and for our work at Hearth Science, was that beginning in 2020, we began to treat the inherited neuro-anatomical maps as provisional at best. Over the past five years, we have re-mapped most of the Autonomic Nervous System. Its physiology is not what is generally taught, even in specialist circles.

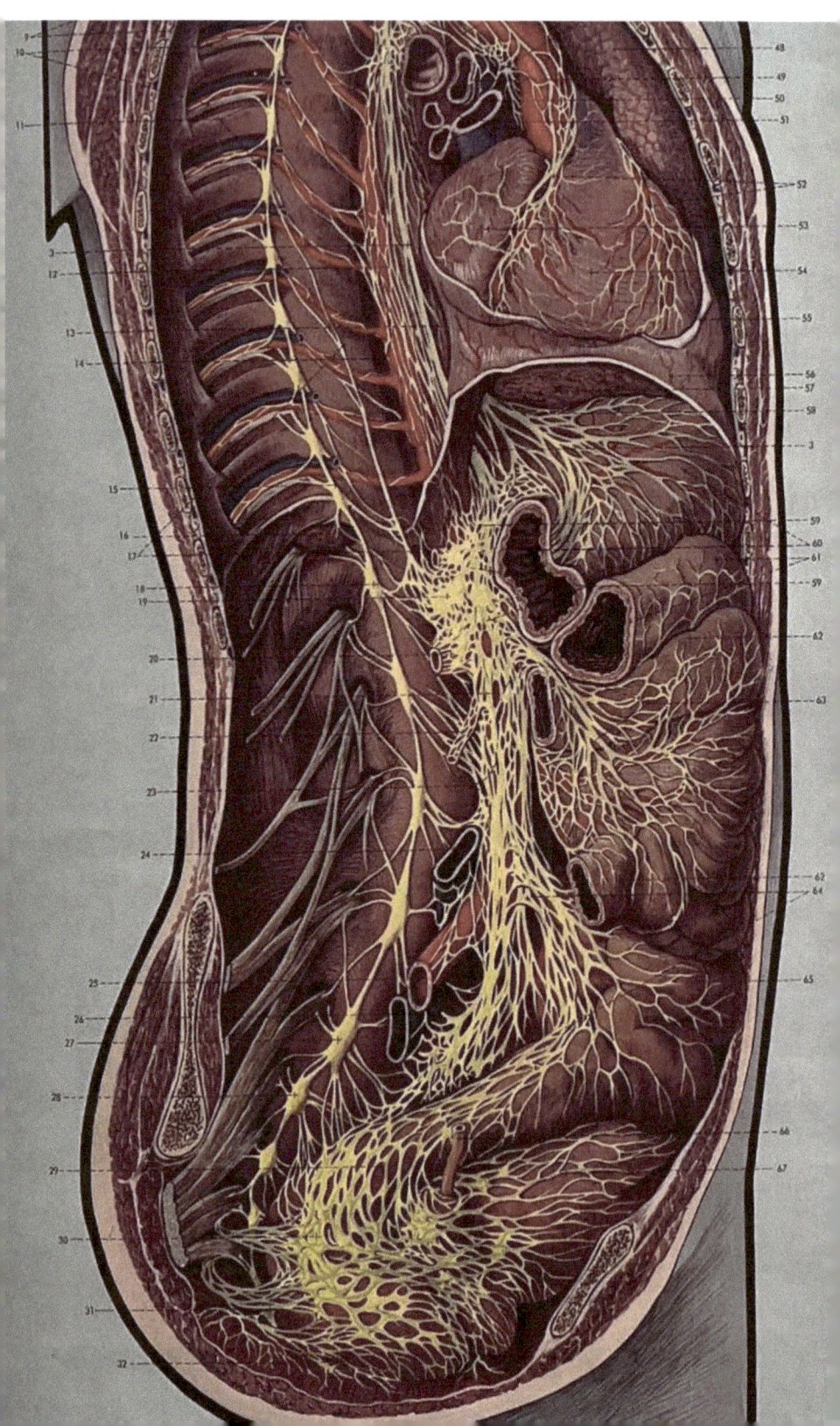

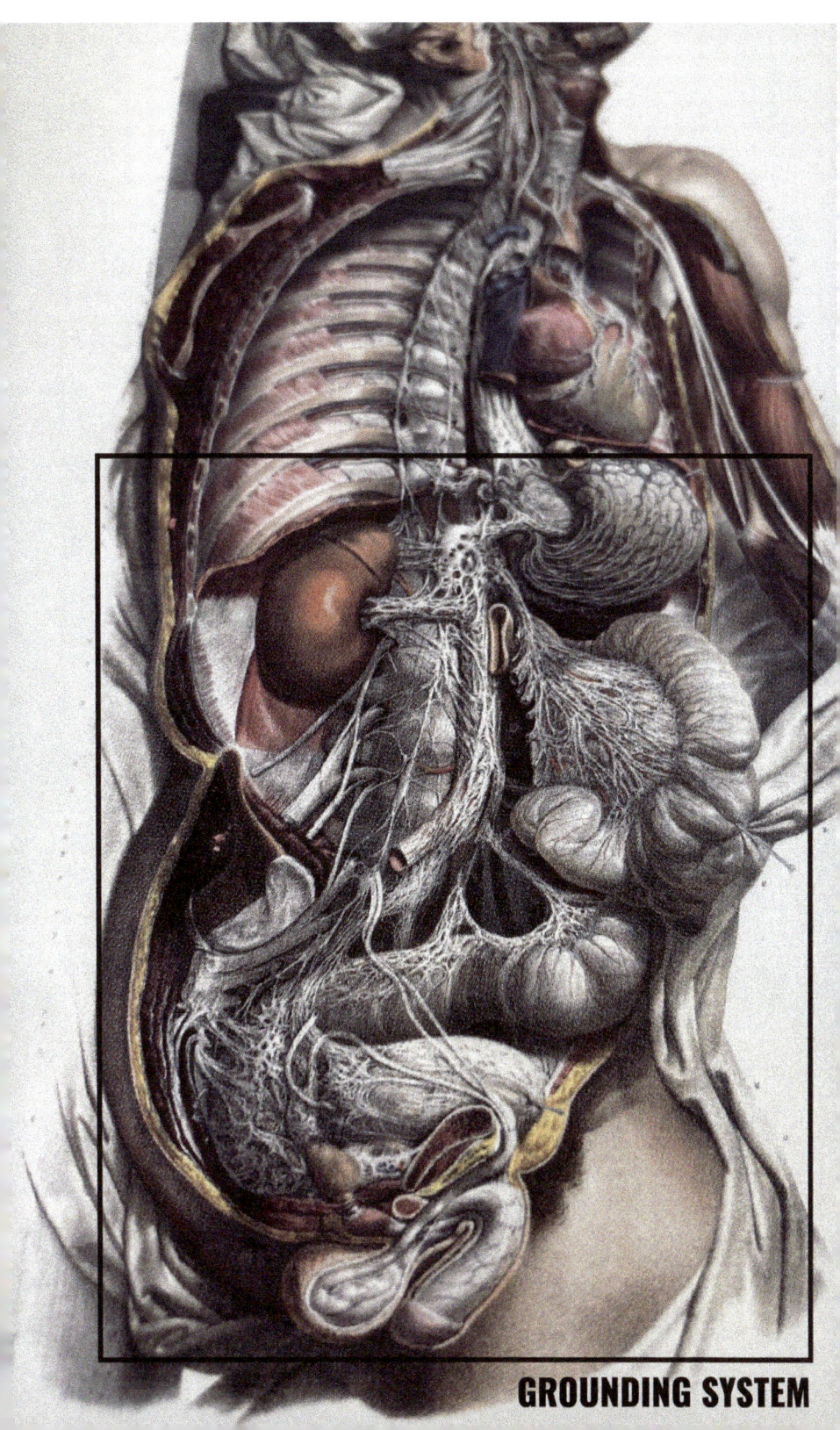

GROUNDING SYSTEM

05 - Grounding System

When someone talks about feeling grounded, what do they mean? Is this just California New Age speak? Or is there something more fundamental, and more *physiological* at play?

Your neurology and circulatory systems develop together. Neurogenesis and angiogenesis are twinned, which means that as neural conduit develops it brings its own blood supply with it, always. Your heart is, among other things, an oscillator. Your blood system is a closed system of liquid pressure in contact proximity to an electrical system: your nervous system. A liquid pressure system connected to an oscillator in contact with an electrical field generates an electro-magnetic field. The one generated by your heart is detectable by a magnetometer eight feet away from you.[1]

So, like any good electrical circuit, does being grounded simply mean that your neuro-electrical system is connected to the earth? If so, what is the neurology undergirding this connection?

And here is where this gets interesting autonomically. *The Grounding System IS the sub-diaphragmatic vagal system.* And it has three configurations. 1) A configuration when there is sufficient safety for it to coordinate with your other autonom-

---

[1] McCraty, Rollin. (2016). Science of the Heart, Volume 2 Exploring the Role of the Heart in Human Performance An Overview of Research Conducted by the HeartMath Institute. 10.13140/RG.2.1.3873.5128.

ic systems, giving you access to the synchrony of all of your autonomic circuitry. 2) A configuration where there is enough danger that your social Connection System down-regulates and it coordinates with a mobilized version of your spinal Movement System.[2] 3) And a configuration under lifethreat, where it moves into being the sole autonomic system functioning, yet no longer connected to the earth. In this final, or lifethreat configuration, you can think of it as your *Ungrounding* System.

The same autonomic system, under conditions of safety, danger, and lifethreat, undergirds a highly differentiated range of visceral states. On the salutogenic (health-creating) end of the continuum, it gives us access to gut knowing, and a sense of being deeply grounded. Intuitive earth-based creatures, rooted, connected to Place. Yet this is not the configuration in which most modern people reside. Most modern people's Grounding Systems are stuck in a traumatic configuration, the origins of which are several thousand years of multi-generational trauma. It is important and revealing that eastern systems understand the Grounding System in its health-creating manifestation, while Polyvagal Theory (a leading edge of autonomic physiology in the West) understands it in its traumatic configuration, where it undergirds shutdown. Neither system understands that they are talking about the same system under differentiated conditions (e.g., safety versus lifethreat).

In the presence or absence of safety, danger, or lifethreat, of the other autonomic systems (Connection and Movement), and of their respective neurochemistries of connection, activation, or shutdown, this system behaves totally differently.

What I would like to continue to explore in this book is how we came to inherit a collective soma where for most modern

---

[2] This mobilized version of the Spinal Movement System in the presence of the activation chemistry of adrenaline and cortisol is what traditional neuroscience calls your 'Sympathetic Nervous System' and gives rise to fight-or-flight responses.

people the Grounding System has become the *Ungrounding System*. If we do not have access to the Grounding System, in its health-creating manifestation, we do not feel the ground.

> *"If we do not have access to the Grounding System, in its health-creating manifestation, we do not feel the ground."*

And we are not aware of it. Our embodied awareness resides northward of this contact, floating, untethered. We experience ourselves as a head on a stick, like Descartes. As both a cause and effect of this, most modern people spend most of their lives wearing shoes that interpose a non-conductive rubber sole between our feet and the earth. We are acculturated to do this pretty early in life, but if we were more grounded, we wouldn't like the way it feels and we would object. If our Grounding Systems are available, we will enjoy the feeling of contact we experience with the ground in most places, and will find ourselves wanting to be barefoot, or in shoes through which we can feel the ground viscerally. The more grounded people get, the more they want their feet in and on the living earth.

When we experience trauma- unmetabolized overwhelming experience- much of this allostatic load is generally archived in the psoas muscles, which are a set of long, spindle-shaped muscles running from the transverse processes and vertebral bodies of T12-L5 (your lower spine) down to the lesser trochanter of the femur. The psoas effectively connects the vertebral column with the inside of your hip joint. When you contract into defense, it tightens, cutting off visceral sensory contact with the ground. This situation is so deeply normalized that we can spend a good part of our lives not making any kind of visceral contact with the ground without realizing it. (I did.)

What I would like to propose to you is that this truncation, this *being cut off*, has been normalized by imperial systems for the past several thousand years. Empire does not want you to

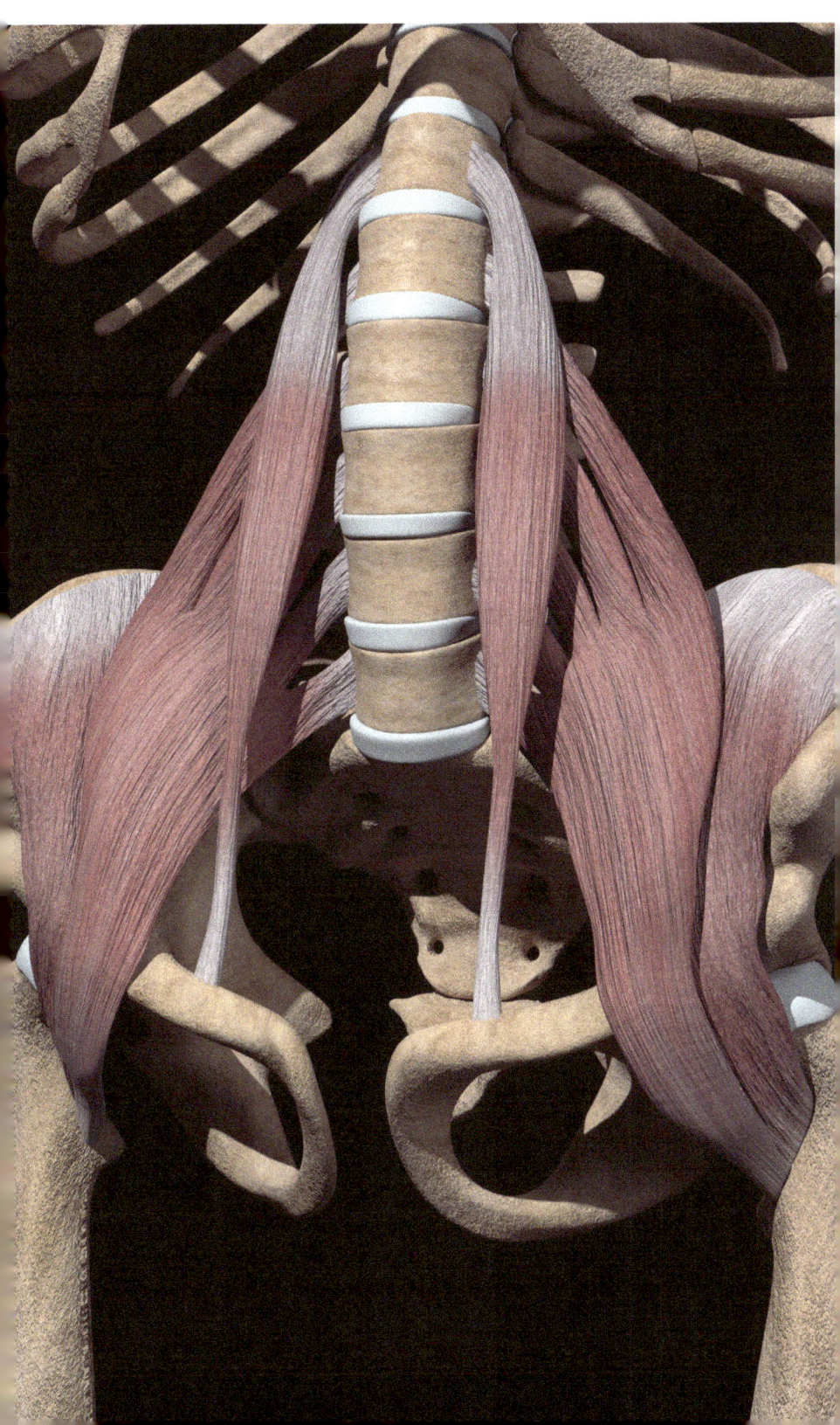

be deeply connected with the Earth. It does not want you to feel your feet on the ground, be deeply connected to your intuition, reside in gut knowing, communicate with the ancestors beneath your feet. From the point of view of domination, it is much more convenient if you *cannot* feel the ground. You are much easier to control.

We also learn this cutting off from our families. Growing up in familial systems where people are cut off from the ways of knowing coming up from the earth teaches us not to be grounded, both because as children we embody the autonomic composition of those to whom we are attached (epi-autonomics), and because these normalized modes of disconnection preclude our developing a vocabulary of felt awareness to describe them.

And then there is the individual physiological layer, where our lack of understanding shutdown processes, the way that they function autonomically, and how to metabolize the energies that get tangled up in them prevents us from doing our own work to thaw these systems.

Like moving trees whose roots have been hacked, we moderns have been denatured of our earth-based and chthonic inheritance.

With this as preamble, I would like to structure this book working from the oldest, deepest, and broadest truncation of rootedness, that of empire, to sociological truncation of rootedness through colonialism and white supremacy, to familial lineages of truncation (multi-generational trauma), to the individual physiology.

As this path unveils, we will continue to contemplate how to transform our relationship to each of these nested contexts, and what is likely to arise when we do. In this way, I would like to formulate this text as a verbal liquid rooting concentrate. Your job, dear reader, as you progress through the text, is to grow deeper roots.

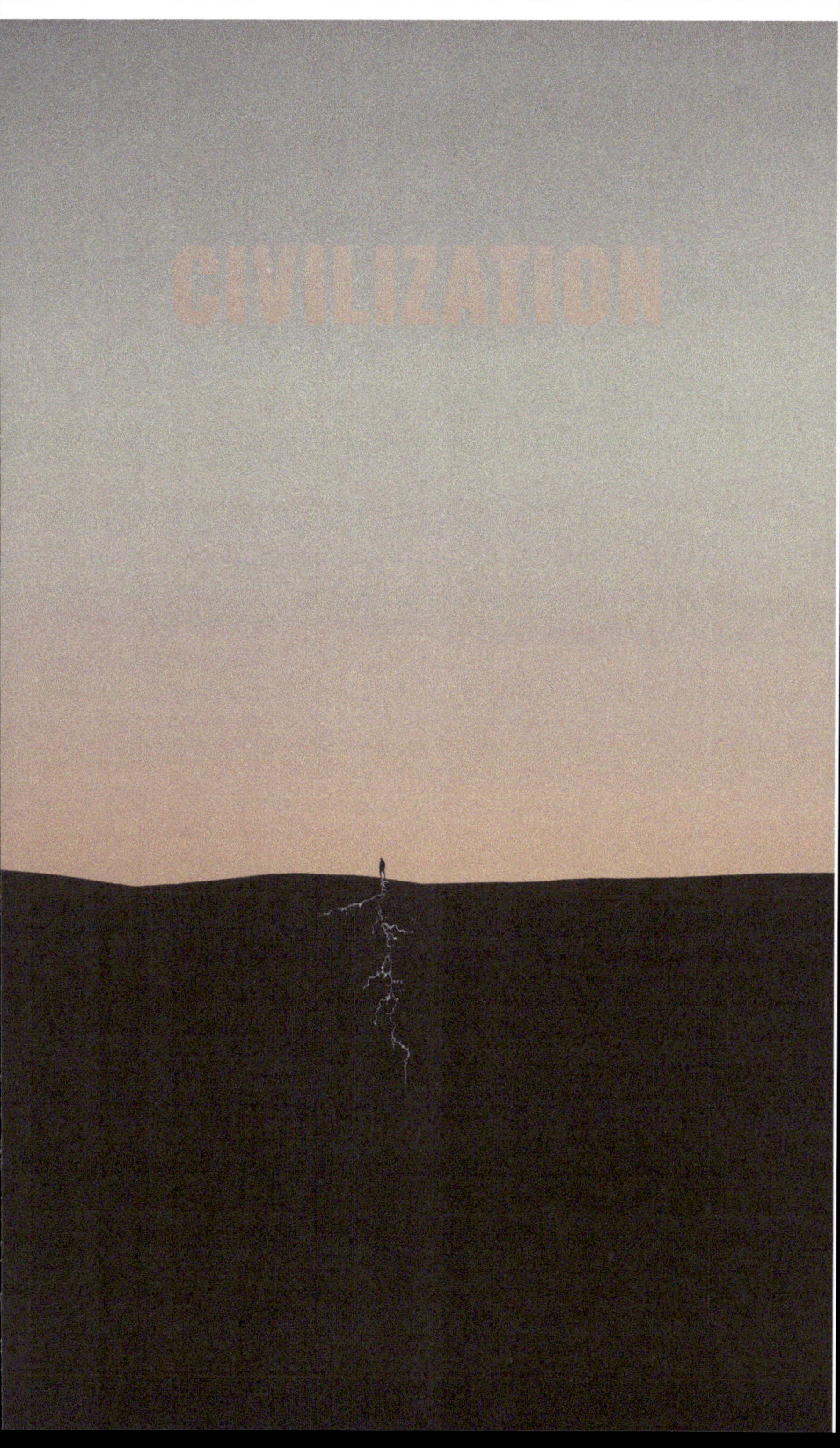

06- A Yoga Class

Two days ago I was teaching a brief workshop with a colleague and friend, a yoga and movement teacher with a fifty year practice of yoga. At the beginning of the talk, which we held with about sixty people online, she led an embodiment practice, which began with her balling her fists and pounding on her thighs for several minutes, encouraging us to do the same. I enjoyed this. At a certain point several minutes into this process, she asked me if I wanted to take over. I started to speak, and then discovered that my microphone was muted.

Before we had begun, she had asked me to lead a grounding practice. And because we were offering a short workshop, and because she is an Elder and I wanted to be amenable, I agreed. But in the moment that she handed me the microphone, had I had the presence of mind to say what I was feeling, had I not wanted to accommodate her request, I would have done something else.

We cannot do a five minute movement meditation exercise and get grounded. That's not how it works. When I say 'get grounded' I'm not even confident that most people have any idea what I'm talking about. I mean, sure, it's part of our California lexicon. It is part of the cultural ethos of yoga, and meditation, worlds and work that I frequent. There are grounding mats, and grounding sheets, and a field called grounding that was 'discovered' by a white guy, just like America.[1]

---

[1] to the Christopher Columbus of grounding: go fuck yourself

We talk about getting grounded like we know how to do it. As though we can take off our shoes, and direct our attention to the sensation of contact between our feet and the floor, as though we can visualize ourselves dropping roots into the earth, and as a result of this she will simply dissolve twelve thousand years of alienation, turn on the beneficent flow of ions into the substrate of our bodies, and re-animate us with lifestuff and kinship worldview.

And yet, forgive me for pointing out the obvious here- nearly all of us moderns are standing on lands thieved at knife and gunpoint from their rightful indigenous stewards, many of whom have been genocided. The place where you live, the land on which your house sits, speaks a primal indigenous language that you do not know, do not realize exists, and that it has never occurred to you to study. Its thought and word-forms were likely en-mouthed in the Indigenous dialect of that place, because many Indigenous languages emerged out of the earth. And you've never thought of this once until now. The local indigenous language of your place, which is likely endangered if not extinct, probably encodes the place names of major geologic features- mountains, rivers, watersheds- in the names by which they know themselves. Needless to say, you do not know those names.

To ask the earth that we are raping and pillaging as a daily matter of course, whose air we shit into every time we start up our cars, whose watercourses we poison with waste effluvients from our sewers, whose precious fields we entomb in forever chemicals, whose oceans we fill with microplastics that are making their way back into our deepest inwardness, and whose lands we have thieved from their rightful and responsible aboriginal stewards to ground us, reminds me of the slave owners who whipped their slaves for laughing at prayers.

What right do you have, you who are actively engaged in the

destruction of biotic life, to presume to plant your roots into the soil of the earth your entire civilization is hellbent on destroying? Who the fuck do you think you are?

And yet, here's the amazing thing. The Good Earth, precisely because she is in fact your Mother, allows us to do just this. Ignorant, ungrateful, crumb-snatching children that we are, bickering at her fireplace, she nonetheless with a grace that we do not deserve, permits us, should we show any inkling of interest, to drape ourselves in her raiment of majesty and mystery. To root down and root home into her baseline of terrestrial vitality.

For this is what happened in the workshop. I unmuted my microphone, encouraged people to begin to sense the contact between their feet and the floor– not as an idea, not as a thought, but as a visceral experience of flow– to ask the earth permission to connect with her, and then to allow themselves to soften into the information rising up from her.

We modern people don't know a goddam thing about this, but the Lakota culture, which is 200,000 years old, has a group of words for the information that the earth uploads to us. One of these words, *anamagoptanye*, has been translated for me as, "The earth is constantly uploading information to you."

What I did, in the workshop, was invite people into contact with this way-of-relating. The earth is, how can I say this – *alive*. Sentient. Aware. A Being. An Entity. An Identity. Your Mother.

If you suddenly realized that you were walking around on someone or something that was alive…I mean, if you really radically viscerally understood the truth of this, not as a thought, but as a feeling, my guess is that you would stop trying to kill her. My guess is that, if you really deeply realized that the entire ensphering matrix of the earth, her surface, her soil, her geologic depths, her mountains, her forests, her oceans, her atmosphere, every object you have ever seen, the entire field of your sensory knowing, was animate, was the face and body of your original mother, that you would suddenly be quite ashamed that many of your daily actions were complicit in her drawn-out millenias-long murder. You would be embarrassed. You might possibly burst into tears. It is conceivable that you would be unable to stop weeping.

I am reminded of a story that Tiokasin Ghosthorse, the Lakota Elder who taught us the word *anamogoptanye* shared with a group of us gathered in a seminar with him in October of 2022. It was a story about the contact between arriving Europeans and the Indigenous peoples of North America. He said that when the Europeans arrived, they walked into the forest, and began cutting down trees. A huge number of them. They denuded a vast area until it was bare, and then they set about building a giant structure with this timber, and then they all disappeared inside of it.

The Indigenous Elders approached the Europeans, and asked them– *We have seen you come to this beautiful place, cut down all of the trees, build a building, and disappear inside of it for a very long time. What are you doing in there?*

To which the Europeans replied: *We have built a house of worship and are praying.*

The Indigenous Elders, who had been praying continuously the entire time, because their way-of-being is a form of prayer, were extremely confused by these actions and this attitude.

07 - War

I find myself, this morning of February fourth, emerging from a year's-long war. The image I have is of a battlefield, rife with the keening of gulls, the shrill calling of hawks, the circling of carrion birds. I can see the piercing blue of the sky; puffs of white cloud soft as cotton balls.

The year is 171 BC, the place Callinicus, five kilometres north of Larissa on the Thermaic Gulf of the Mediterranean, in what is now, over two thousand years later, Greece, but was at the time Macedonia.

There is smoke rising from the battlefield, which is strewn with corpses of people I have known as well as those unfamiliar to me. Some wear the colors of my side, some the colors of the Roman legions. We are unpleasing to look at in death, particularly the grisly death of the battlefield. This is long before the remote death of drones- we did not have the alienated luxury of watching on cameras from a distance then. Of blowing people up mute, without knowing their screams. This is up-close, personal, reeking of vomit, stenches of the earth, horses gutted by lances, their hot viscera exposed. Vultures peck out eyeballs, tug on entrails, grapple over severed limbs. The chaos of battle is evident in the scrapes on the earth, which is rutted and stamped and scarred with footprints of men and beasts; bodies that have been dragged, brakish water.

I know many of the men still alive, walking the field, finishing off the wounded. Coagulated blood is what adorns most of us, black as it has dried, a skin over the armor that we are wearing. I hold my sword in both hands. I am hacking off people's heads. Some of them are already dead. Some of them are not. In some cases I take my helmet off so they can look in my eyes as I take their heads. In some cases I put my helmet on so that they stare, instead, into Death's head. The mask I wear is of the fanged jaws of a rattlesnake. It is the last thing they will see on earth.

I am in two times. This battle, two thousand and some odd years ago, is one that I fought in another lifetime.

In this lifetime, a modern person, living another set of endtimes in California circa 2025, the battle is more chimerical. It plays out in my mind, imaginal. I am meditating, lying on our couch, getting ready to move.

The townhome in which we have lived for the past six years, from June 2018 to February 2025 goes on the market in a few days. We have just signed a lease on a new place. I am washing the inward walls of my psyche, cleaning out the gore from my heart, drawing the disgust to the surface so that I can purge it.

I have survived, yesterday, an astonishing high-speed high-impact car crash that totaled the Tesla Model 3 I was driving, reduced the front of the car to a screaming compression of wracked metal, splintered plastic, and crunched circuit boards while I was sitting in its cockpit, thankfully solo in the vehicle. The accident, which happened at about 2:30 on a Sunday afternoon, in the rain, occurred on a highway notorious for flooding when my car, traveling at sixty miles per hour and headed north, lost contact with the road, began to fishtail, then went into a flat spin, performed two full rotations, was struck by another vehicle from behind, smashed head-on into the median, ricocheted off and spun yet again, completing a 1080 degree turning by my calculation, then came to a stop facing the same direction I had been when the car began to wobble. The move into the flatspin occurred as a result, I believe, of steering auto-correction applied by the vehicle itself, rather than me. The auto-correct made the fishtail worse. In that sense, the car tried to kill me. The vehicle then, honorably, took 99% of the impact of the crash by the particular manner in which it accordioned, for which I am deeply grateful. Autonomous machine steering may have caused the crash, crash-test engineering prevented it from killing me.

In the flat spin, for several seconds, I was aware that I had no control whatsoever over the vehicle's trajectory. Electric vehicles are heavy, and I was traveling at highway speed. The laws of physics took over: I was strapped into the cockpit of a vehicle weighing about 4300 pounds, spinning up a slight incline at sixty-miles per hour. It was going to move inertially according to Newton's first law of motion until that motion was interrupted by something. First I clipped another car, then I collided head-on with the median: enough to bring the forward movement to a halt.

There was a moment, emerging from the wreck– both airbags deployed, my glasses thrown from my face, my body canted forward into a crash position with my head in my hands, the cabin filling with the sudden reek of scorched plastic and crushed metal where, when I was able to locate my glasses around my feet, check my body from inside to make sure it was intact– I jumped out of the car and found myself standing, in the rain, on the windswept highway, watching hundreds of cars rear up before me. The crash was spread across three lanes of traffic fully blocking the arterial flow of the northbound lanes. In the whip of wind and rain I watched the fire engines snaking toward us from the south, their prismatic red lights spinning like ruby cut glass, splintering on the water droplets beading on my glasses, and it occurred to me that I was familiar with the ancient contours of this same scene.

I carry the memory of war down deep, and up close. For the past six years I have been engaged in another kind of modern warfare called entrepreneurship. It has left a foul taste in my mouth. It has almost made me hate modern humans. Almost.

I have been cheated, stolen from in broad daylight. I have watched one of the most famous medical schools in the world thieve an entire body of our work with no consequences and come back to try it a second time. I have watched the owners of an elite executive coaching firm lie baldly to my face about the entire premise of their intentions in collaborating with us, then get caught red-handed in the lie. I have watched the Managing Director of a hundred million dollar impact venture fund go into cognitive decline while running the fund, spend years hiding it from the companies in which he invested and his bosses who were too rich and otherwise absorbed to notice. I have watched grift and greed and corruption and arrogance all play out in my tiny corner of the world of 'conscious capitalism', and I have found it revolting. I have encountered grifters and charlatans and all the usual suspects in the perverse carnival of commerce and transaction, the province of the art of the deal.

But not only that. If my disgust was confined to the world of commerce, of transaction, it would be one thing. But I have also, during this time, discerned that a Brazilian spiritual group of which I was a part for nearly fourteen years is a cult. I have watched people I used to respect say and do things I find abhorrent, and I have watched the bile rise in myself again and again and again. Like the battlefield in my mind, I see six years strewn with the wreckage of bodies and relationships I have discarded. I walk back through their faces- through the many moments I spent on building those relationships, the disgust that led me to abandon most of them. I walk through the past six years of relatings in my mind, my sword drawn, severing heads from bodies. In most cases I take my helmet off before cleaving their heads from their necks in my mind. I want to look them in the eyes. Behind me, the wreckage of corpses piles up; accrues.

I am not a saint, to be sure, but I have made it an objective to which I am accountable in this life to exit the domination paradigm I was born into, yet all around me are those infected by domination. The medical establishment is infected by domination. The world of leadership coaching, which serves the world of leadership, is infected by domination. These conscious capitalists are infected by domination. The spiritual group I was part of became infected by domination. My grandfather was infected by domination. My father was victimized by domination and then infected by its festering aftermath.

Domination is an illness: the very illness that gave birth to the modern world. This battle at Callinicus in 171 BC is between the Macedonians and the Romans, part of what will come to be known as the Third Macedonian War. The Romans were infected by domination, and in a series of battles that would culminate with their decisive victory at Pydna three years later, they would manage to subdue the sovereign Macedonian culture, which was not infected thusly, and terminate its dynastic line.

I have faced the Romans before: I have been facing down domination for lifetimes.

Yesterday a close colleague confronts me, shakes me as if I am in a trance. *Snap out of it*, she says, *you are acting like you are in a war. Your heat is scaring people. You wear fangs.*

I step back to look at myself, battle-hardened, mask of the Death's head over my own, blade in my hands, and I realize she is speaking truthfully.

The death cult has trained me as well. I must be careful not to become part of what disgusts me, what I abhor. It is a danger.

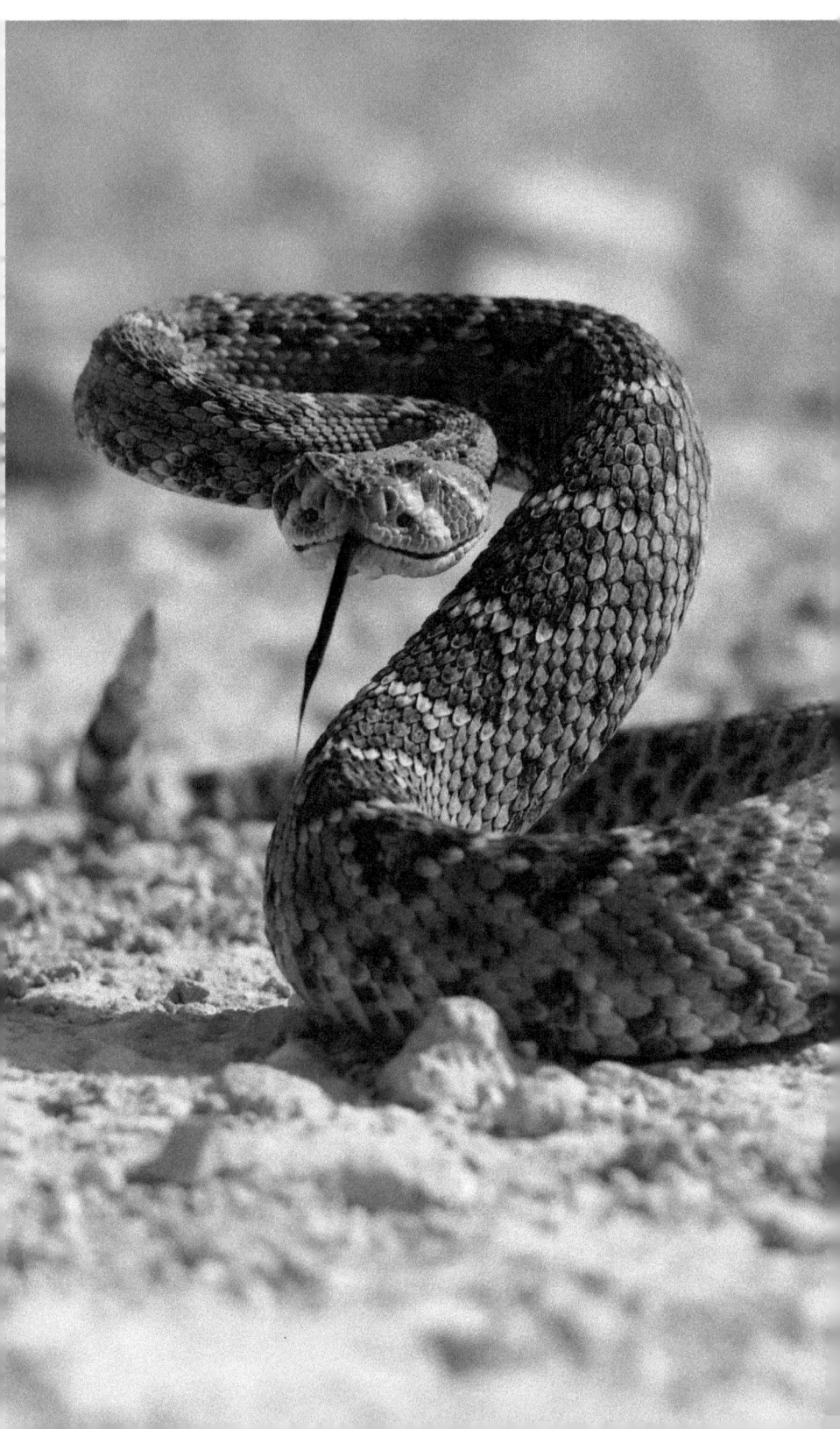

08 - Death's Head

On a day a moon ago I woke after having worked thirty-one days in a row, and, taking a shower, realized the last time I had worked at this intensity for so many days was during a war. The moment I thought this there appeared so vividly in my mind's eye the image of a battle, replete with sounds and smells, shouting and metal scraping and guttural screams and the salt smell of the sea, the colors of it, many troops in crimson, the close proximity of people fighting hand-to-hand, that I was, for the better part of a minute, simply transported there.

Later in the day, driving to our nature preserve, I ran over a rattlesnake. It was stretched out in the road, and I was going too fast to stop. I got out of the car, a hawk called, and when I got close to the creature I saw from the arrowhead shape of its skull that the snake was venomous. Then I saw the rattle. I returned to my car, took an axe from the trunk and cut the snake in two. I picked up the head, and was astonished by how soft, how supple the skin was. It was deeply beautiful. I had never held a rattlesnake before. They are not something you generally pick up.

I have held other snakes in my life, but they were scalier, none with a velvet skin like this. With a diamond-patterned beauty, fawns and browns, and its softness, it was lovely to hold. Bewitching, I would say. Deeply strange. How could something so dangerous be so soft? I stroked it with a finger, and I wanted to study the head as well. I wanted to look into the snake's eyes, which were wide open, to see what might be writ there-

was its gaze merely cold? I took the head and I put it in the back of my car, on the seat, and I finished the drive.

About ten minutes later, after unloading the lumber I had brought to the land, I went back to retrieve the head. I was looking at it, the pale yellow-whitish underbelly with its intricate tesselations of scale lying on the seat, the elaborate tilework of the underside of the jaw, when it flipped over and revived. This was so eerie I stopped breathing.

The snake had a gaping tubular hole at the end where the body had been: I could see straight into the body cavity, which oddly, in retrospect, was not bleeding. There had been, in fact, almost no blood at any time. The snake's eyes had been, and remained, wide open. I took a broom from the trunk of my car and knocked the snake out onto the grass. Then I got the axe and killed it a second time. This time I cut the head off just behind the skull. Again, almost no blood.

Unnerved and jangly, I took the axe, and hiked, bare-chested, the quarter-mile back to where I had killed the snake the first time. I knelt in the dirt road, and cleaved off the rattle in a stroke. This I picked up, and brought back to the car, where I set both the head and the rattle on a wooden board on the ground. I wasn't going to touch the head again until I was damn sure it was *dead* dead. I found myself pacing around for some time, restless. I was suddenly the possessor of the head of a rattle snake, and its rattle, and though I had some sense of their talismanic import, and also some sense of their relatedness to being at war, and my reverie in the shower, I confess that I wasn't sure what to do with them.

I went and sat on the land and breathed into my feet and through the earth until I could feel myself on the inside without shaking and became still enough that my thoughts stopped. And then, for some reason, it became obvious to me that I needed to place the objects in a sacred box.

A couple of hours later, when I was convinced the snake was

actually dead I picked up the head. Using my finger and thumb I squeezed it from behind, laterally, and when I did so the jaws opened and the fangs, as though they were spring loaded, rotated out into striking position. It had a premonitory quality, this hinge-like motion. It accorded with the visual I have either seen or inherited, through primal ancestral memory, of the position a venomous snake takes before striking, with the mouth open. The inside of the creature's mouth was soft pink, the forked tongue black. Primal memories unspooled, unbeckoned.

We have history, you and I, some ancient part of myself thought towards the snake. *This is not our first encounter.*

The fangs, when the mouth is closed, rest folded up against the roof of the creature's mouth. If they did not it would stab itself every time it closed its jaw. As I held the jaw up in the forest sunlight, studying death at such close proximity I saw something astonishing. Behind each fang was another structure. It twinned the fang, with the same arc, but this needle was no wider than a human hair.

The fang is the bite, and the fangs are hollow on the front side, which is the mechanism by which the venom is conveyed. But what was this other structure, a structure only visible in certain light, fine as a hair? A structure no one had ever told me existed. I have scoured the literature now, a library of images, and there are no pictures I can find of this second set of structures. They do not exist. Yet there they were, a pair of them, just behind the fangs, clear and obvious on very close inspection, vivid as life. Unforgettable. Unmistakeable.

And so I ask you, how is this like the modern world? What is the death's head that must be killed twice? And if modernity, in its necrophiliac incarnation in the death cult of capitalism, this empire inherited from Rome, this great destroyer of life, wounds with the fangs, what is the role of the nearly invisible hairlike needle behind it? What role does it play?

The head, after several days in the box began to stink, and so I boiled it and scraped all of the flesh off. It sits now in a sacred box on my computer, begging the question, each time I sit down to write– can you not get seduced by the modern world? Can you remember that at its center is a death's head?

How many times will you have to kill it before it is dead?

09- Digging out the Taproot of Supremacy

For the past several years, I have been harvesting and planting California Buckeyes during the winter rains. The trees sprout from the buckeye itself, which is about the size of a seven-year-old child's balled-up fist. Each mature Buckeye, in the fall, becomes enrobed in a profusion of these nuts. When they drop, *en masse*, in mid-winter the ground is littered with them; they are everywhere. Some of them are eaten by squirrels, some of them land or roll into places where they cannot find the soil beneath them. Yet many begin to root, resting on the earth. They don't need to be planted beneath the surface. They attach where they land and simply begin to root down.

With the correct temperatures and enough rain, a taproot breaks out from the body of the nut, extending like a narrow white tail, its knobbly extension dropping straight down. After it has grown several inches, and become convinced it has encountered suitable soil, the trunk of the root birfurcates in a vivid fuchsia split at the edge of the nut, and the tree's first leaves, and what will become its stalk, and later its trunk, unfurl upward from here.

Having done this several times now, I learned this year that the seedlings need to be planted in very deep containers. In the first several months of growth, the taproot drops straight down with the same velocity the leaves and stalk rise up. This is different than many other plants, many other trees, which develop broader spreading root systems. Nourished by the hulking nut, the tree's first year of growth is in hyperdrive. If the container holding the Buckeye is too shallow the taproot smashes into its bottom, get frustrated, circles, coils back on itself. It wants to grow straight down. It is seeking the depths.

When does the modern era begin? What is the dawn of the modern world, the age we know? What are the mental figurations that give rise to it? Humans have been here for at least two hundred thousand years, and yet our recorded history reaches back less than five. The history you were taught in school (the history I was taught in school) began with Mesopotamia, a few thousand years back.

This means that at least ninety-seven percent of our lineage history is veiled in the shadows of deep time; unrecorded history. How can a creature intent upon knowing itself understand what has given rise to its modern form if it does not know 97% of its lineage history?[1]

If we turn toward the origin stories of western civilization, and listen with the ears of trackers, we may yet hear echoes of something older. The stories we have inherited that claim to be 'In the beginning...' aren't nearly ancient enough to be so. Let us pick up the trail, and walk it back, until it dissolves into mist. Possibly, if our senses are sharp enough, our ways of knowing and listening more embodied and nuanced, our sensory radar will penetrate the fog and we will catch a glimpse of the pattern behind the pattern and be able to follow it long after we can see it, long after it has disappeared into the mists that predate recorded history. I am seeking out the taproot of supremacy. I can see the tree in full form, planted squarely in the psyche of the modern world, the strange fruit of its bloom and ripening. I know it came from some seed, some nut: that it grew in us, wasn't always this way. It is an import, an invasive species: the product of alienation.

---

1 As a relevant aside, our deepest oldest autonomic systems are 500 million years old.

I assert that we can decolonize the world all we want, but if we don't decolonize consciousness, nothing will change. We will simply exchange one set of oppressions for another. From where was it birthed, this taproot of supremacy, and what did it engender? How did things come to be this way? Come, listen in your body with me to the background radiation in the white space behind our origin stories. Let us point our listening at the origin of things.

Some facts that can be set out:

March 30, 2023: the Vatican formally repudiates the Doctrine of Discovery, 571 years after the papal bull *Dum Diversas* (1452) authorized Alfonso V of Portugal to reduce any "Saracens (Muslims) and pagans and any other unbelievers" to perpetual enslavement. This papal bull, written nearly six hundred years ago, was one of a trio of authorizations granted by the Vatican to Christian kings that gave the Catholic churches the imprimatur to colonize the non-European (non-Christian) world, and established the legal basis for the enslavement of other people, and the concept of *terra nullius* (empty lands). When I was in elementary school, a mere forty years ago, I was told straight-facedly that Christopher Columbus discovered America, which is problematic due to the fact that indigenous peoples had been here for tens if not hundreds of thousands of years before that. Christopher Columbus did not *discover* anything. He opened the Americas to European exploitation. The papal bull *Inter Caetara* (1493) explicitly grants to the Christian kings land and title to all lands extending in all directions out from Europe not occupied or governed by Christians. It says:

"And, in order that you may enter upon so great an undertaking with greater readiness and heartiness endowed with the benefit of our apostolic favor, we, [the Vatican] of our own accord, not at your instance nor the request of anyone else in your regard, but of our own sole largess and certain knowledge and out of the fullness of our apostolic power, by the authority of Almighty God conferred upon us in blessed Peter and of the vicarship of Jesus Christ, which we hold on

earth, do by tenor of these presents, should any of said islands have been found by your envoys and captains, give, grant, and assign to you and your heirs and successors, kings of Castile and Leon, forever, together with all their dominions, cities, camps, places, and villages, and all rights, jurisdictions, and appurtenances, all islands and mainlands found and to be found, discovered and to be discovered towards the west and south, by drawing and establishing a line from the Arctic pole, namely the north, to the Antarctic pole, namely the south, no matter whether the said mainlands and islands are found and to be found in the direction of India or towards any other quarter, the said line to be distant one hundred leagues towards the west and south from any of the islands commonly known as the Azores and Cape Verde."

-Inter Caetara, Pontifex (Pope) Alexander VI (1493)

Upon what premise does the Vatican exert this 'moral' authority to grant land and title to the Earth to the kings of Castile and León? Straightforwardly, because non-christians are not fully human. Here is the signature that we are looking for, the stamp of supremacy. The sanctioned church declares: *We christians are human, you pagans are not.* Pope Francis, writing in 2023, acknowledges it directly: "Never again can the Christian community allow itself to be infected by the idea that one culture is superior to others, or that it is legitimate to employ ways of coercing others."

I call your attention, here at our beginnings in the present moment to one other place, a photograph in a newspaper article, seemingly unrelated. Here is a white woman in Iowa, in her thirties, who works in a hair salon, speaking about her views of Donald Trump. From her own diction, we can infer that she is not highly educated. "There's not enough Republicans supporting him," she says. "He's just very rude. And he doesn't talk like a president is supposed to." I bring your attention to the facial expression. What does supremacy look like? A smirk.

I am not speaking of white supremacy specifically, because

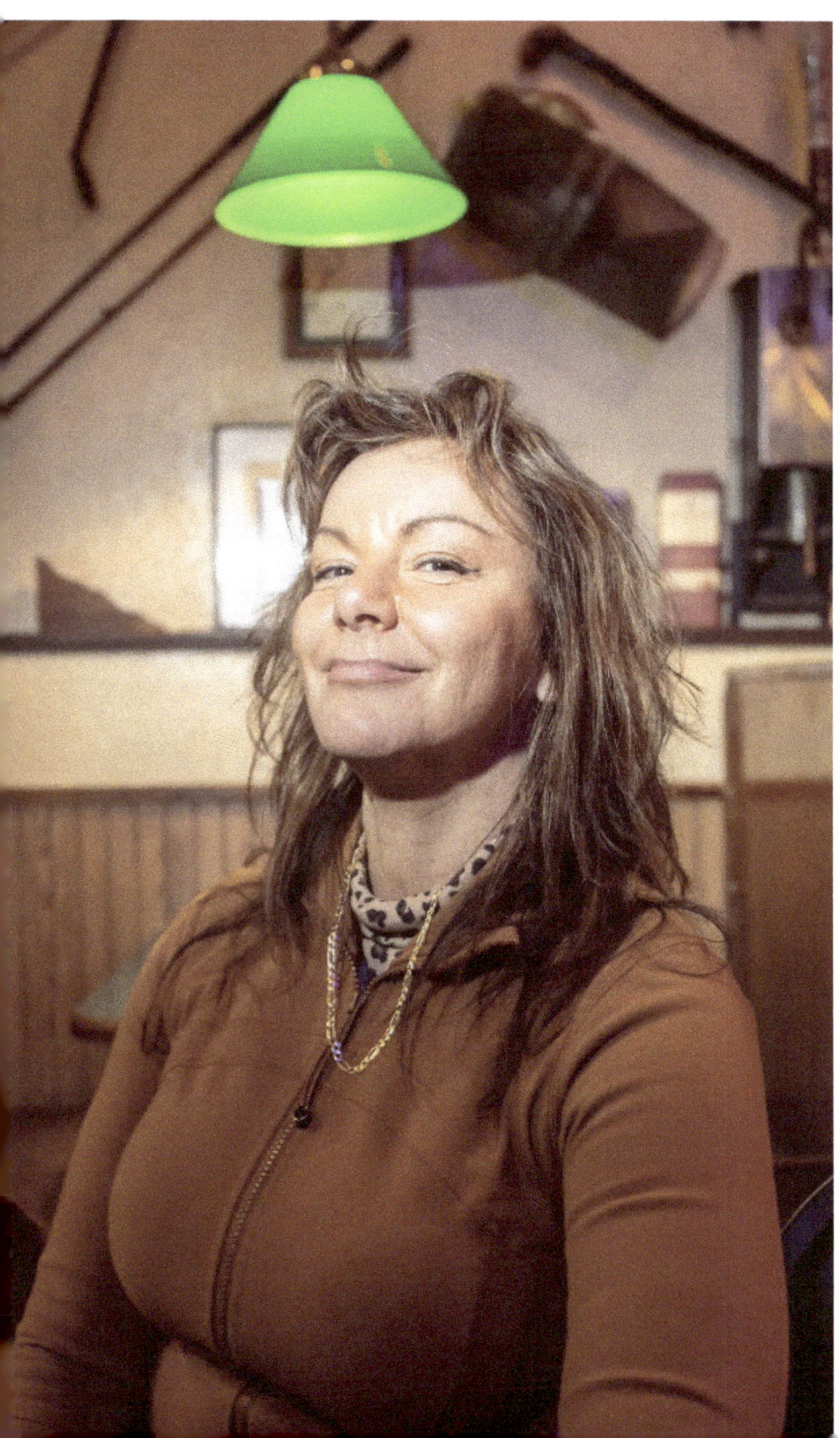

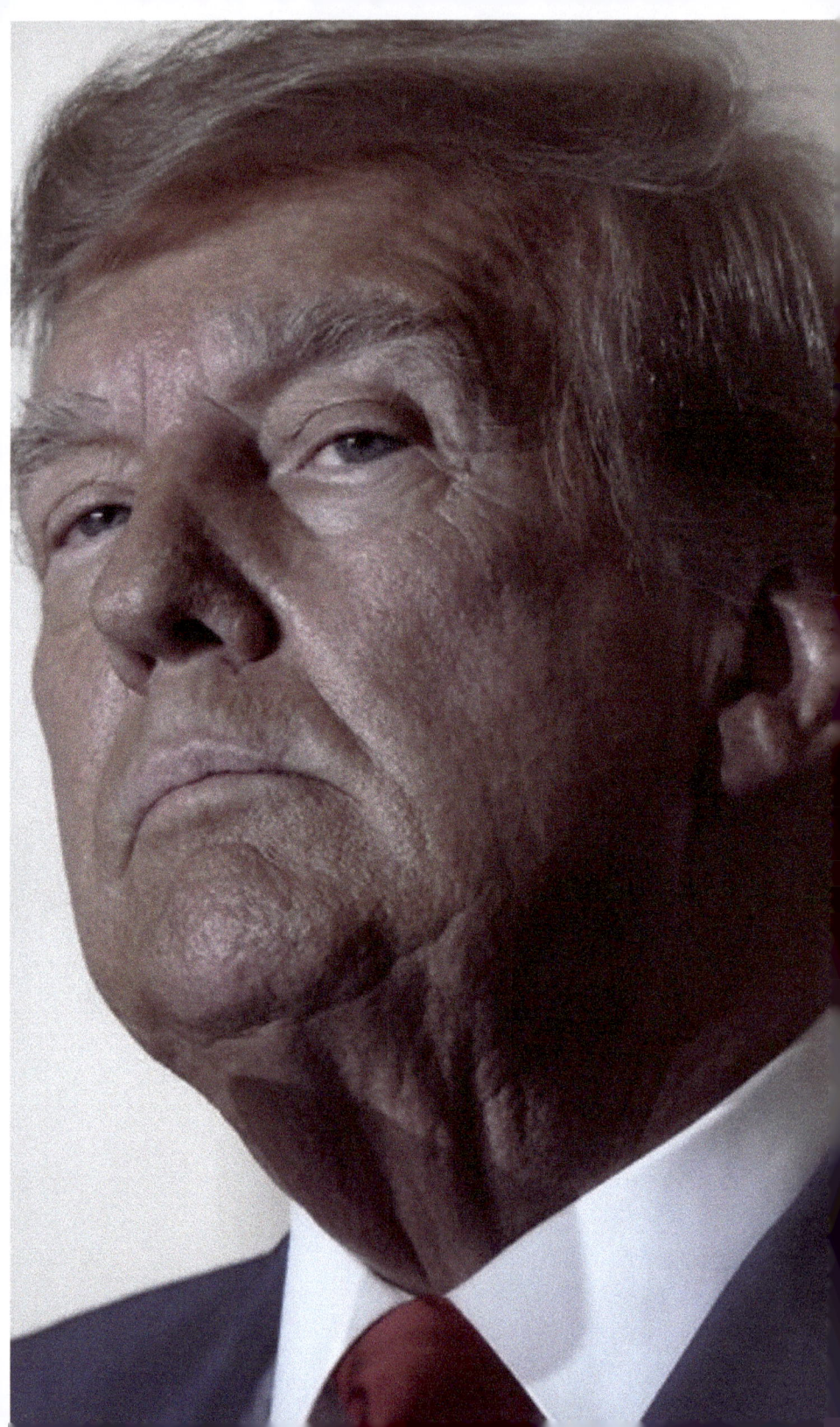

white supremacy is a flavor, a sub-category I would propose to you, of this larger phenomenon of supremacy. Yet supremacy itself, in all its variants, is a form of smugness. A smirk of dismissal. Notice the tilt of the head: she is looking at us askance, from off to the side. The slight uplift of the chin so that she can look down at us. The squint. We are in the realm of archetypes. I mean no disrespect to this particular lady: I am looking through her at the gesture; the place in consciousness from which she addresses us. Now here is the gaze of the man for whom she disdains allegiance.

Again, notice the gaze, and from where it is directed.

So let us begin with these portraits: the Vatican's repudiation of the Doctrine of Discovery, 571 years after they enshrined it in papal authority, and the smirk of a thirty-something woman in Iowa looking down her nose at us. The act and its expression.

10 - Hierarchy

I remember the first time I ever became conscious of social hierarchy. I was seven years old, and had just been displaced from my home, community, and place. I grew up in a small town in rural New Hampshire, in the Connecticut River valley. My father was a landscape architect, and at this time my mother did not yet work. We lived in a house that was probably 800 square feet, and several hundred years old. The stairs creaked dutifully every time they were ascended or descended. Downstairs was a kitchen with a screened-in porch, and a living room. Upstairs my parents bedroom, my bedroom, a single bathroom. Outside the house were other colonial homes like it, 250 years old, some stately and some dilapidated, and a grid of streets that led up into the forested hills. In five minutes I could be out of the neighborhood and into field and forest. Possibly the town consisted of a thousand inhabitants; it might have been fewer. There was a central square with a cannon that dated back to the Revolutionary war. A bank, a post office, a couple of restaurants including a Greek (for some reason) pizza parlor called Athens Pizzeria. A small, out-of-the way New England town. The kind memorialized now in calendars with glossy photographs of covered bridges at peak autumn foliage. No one we knew had any money. But we were rich in belonging, my roots were in the earth, and in that place. I was not aware of class, of status. Didn't know it existed.

From this place, this background, this originating context I remember moving to the suburbs of St. Louis in November 1982. I remember arriving in elementary school, into the second grade. I remember meeting Lamar Macklin, and Danny Lipsitz, and Joey Mitchell, and I remember going over to Joey's house one day after school and realizing that they had more money than we did. I'm quite sure that no one said anything about this to me: they were not tacky. I think I just remember walking around in his house and sort of marveling at how nice everything was. The house seemed enormous to me: it contained endless rooms; more bedrooms than there were members of their family. *Why?* I thought. *Guest bedrooms?*

I recall noticing how nice the houses on their street were. This was not something overt. No one said or did anything to make me feel diminished. I just remember standing there, on the side of his house, between their driveway and the next, looking at the manicured lawns, gazing at the stately colonial houses on the street and realizing, *Oh wait, we could not afford to live here. These houses are much nicer than our house.*

Money had never occurred to me before that. I'm sure I had seen it, I must have. I know we bought things in New Hampshire. I just don't remember ever having thought about it once. Part of what I remember about being in St. Louis that year, being seven years old, being eight years old, was this rapidly dawning realization that there was a sort of hierarchy of class: a ladder. And that there were signifiers of what rungs a person occupied on the ladder. That this was a kind of social code.

You could utilize certain signifiers to decode where a person stood in terms of class. The clothes they wore, the cars they drove, the neighborhoods they lived in: all of these were signifiers of status. I remember realizing that certain neighborhoods had more status than others. That the houses here were nicer than over there. That this side of Olive Boulevard was wealthier than that side of Olive Boulevard. But it was deeper than this, I remember thinking, because it wasn't simply about money: it was about worth.

The good, the virtuous, the desirable: that is the top of the ladder. What we are programmed to emulate.

And although I did not have the language for it at the time, wouldn't have been able to frame the thought in terms of social location, I could see that there were ladders of class, and ethnicity, and religion. That some places on the ladder had more value than others, and that this was even existential.

That what was good and virtuous and desirable was white, and male, and rich. White was better than brown and brown was better than black. Before I had even consciously realized what I was doing, I had ranked my classmates according to this schema. I had ranked the religions. I had ranked the neighborhoods.

I remember looking at my own life, suddenly, through this lens. The rusting orange Volkswagen Rabbit my father was driving– how had I never before noticed how beat-up it was? I felt suddenly embarrassed. The strange and ancient farmhouse we had moved into with the mouldering foundation. It was a bit shameful, no? The clothes I was wearing that were not branded? I remember realizing, quite suddenly, that I was nowhere near the top of the ladder.

I became rapidly rabidly obsessed with the signifiers of status. My earliest memories of cars came from ranking them with a view to their class implications. At the top of the rankings were the Mercedes-Benz, the BMW, the Jaguar. These cars exuded effortless luxury, signified easy affluence. Each of them, in my childhood memory, is tinged with slightly different emotional evocations. The Benz was royal. The BMW understated. The Jaguar daring. In the middle were things like the Ford Taurus, the Toyota Camry: solidly middle-class. And then there were the cars in the lower third: the Toyota Corolla, and the yet lowlier Ford Escort. At this time you still saw, from time to time, the humblest of automobiles: the Yugo. Goodness, I still remember the sense of pride I felt when my family graduated from driving a lowly Toyota Tercel to driving a solidly middle-class Camry. I remember the kind of existential relief this granted me: a boost of confidence, a sense of arrival I remember feeling in my body. I did not have the temerity, even in my own private mind, to wish for a Mercedes– that was simply in another league, remote, for someone else. Unimaginable. An affront to the order of things.

Looking back, the emotional significance of this seems absurd. I imagine a Greek chorus. I imagine them harmonizing around me, singing my relief, memorializing my shame. I remember the moment that Joey Mitchell's mother showed up to pick us up from school driving a BMW. I felt betrayed somehow that he hadn't bothered to tell me they bought one. As I climbed in, the greek chorus sings its astonishment. I had never sat in one before, and I remember memorizing the contours of the leather seats, studying this luxury up close, running a finger over the stitching and thinking, *He moves in an orbit that I will never know, this child who resembles me in so many other ways.* I remember thinking, *Wow, he's really got it made now. What isn't out of reach for a boy whose mother drives a BMW?*

From the time I was about eight years old, and became aware of status, you would likely find my closet filled with off-color garments. I put together a collection of purple and yellow striped, pink and mint green shirts. You might have thought I was color-blind if you hadn't realized that all of them were Polo by Ralph Lauren. Since we couldn't afford to buy Polo, I scoured the racks at Marshalls.

These were the shirts from the previous season that had started at Nordstrom, and failed to sell, started at Macy's, and failed to sell, and had then wound their way downward through the retail ecology, getting progressively picked off, their prices falling at each round, until they had ended up on the lowly racks of the deep discounter Marshalls, from which they made their way into my closet. These were truly the dregs of the fashion world; garments so odd that no one wanted them. But I didn't care that the shirt was royal purple and canary yellow, that it looked like the plumage of a tropical bird. I cared that in the corner of the chest was the stitched insignia of a tiny polo player on a horse, at two centimeters tall exuding the quiet confidence of luxury that I required to feel better about myself, now that I could not longer feel the earth under my feet.

Because, in reality, this is what had happened. I had grown alienated, without realizing it. I did not feel anymore that deep sense of belonging. And without it, without being able to find my way into the forest, to feel myself a part of her, to find any coherent sense of village, I had my nose pressed up against the glass of the party that I couldn't get into. All of this status-mongering, all of this ranking, all of this hierarchy was a substitute, the psychic displacement of no longer feeling at home, no longer feeling that I belonged. Without tribe, without village, without place, without roots, to whom did I belong? Who would take me in, adopt me as son? Was it Ralph Lauren? Was it BMW? Could I buy my way into belonging? In the absence of the wild mother, who would adopt me?

It was – it is – that simple.

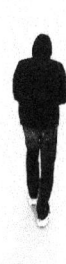

11 - Tragic Exiles

As an exercise in awareness, I like to attempt to reach back into the heartspace and mindview of our earliest human ancestors, to attempt to place myself at the origin of our species in the Kalahari two hundred thousand years ago. Because some of the culture of the Kalahari is still intact, this exercise is not as fanciful as it seems, as we have experiential contact yet with this source culture.

What we think of as alienation, is, functionally, an absence of belonging. In language, a *lacuna* or *lexical gap* is a hole in a language: the absence of a word or phrase in a particular language where it could be reasonably expected to exist. In Japanese, for example, the word *komorebi* refers to the color of sunlight filtered through the leaves of the forest. In English, we cannot speak directly of this green-gold, as there is no word for it, despite the fact that this very color is the hue of our deepest ancestral dreaming: the primal homescreen. Now that you know there is a word for it; you cannot unsee or unfeel this. This filtered forest light becomes its own thing: accretes beingness by being named.

Ludwig Wittgenstein asserted famously, in the *Tractatus Logico-Philosophicus*, that language is essentially a net inside of which we live: *The limits of my language mean the limits of my world.* He asserts that what is beyond language is not available to imagination.

Yet there is an embodied progenitor to linguistic absence, as language maps our experience. And the *lacuna* in experience, the hole in the fabric of the felt wrought by alienation, is beneath and before the holes in language, because what cannot be felt will never be known to be missing and we will therefore never attempt to describe it.

Except that we have felt its absence as an ache since always. We have felt its ache since Homer spoke *The Odyssey*, imbuing its titular protagonist with *nostos*: the longing for home, as his principal engine. It is an absence that pains us, not a simple void. It has a gravitational force; it sucks at us inwardly. It is not simply an absence; it is a black hole. We know, even without the language to identify it, even without the interoceptive vocabulary to point to it, that there is something fundamental missing. Something that we have lost, or that has been thieved from us. All of our origin stories attempt to explain why we deserve this painful destiny; why we have been sired into the agony of this lack.

In an existence where we belong to the Universe, where we are part of it and viscerally experience our relatedness, our kinship with *All There Is*, we are woven together with all of Life. Through the lens of this sacred unity, nothing is alien, nothing is untethered. Through the ropes of relating we have access to all the information in the universe: in-formation. Information is energy in formation. Within this mode of belonging, there is no need for the kind of God that monotheism proposes, because God is experienced in everything, including us. This experience of belonging is down beneath language, beneath sensation. It is a visceral immersion in *with*. A music of which we are a part; within which we move. An animism.

What moderns call God is an artifact of our alienation. The name we give to the antidote to the empty place that sucks inwardly at us. The way we think about the Creator is confused. Something benign yet not human, unfathomable, accessible possibly through altered states, mediated by trained initiates. It supposes that we are somewhere down here, and there is someone up there running things. The hegemony of European rationalism, so called, which rejects as irrational those things that cannot be explained 'scientifically'–and therefore relegates religion to the realm of the antique–misses the point entirely, which is that religion expresses a yearning. It is right there in the etymology of the word. A yearning to be tied back to the creative wellspring, the Source *(re-ligio)*. A yearning to have that aching void filled with what is supposed to be at the center of us, were it not this emptiness. What we call God–and assuredly our attempts to illustrate this, constrain it in human form, put a beard on it and paint it on a chapel ceiling are much deeper a reflection of the hall of mirrors of our own narcissism than anything approaching reality–arises from the felt intuition that we have been cut off from the wellspring of reality, and long for a relationship with it. The problem is that we've become consumed with what this looks like, and forgotten how it feels.

This yearning for God–and to be crystal clear I heartily endorse as crucial both this yearning, and its consummation–is the yearning to not be alienated, not an orphan of an uncaring universe, but a child of belonging. The yearning for God, its essence, its distillate, is a yearning for belonging, in a cosmic sense. To FEEL part of the divine reality, the divine family, the eternal flux.

I'm driving toward the taproot of Supremacy, and it has brought me here, to this contemplation of the Divine, which is generally clothed in the poor cloth of our own minds, our own gaze, and our own thinking, and has been formalized over millennia into the varied yet static forms we generally are made aware of by religion.

Yet I direct my attention back, further, to tribal wanderings, to the Jews in the desert, ye brethren of mine, ye wandering tribes of Israel. The old testament God, to whom they entrusted worship, the *tetragrammaton*, is a God to whom they prayed for what? For a good harvest, for peaceful hearts, for a glimpse at the fabric of the real, for harmony in the home and hearth, for blessing. And the common denominator of all these worthy prayers? Belonging.

Jesus has been as intentionally mistranslated as anyone in history. Yet of crucial import to this conversation (I say this based on having studied, through books, the Aramaic language he spoke) is the fact that contrary to both popular conception and to established church doctrine, Jesus did not say, "Pray to me." He said, "Pray as I pray." He was teaching people how to come back into relationship with the Cosmos. How to feel kinship. This is not written in some book. Relatedness is not in a text, in a scripture, be it a torah or otherwise.

"Seek not the law in your scriptures, for the law is life, whereas the scripture is dead. I tell you truly, Moses received not his laws from God in writing, but through the living word. The law is living word of living God to living prophets for living men.

In everything that is life is the law written. You find it in the grass, in the tree, in the river, in the mountain, in the birds of heaven, in the fishes of the sea; but seek it chiefly in yourselves. For I tell you truly, all living things are nearer to God than the scripture which is without life.

God so made life and all living things that they might by the everlasting word teach the laws of the true God to man. God wrote not the laws in the pages of books, but in your heart and in your spirit. They are in your breath, your blood, your bone; in your flesh, your bowels, your eyes, your ears, and in every little part of your body.

They are present in the air, in the water, in the earth, in the plants, in the sunbeams, in the depths and in the heights. They all speak to you that you may understand the tongue and the will of the living God.

But you shut your eyes that you may not see, and you shut your ears that you may not hear. I tell you truly, that the scripture is the work of man, but life and all its hosts are the work of our God. Wherefore do you not listen to the words of God which are written in His works? And wherefore do you study the dead scriptures which are the work of the hands of men?"

-The Essene Gospel of Peace

When then, did we lose this experience of relatedness? When did we stop reading the book of life in the Living World, studying this living law, and why? When did we cut down the forest to build a church to enter into and worship?

Somewhere between the Original Fire tended by the Black Mother of Us All, the matrilineal line with the circle of the village organized around it, and the ritualized alienation of modernity, there are a series of denaturing catastrophes. What were they?

These catastrophes are stories of being cast out. A sequence of tragic exiles. A repetition of removal from kinship: damning blasts of expulsion. First from the garden of relatedness to all (Eden), then from relatedness with our human brothers and sisters.

12 - Original Exile

Origin stories are important. We humans are meaning-making creatures, and we have a primal and existential need to know how things came to be the way they are. Yet it is probably important to notice that the origin stories that we are told are retro-active. They weren't penned at the origins, but significantly later. They are stories about something that happened a long time ago, and as we receive them it is important to ask ourselves who they were composed by, and whose purposes they serve, and to what ends.

There are numerous origin stories of the modern world, yet perhaps none so pervasive in its configurings of the world we have inherited as *The Bible*. And the first book of the Bible, Genesis, is concerned with the origin of the cosmos, and the origin of humanity. The story it tells is deeply and discomfitingly strange.

In the first three books of Genesis, the world as we know it is created by God, it is peopled by the first human, Adam, who is placed as a King, in the likeness of God, that he may "rule over the fish in the sea and the birds in the sky, over the livestock and all the wild animals, and over all the creatures that move along the ground." [Genesis 1:26]

Lacking a suitable companion, he is gifted woman [Genesis 2] who is drawn from one of his ribs.

18 The Lord God said, "It is not good for the man to be alone. I will make a helper suitable for him."

19 Now the Lord God had formed out of the ground all the wild animals and all the birds in the sky. He brought them to the man to see what he would name them; and whatever the man called each living creature, that was its name. 20 So the man gave names to all the livestock, the birds in the sky and all the wild animals.

But for Adam no suitable helper was found. 21 So the Lord God caused the man to fall into a deep sleep; and while he was sleeping, he took one of the man's ribs and then closed up the place with flesh. 22 Then the Lord God made a woman from the rib[1] he had taken out of the man, and he brought her to the man.

23 The man said, "This is now bone of my bones and flesh of my flesh; she shall be called 'woman,' for she was taken out of man."

Adam and Eve reside in the Garden of Eden, an earthly paradise. They are commanded not to eat of a certain tree, "You are free to eat from any tree in the garden; 17 but you must not eat from the tree of the knowledge of good and evil, for when you eat from it you will certainly die." (Genesis 2:17)

Genesis 3, which describes the Fall of Man, explains:

Now the serpent was more crafty than any of the wild animals the Lord God had made. He said to the woman, "Did God really say, 'You

---

1 This is probably, for a whole host of reasons, a mis-translation. There is no word for 'rib' in either ancient Hebrew or Aramaic. The ancient Hebrew word is *Tzela*, which means rib, side, or tail. There is another way of understanding the word tzela, based on Midrash (Bereishit Rabbah 8:1; Vayikra Rabbah 14:1); the Gemara (Berachot 61a) and the Zohar (Bereishit 34b-35a; Shemot 55a; 231a). As is known, there are two narratives detailing the creation of mankind—the first in chapter one of Bereishit, the second in chapter two. In the first account, according to some commentators, it appears that the Adam was not solely a male, but was rather a being consisting of both male and female halves. In chapter two, according to this explanation, this two-sided human was separated into the two genders, and it is this surgical procedure that is described in the verse.

must not eat from any tree in the garden'?"

2 The woman said to the serpent, "We may eat fruit from the trees in the garden, 3 but God did say, 'You must not eat fruit from the tree that is in the middle of the garden, and you must not touch it, or you will die.'"

4 "You will certainly not die,"[2] the serpent said to the woman. 5 "For God knows that when you eat from it your eyes will be opened, and you will be like God, knowing good and evil."

6 When the woman saw that the fruit of the tree was good for food and pleasing to the eye, and also desirable for gaining wisdom, she took some and ate it. She also gave some to her husband, who was with her, and he ate it. 7 Then the eyes of both of them were opened, and they realized they were naked; so they sewed fig leaves together and made coverings for themselves.

The way that the story is told, the first humans, Adam and Eve, are almost immediately after their creation banished from the earthy paradise in which God has placed them.

The way that the story is told, God lies to Adam about the Tree of the Knowledge of Good and Evil, telling him– *when you eat from it you will certainly die.*

The way that the story is told, the crafty serpent, whose belly is on the ground, deceives Eve, who in turn deceives her husband: both disobey God. As a result of this disobedience, both are cast from the Garden of Eden, and forced to work by the sweat of their brows.

Much of the Christian interpretation of the world hinges upon this origin story, which purports to explain Original Sin,

---

[2] The King James Version says, 'You will not certainly die,' however this places the emphasis in the wrong place in the sentence. What is certain is the serpent's assertion, not the death. Thus the slight alteration, which is present in other versions as well.

which in christian theology refers to the condition of sinfulness that all humans share, inherited from Adam and Eve due to the Fall. The Catholic church then teaches that baptism removes original sin.

So, let me get this straight. Immediately after creating humanity in the image of the Divine, God tells a bald-faced lie to the first humans, who despite being made in the image of the Divine straightaway deceive him, and are then expelled from his Grace? And the only route back to this grace is by becoming a paying member of the Church that tells the story of this occurrence, for this church has the power, by permitting you to become a member of it, to wash away this original stain?

You've inherited an intransigent deep ancestral blemish that you did not know existed that can only be removed by joining our cult right now? That's the story?

Yet what is the story attempting to explain? Alienation.

If we can set down the absurdity of it for a moment, and regard it not as a set of facts but as an attempt to solve some very fundamental problems, the list of problems looks something like this:

1. We need an explanation for why humans at the time of the writing of this story experienced themselves as alienated. If they did not experience themselves as alienated, this story would not have resonated with them, as it did and does not resonate with most animists and Indigenous people. A precondition for this story to make any sense whatsoever is that we feel remote from an embodied experience of union with the Divine. We need a reason why.

2. We need someone to blame this alienation on. One way to put this is that the writers of this story had discovered that the best way to bring people together is to give them a common enemy. A scapegoat.

3. It is expedient to blame this on a woman, and to tell the story that women, who give birth to all humans, actually came from men. Sorry. Just a moment here. Have you ever met a person who was not born of a woman? No, you haven't. But the first woman came from the rib of a man?

4. And it is expedient to blame this on a snake: no one likes snakes anyway. Also, they do not talk and therefore cannot defend themselves.

Let me tell this story in a different way. Let me reconfigure it for you.

Let us start with the experience of alienation, *a priori*. Let us just say that, yes, humanity experiences itself as alienated from the Source, and has no idea why. In the absence of an explanation for this alienation, we are powerless to attempt to solve it. So the origin story is necessary in order to configure the problem in such a way that it can be solved. The argument of the Bible is that the solution to the problem is Christianity. The problem is alienation: the solution is Christianity. This is what *The Bible* is selling you.

But what if the alienation of man (this is who we are solving the problem for, the sons of Adam, if you haven't realized this) is actually due to Adam's alienation from both his feminine nature (woman), and his indigenous nature (the belly-on-the-ground serpent).

What if the story is correct in the following and specific sense: Adam is, yes, alienated. This alienation is the result of something that has happened in relation to parts of self becoming cut off. The parts of self that have become cut off are feminine ways of knowing (knowing-through-feeling) and indigenous ways of knowing (chthonic, grounding, knowing-through-earth).

And so what if, rather than needing the intercession of a skygod through the intermediaries of a death cult, we might rather need to turn inward toward feeling (the feminine), and downward toward the earth (the Indigenous)?

There is something else in the story that suggests to me that this is so. A line in Genesis 2 explains that God has placed two trees in the garden that are not intended for Adam: the Tree of Knowledge, and the Tree of Life. I think it is useful for us to understand the Garden of Eden not as a circumscribed geography at the confluence of four rivers, but as a mode of being. The psychic landscape at which the story points, clearly, is our deep ancestral baseline: the small band hunter gatherer lifestyle. This was a lifestyle where we moved, seasonally, with the migration patterns of the animals, hunting and gathering as we moved across the surface of the earth. We did not earn our livings by the sweat of our brows, did not plant crops. We were not stationary. Rather, as in the Garden, we navigated a world of abundance, where operating through faith we did not require storing up provisions against loss. This is the state of innocence to which the story refers: we did not know that we were naked. The nakedness is not clothing: it is that we are holding nothing back. There is no part of us that is held in reserve: set aside. Our immersion in experience is complete. We are fully present. No part of us is veiled inwardly or outwardly.

The thing that occurs to me about this lifestyle, this mode of being, if you will, is that it is centered in kinship, centered in relating, and from this mode *power over* is not particularly interesting or appealing. What people operating in this mode are questing for is not the knowledge of good and evil. If you can talk to the birds and the wind and the trees and the earth, and if everything is provided for you, what knowledge of good and evil do you need?

No, this temptation of which the story speaks, this whisper from the snake – *when you eat of that fruit your eyes will be opened* – this temptation calls out to a part of the psyche that in small band hunter gatherers probably did not exist. It is the writers of the story who feel the pull of that temptation because they have already been invaded by alienation. Again, it is a story told backward, a story required to explain something that has happened *to the people writing the story.* And what it is pointing at is the origin of moving up out of direct experience into cognition. The knowledge of good and evil is the relocation, the re-homing of self into thinking. Frankly, if you are living in Union with *All That Is*, this prospect is both bleak and unappealing.

Small band hunter gatherer peoples, if offered the Tree of the Knowledge of Good and Evil by the crafty serpent, did such a creature exist, were probably pretty likely to say, *No thanks, we're good.*

What you are proposing here is likely to get us into a mess of trouble, and what need have we for it anyhow? Here, in consciousness of relatedness, in the experience of Union, we have access to the language of celestial musics all. We confabulate with all the creatures, know their true names, and have kinship with them. We talk to the rivers and know their true names. We converse with the stones about the nature of time and impermanence. We dance with the elements. We are at One. What need have we for static hierarchizing knowledge? It doesn't even appeal.

The very notion in the story that Adam and Eve would be tempted by this is the backcast figuration of someone power-hungry and mapping this back onto ancestors who did not have the same acquisitive and domination-oriented thrust. It is confusion of cause and effect: to translocate the illness of alienation backwards onto people who had it not. This is, dare I say it, insane.

13 - Cain and Abel

If we, again, turn our attention back to the Bible, that source document of origin stories that are not really so, we find the story of Cain and Abel. This is still early in the book, Genesis Chapter Four, just after the story of Adam and Eve. We are one generation after having been cast out of the garden.

Cain, the first born, is a farmer. Abel, second-born, is a shepherd. Each makes a sacrifice to God: Cain of herbs of the field, Abel of a lambling. In the story God accepts Abel's sacrifice, while disdaining Cain's. Cain rises up and kills his brother, is marked, and cast out (again, the second damning blast from this divine trumpet, for his parents have already been cast out once), and forced to wander.

If we apply the same method we have applied in our analysis of Adam and Eve, seeing this as a sort of fractal radioactive ember of some deeper older story that carries yet throughlines and undercurrents of meaning, applying our tracking skills, listening for the pattern of the story beneath the story, we can ask also who wrote this story, and whom did it benefit, and to what end, and perhaps some useful things will come into clearer view out of the mist.

The first alienation is from original belonging, which has been blamed on a woman (the feminine) in partnership with a snake (our Indigeneity). If we unlock this story, and open it, we find that contrary to established meanings, the turn toward belonging is back toward the feminine, and toward contact with the ground (Indigenous people are earth-based [chthonic] people).

The second story, the story of Cain and Abel, narrates the entrance of war into the human story. Both children of the original mother, brother turns against brother. This is a story of the generation of tribal [civilizational] lines. It is attempting to explain a diaspora in the human family as a result of murder. Again, let us take as accurate the essence of its effect, as we have taken as accurate the essence of the effect of the story of Adam and Eve. Through the story of Adam and Eve, we arrive *en medias res*, in the middle of the play, as it were, in a world where people are alienated from Nature. The story is attempting to tell us how things got to be this way. So too, in the story of Cain and Abel, we arrive in a world of diverse civilizations in diverse places, with different skins, where brother murders brother. People are alienated from other people. The children of the original mother no longer know they are of the same family. Crumbsnatchers from the original fireplace scattered to the wind. Some of them are farming peoples, tied to place. Some of them are herding peoples, nomadic. They have lost the remembrance of their shared roots, their common origin, their shared mother, the common hearth.

What is missing from either of these forms are the original peoples, the hunter gatherers, so we know that this is a story whose origin is within the past 12,000 years. A story situated after the birth of agriculture. By the time Cain and Abel happens, the diaspora from the Kalahari is a fact lost already to ancient history, beyond the pale of the backcast gaze, forgotten. Civilizations in this next era have organized themselves around two principles: that of tilling the soil, and that of herding animals. Tilling cultures, which are anchored to place, have become more urban, and seats therefore of technology. The etymology of the word Cain, in Aramaic (*kain*), links it to 'forge' or 'smith'. Cain is a farmer, but also a metal worker: a skilled artisan, a city-dweller. Cain's sacrifice is rejected, and he kills Abel. In the story he does this with a rock, but I find myself wondering about this. Here is a smith, a bronze-age artisan, killing a shepherd. I find it hard to believe he would not have done so with a weapon forged by his own hand.

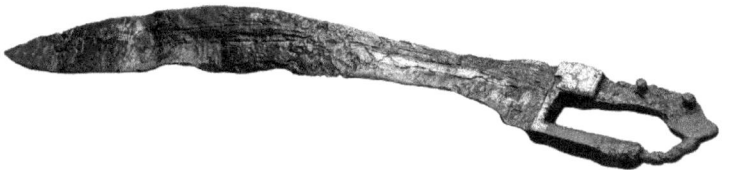

A bronze-age sword

It is my intuition that with the same forge that bronze-age humans have shaped the plow, they shaped also the sword. We have come into the era of intensified fire, the era of the forge, and with this ability to liquify and shape metal we have figured out how to smith tools that will break open the earth and break open bodies. We can shatter stone and bone, now. We have crossed a technical threshold of intrusion.

This technical wherewithal has been harnessed to tilling the soil, as well as to defending the city. This culture has begun to stockpile grain, to reserve it against the coming of winter, against the possibility of drought or flood. We guard against famine. In the movement that precedes this, thousands of years before, the movement that gives birth to settled agriculture, there is the transition from hunter gatherer lifestyles–utterly dependent on the Living World–to planting.

Let us view this as a continuum. Someone, we can imagine, realizes that the fruit they eat has seeds, begins to understand that from these seeds grow new plants, and with them more fruit. It is not difficult to imagine an interim phase, a phase where our ancestors were hunting and gathering, yet also planting along the migration routes. We were following the animals, moving with them in cycles. Why not enrich the routes with the seeds of the plants we wish to harvest? Would there have been some kind of interdiction in this? Would this have felt like a violation of the original pattern? Disrespect to some form of belonging?

I don't see how. I can imagine the original peoples traveling- and this is in deeptime yet- let us say a hundred thousand years ago, through landscapes, savannah, with features that change, annually, and yet slowly so. I can imagine the animals stopping to drink at a lake here, a watering hole. I can imagine my uber-grandparents pausing by the water to drink, I can imagine them planting some of the seeds they had gathered a little distance off from the water's edge, and telling their children. I imagine those same children, some generation later, harvesting fruit from these trees as they too follow the animals.

In order for this to happen-the psychic innovation of altering the landscape-shaping it to better provision them, something has already happened in the consciousness of the human. Some agency being birthed. Something like *Will*. Some impulse of gardening.

We are, at this time in history, one hundred thousand years ago, all trackers. Our sensory capabilities are so far beyond present-day imagining as to be almost unfathomable. We possess possibly not quite our current level of finger-level dexterity, for our hands then were likely not spending much time writing, scrolling, playing piano, tapping on keys. But the body, in general, would have been fit-packed dense with muscle, and agile-at a level hardly imaginable to anyone but the most extremely elite athletes. This physicality, developed through the everyday necessity of migrating, through the sheer physicality of surviving, is paired with an agility that again we would find remarkable. The quickness of hand, the quickness of mind of the hunter. These are people with no stress whatsoever in our contemporary definition of it. There are no deadlines, no bills to pay, no jobs, no bosses. The economy doesn't expand and contract. We are all part of the ancestral village: no one struggles with isolation, there are no single mothers, no one doing it on their own. In this absence of stress, the people are at home in relating: their Connection

Systems are online all of the time, their Autonomic Nervous Systems fully available. Their ability therefore, the performance of these humans, their neurobiological fluidity, is off the charts.

Animals are psychic. Did you know that? They can read your thoughts. And so the people are expert, also, in veiling their minds, quieting them down to nothing. They reside in a continual present, masters of what we would call mindfulness all. And their attention flows through the senses synaesthetically.

They are barefoot, always, with feet that read the laylines of energy in the earth, feet that aid in navigation. Hands and skin that read the meaning, scent, and humidity of wind. Hands that sense for energy, sense for tracks, sense for water like dowsing wands. Radar hands. Beings reading, through their profound embodiment, the energy landscape just barely veiled by matter. I would propose to you that at this time in our evolutionary history, the hegemony of visuality was not yet in place. People did not primarily *see* the world. The conscience was not, as Richard Sennet would later assert, of the eye. The refinement of senses was oriented into the felt. We were using the original intelligences with which the human organism is so richly endowed, which arises when the autonomic physiology is stabilized in its baseline state of social engagement. We possessed, at this time, original integrated sensing. We felt everything. And within this feeling, we are people who speak bird language, people who have built ropes with all of the Creation, inhabiting a landscape humming with meaning, with conversation, where we, at will, can pick up and try on the minds of the animals, step into the mind of the cheetah, possibly see through his eyes. Energy beings feeling our way through the pattern language of the Living World.

We, part of the fabric of unity, step through the doorways of individual identity and across the chain of being, becoming the rocks, the sun-baked mud, wearing the mind of the acacia trees, the impala. These uber-grandparents of us all, sensorily and bodily awake in a manner that exceeds our definitions of alertness and embodiment, connected to everything, reading the great book of nature. These are our parent's parents, all of us.

Some, we can imagine, over the spans of deep-time, might have a proclivity to walk less. Might have more stationary attitudes, might have been more meditatively inclined. Might have wanted to sit in one spot. Might have elected, or been asked to stay in one place and tend to the trees. Might have been injured and needed to rest. There are many reasons, perhaps, why some might not have been able, or inclined, to migrate. Perhaps the passing groups bring them food. Perhaps those who stay those ancient winters starve to death, and their skeletons, picked clean by carrion, are encountered the following spring on a reverse migration and revered. Under the first orchards I imagine the bones of some of these early ancestors who could not accumulate enough calories in certain seasons to make it across. I can imagine the bones draped with flowers picked by the tribe wandering past.

A failed crop and the early farmers fall. An early stationary village winks out, like the last ember of a fire.

Is this why God is not pleased with Cain? Because Cain's way of life, at its beginnings, is tenuous?

Abel, the shepherd...Is Abel the original tribe, the hunter gatherer ancestry, murdered? Is this what the story means?

Who wrote this story?

From this same ancestral line are there people who, rather than continually following the animals–how much work it is!–capture some rather than kill them and then begin to travel with those? Would these have been sheep? I doubt it, though I don't know. Some kind of four-legged that could have been eaten. Someone suggests, it seems inevitable in hindsight...

we're walking our entire lives, following the herd. Let's keep the herd with us.

I can imagine, once again, early experiments. How do you keep the herd near you? Do you hobble some animals? Choose an animal that cannot run away? Looking back into these mists of deep time I wonder. At some point, there are people with herds. I don't know if they are stationary. I doubt it. The animals follow the available food, accompanied by humans or no.

Abel is from this lineage. These lines, both of them, Cain and Abel, have opted for easier lives. Acquired some form of food insurance. Have opted to not depend utterly on Nature, and by the time of their story I believe that both of them have already put on supremacy mind and are having trouble taking it off. In what particular sense?

There is a kind of profound humility that comes when you depend entirely upon Nature for your survival. It is co-extant with the bone-deep knowledge of starvation. We moderns, consumers of empty calories, of Cheetos and Coca-cola, have lost contact with this, but our ancestors were experts in deprivation. We know, we *knew* what it meant to starve. Our small band hunter gatherer ancestors did not have refrigerators, storehouses, walls to keep out marauding others be they animal or human.

There is a kind of profound humility that comes from the daily forced reminder that being alive is a gift, and that this gift can be withheld. Nature has no bankruptcy protection: doesn't make loans. Go negative with calories for long enough and you will die. There are no government bailouts for biology.

Both emerging lines, that of the farmer, and that of the shepherd, seem to me like bets to try to change the odds, to try to sweeten the deal. Insurance against hardship.

Here, in Cain and Abel, is a story we have turned into an inverted kaleidoscope, an attempt to see through jumbled patterns and construct an instrument to look backwards into deep time.

By virtue of this insurance do we necessarily step in the direction of supremacy? Is it possible to have some form of abundance and not accumulate the gain and accrue it to ourselves? Not come to the conclusion that we are somehow better than those who do not have? Not move out of the present moment?

Conclude that we are more intelligent? Closer to God? More blessed? Do we not tell stories that confirm us in our biases? Happy is the one who does not attribute success to himself, but rather increases their gratitude. How many 'successful' and I put the word in quotes, as I interrogate it here...how many successful modern people do you know who will look you in the eye if you ask them about their flourishing and tell you it was luck? Most of the people I know attribute it to their own talents. Even born on third base, when they score they narrate stories about hitting home runs.

Is this the origin of supremacy? A shift in the manner of living, aeons ago, that took us out of direct contact with the necessity of the now? Out of being provided for by a benevolent universe? The first hedging of bets, the first accumulation, and then a need, retrospectively, to explain why we had food and someone else did not? To story this in a hierarchy and declare that one mode of living was more pleasing to God?

14 - Deepest Belly of Forsaken

The origin stories at the birth of a culture are not just stories. They are expressions of the way that we feel. The Bible wouldn't have gone viral, wouldn't have become simply *The Book*, if its telling of how things got to be the way that they are did not serve to carry the experience of the people. The stories have to resonate to be internalized.

If we are going to work our way back into the Garden, capital G, we have to pass back through the stories of exile in reverse, which is to say that we have to find a way to re-factor those equations of loss, of which we are the deep descendants, working them backwards until we arrive at their *before*.

In the Judeo-Christian tradition, I see several of these stories in particular as being palimpsests, written over with many layers of central and accreted meaning. The story of Cain and Abel, first of all, and first because if we are working backwards, following this trail in deep chronology back to the original rift, is the first one that we have to grapple with. Cain is the first born son of Adam, the first man, and the first exile. Abel is his second born.

And so what of this story of brother killing brother? To excavate, I look inward, I look at the struggles I have with my own brother. What of this turning away? In the Biblical story, Abel is a shepherd, and Cain is a farmer. We, the children of Cain, are descendants in his lineage, civilizational and energetic if not literal. We are the city dwellers, the ones whose lifeways pursued settled agriculture, who built up great cities, stored up grain against the coming of winter. Yet of the brothers, it was not our offering to God that was looked upon with favor, but that of our brother, Abel, the shepherd.

Genesis 4:1–16

4 And Adam knew Eve his wife; and she conceived, and bare Cain, and said, I have gotten a man from the Lord.

2 And she again bare his brother Abel. And Abel was a keeper of sheep, but Cain was a tiller of the ground.

3 And in process of time it came to pass, that Cain brought of the fruit of the ground an offering unto the Lord.

4 And Abel, he also brought of the firstlings of his flock and of the fat thereof. And the Lord had respect unto Abel and to his offering:

5 But unto Cain and to his offering he had not respect. **And Cain was very wroth, and his countenance fell.**

6 And the Lord said unto Cain, Why art thou wroth? and why is thy countenance fallen?

7 If thou doest well, shalt thou not be accepted? and if thou doest not well, sin lieth at the door. And unto thee shall be his desire, and thou shalt rule over him.

8 And Cain talked with Abel his brother: and it came to pass, when they were in the field, that Cain rose up against Abel his brother, and slew him.

9 And the Lord said unto Cain, Where is Abel thy brother? And he said, I know not: Am I my brother's keeper?

10 And he said, What hast thou done? **the voice of thy brother's blood crieth unto me from the ground.**

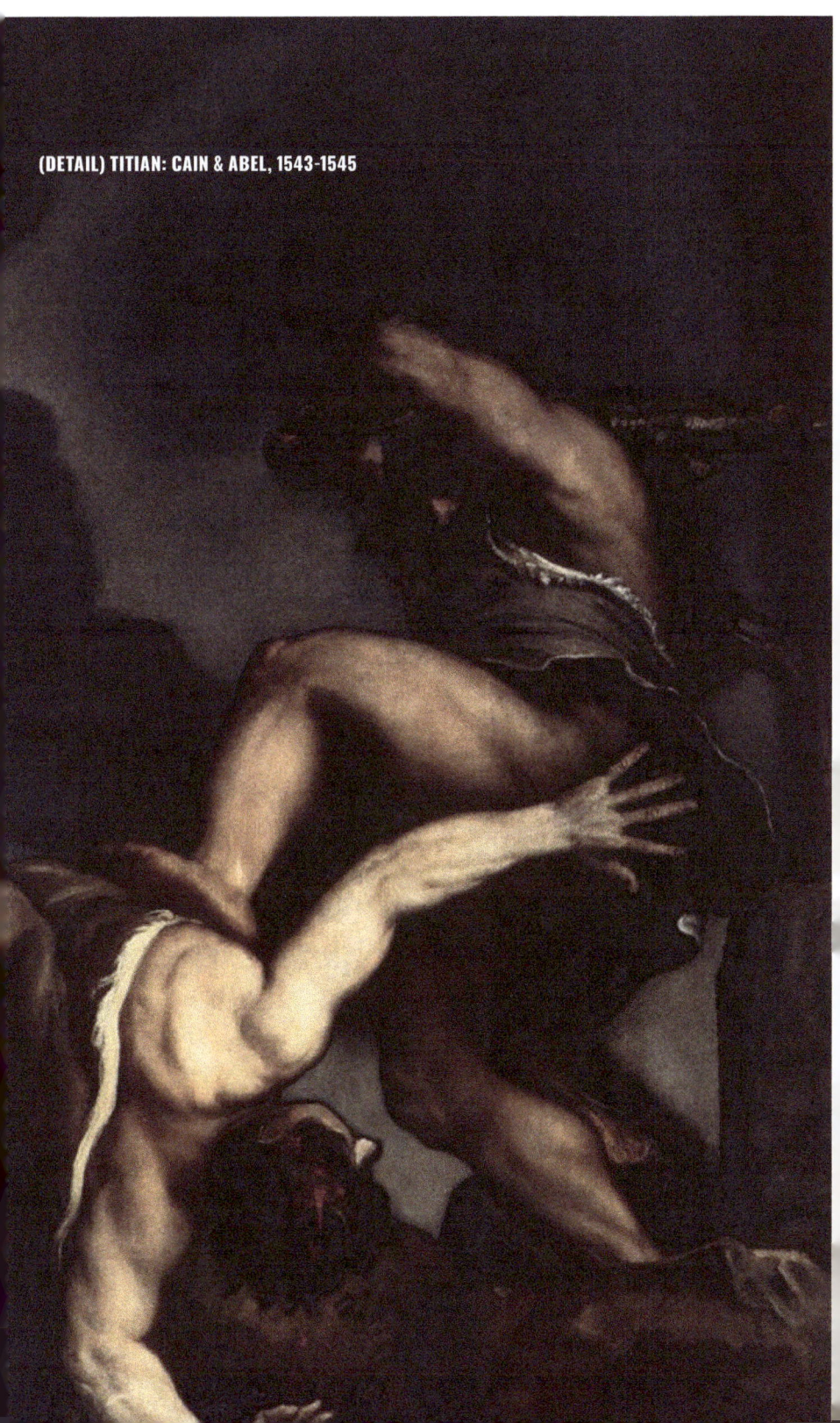
(DETAIL) TITIAN: CAIN & ABEL, 1543-1545

11 *And now art thou cursed from the earth, which hath opened her mouth to receive thy brother's blood from thy hand;*

12 *When thou tillest the ground, it shall not henceforth yield unto thee her strength; a fugitive and a vagabond shalt thou be in the earth.*

13 *And Cain said unto the Lord, My punishment is greater than I can bear.*

14 *Behold, thou hast driven me out this day from the face of the earth; and from thy face shall I be hid; and I shall be a fugitive and a vagabond in the earth; and it shall come to pass, that every one that findeth me shall slay me.*

15 *And the Lord said unto him, Therefore whosoever slayeth Cain, vengeance shall be taken on him sevenfold. And the Lord set a mark upon Cain, lest any finding him should not kill him.*[1]

16 *And Cain went out from the presence of the Lord, and dwelt in the land of Nod, on the east of Eden.*

[Emphasis mine.]

I would like to dwell exegitically upon a few particular elements of the above text, which is taken from the King James version.

First, let us note that when Abel and Cain present their respective sacrifices to the Lord, the passage says of the Lord that, *But unto Cain and to his offering he had not respect. And Cain was very wroth, and his countenance fell.*

The story does not tell us why the Lord does not respect the

---

1 I have added the word 'not'. The original King James version reads, 'lest any finding home should kill him' but it means that the mark is a warning to let people know *not* to kill him.

offering of Cain. I would propose to you that this is because the authors of the story do not know. And I would propose to you that this is because the story is a retelling of a much older tale, of which these authors were dimly and yet incompletely aware. The story of Cain and Abel is attempting to explain something fairly ancient in the lineage history, ancient even at the time the Bible was written, something in deeptime. By the point when the Bible was recorded, there had already been a bifurcation from the original Lifeway, e.g., ancestrally and genetically, which was the Small Band Hunter Gatherer baseline. Adam and Eve are Small Band Hunter Gatherers. Although we have always been tempted to read Eden as a geographic place, a literal garden somewhere near the confluence of the Tigres and Euphrates rivers, Eden is a chronicity more than a geography. Eden is the cadence of Union, before it was interrupted.

The Fall of Man, Adam and Eve's exile from the Garden, is not an exile from a mythical place, it is an exile from the ritual cadence of Union. Eden is a relationship, not a location.

The world of the Small Band Hunter Gatherer (SBHG), which is the cosmo-vision of relatedness enacted, the lineage arrayed in the lap of faith, where one does not store up provisions against the winter but rather travels with the animals cyclically in the Garden, with absolute faith that we shall be provisioned: this is Eden: the quality of this direct relationship with the Divine.

And so by the time Adam and Eve are exiled from this relatedness, again in deeptime, by the time that they conceive descendants, their two children are experimenting with deviations from this original Lifeway.

Abel is experimenting as a shepherd, which is to say that he has continued the wandering lifestyle of the itinerant band, though now he is bringing his flock with him (a form of insurance). Why does Abel wander? He moves with his flock, seeking forage to feed them. And so he yet preserves elements of the 'movement across the face of the earth' characteristic of the SBHG lifestyle.

Cain however has become a farmer. Cain has taken the seeds gathered along the wandering paths and planted them in a single place, seeking to permanize his settlement. And apparently the Lord does not find this pleasing. Or else, or also, there is something characterological about Cain that displeases the Lord. It is hard to say which is the antecedent. Did Cain become a farmer and therefore something characterological in him has changed in a manner displeasing to the Lord? Or is it the other way around? That by ceasing in his motion over the earth, which is in a manner a rejection of the cosmic dance, a rejection of a motion pattern of relatedness, something has shifted in his character? The farmer seems a deeper break with the Small Band Hunter Gatherer lifestyle than the shepherd.

I invite you to read these passages with me not through your cognition, but through the body. I invite you to try them on somatically, these readings, to see if something, anything, within you recognizes what I am speaking toward.

These are brothers, in the story, but they are also different lifeways. What does it mean that the agrarian lifeway has slayed the shepherding lifeway?

When Cain's offering to the Lord is not respected, Cain was very wroth, and his countenance fell. *Wroth* means wrathful, enraged, and it is interesting to note that this is his initial response. It does not seem obvious that one would grow enraged if the Lord did not accept one's offering: dejection seems the more likely choice. The passage, *and his countenance fell* feels important.

Our countenance, our face, is and has been considered, for most of human history, to be the most unique feature of our humanness. If we accept that we are made in the image of the Divine, the face itself, our visage, is generally accepted to represent us most completely. Later in the Bible the Lord permits all manner of disfiguring to test the faith of Job, but his face is left untouched, unmarked, unscathed.

So it is important that when Cain's offering is not accepted, his face falls. Glossed autonomically, we could say that at this moment he is no longer himself. He has shifted inwardly across an autonomic threshold: he is no longer able to look us (and God) in the eye. His face has fallen away from relatedness; he is no longer available. This echoes the moment in the Biblical story of Genesis (3:7) where Adam and Eve realize they are naked, and grow ashamed. The story says that their eyes were opened, but it is the opposite of this.

Perhaps Cain is wroth simply because he is comparing himself to his brother, yet it is worth wondering why he would not have celebrated the acceptance of his brother's offering. Why not be happy for his brother, rather than becoming enraged and murderous? Why not seek to emulate his brother, rather than destroy him? Why not become a shepherd?

Autonomically speaking, we recognize that moving across the threshold into fight-or-flight is a mobilizing and a polarizing response. The body becomes active: we seek to determine who is with me and who is against me. In the grip of rage, Cain blames his rejection on his brother, determines that his brother is against him, and murders him.

In the story, it would be powerful if there was a beat here, a pause, to allow Cain to catch up with himself. We rather have the feeling that at some point, perhaps in a few moments, perhaps in a few days, the horror of what he has just done would arrive to him, in the absence of additional inputs. In a frenzy he has murdered his brother, though his brother has done no wrong other than please the Lord. We can, perhaps, imagine a moment when Cain's rage cools and he experiences remorse. When his autonomic temperature changes from fire to ice. When he sinks into grief, holds his head in his hands, wonders, *What on earth have I done?*

It seems a necessary step, this self-examination. And yet there is no such opportunity, because the Lord is upon him, looking for Abel. Ironically at some level, the Lord's intrusion keeps Cain in the physiology of fight-flight; of defense.

Where is your brother?

I know not: Am I my brother's keeper?

To which the Lord replies: *What hast thou done? the voice of thy brother's blood crieth unto me from the ground. 11 And now art thou cursed from the earth, which hath opened her mouth to receive thy brother's blood from thy hand...*

The exile that comes next, through God, to Cain, and therefore to his descendants (by which I mean us) arrives without delay and with strangeness and specificity.

Thy brother's blood crieth unto me from the ground, which is to say that the soul of the dead brother exists still and is crying to the Lord from within the Ground, which is to say that *the Ground itself can hold the energies of the lamentation of the dead.* That their bodies being buried there does not extinguish the cries of their voices. This is, if you really take it in, a rather unusual pronouncement to modern ears.

And now art thou cursed from the earth, which is to say that the Earth herself, Sovereign Being, has now cursed Cain, such that: *When thou tillest the ground, it shall not henceforth yield unto thee her strength* (e.g., your crops will not nourish you with the force of the earth); *a fugitive and a vagabond shalt thou be in the earth* (you will always be rootless). So here is, very plainly, the figure of our modern conundrum: the stamp of the very subject of this book.

Cain is exiled by his own hand first. He is exiled by his own turning to steam, his own autonomic shift, which causes him to act in way that he would surely regret later, if there was space to face this, which there is not, because he is immediately exiled again by the Lord himself.

There is here a double wound, a double loss.

We could say that there is the very public exile of his mark, and the Lord's disfavor, and the curse.

There is also the private inward exile, his own turning away from self, his own movement into defensiveness that guards the deeper wound of his own inability to grieve what he has done because the punishment of the Father has fallen so swiftly and so hard.

I'm not questioning the judgment of the Lord, I'm simply noticing that there is an inward process within Cain (unless he is simply evil and unrepentant, which then is not an interesting story) that does not get to complete itself because the punishment meted out from on High is so immediate and severe. Cain himself says so: *My punishment is greater than I can bear.*

I'm glossing these stories with a specific objective, which is to figure out how to reverse engineer our way back from the alienation.

All of these stories– and I said this earlier– are attempts to explain how things got to be the way that they are. In order for the stories to continue to have life breathed into them by generations of new readers, they have to speak to current conditions. They have to address something about the way we experience ourselves. Once they fail to do this, they begin to dissipate as cosmology; they become antique; they rust.

Yet of our felt sense of alienation there is no doubt. It is the foundation of the modern. The excavation, the archeology, examines the layers. Examines the way the ball rolls further and further down the hill away from Union.

Underneath Cain's hardness toward his brother, the turning away, is a grief. An existential grief. Can we move to the moment before he strikes his brother down, the moment when he is still in contact with that grief?

In a split-second, walking in the field, he will harden, and strike down his brother. But before he does this, there is something unbearable that he is feeling. Something that, rather than feel, he would destroy the life closest to his own.

What is the nature of this grief?

If we take the story as its own world- if we insist that the grief arises within the frame of the story, that it is not, for example, that Cain has felt the grief of his father, Adam – Adam who is purportedly the first man, who was made by God and promptly disobeyed him, which seems a fairly strange thing to do immediately if you were just made. If we take the frame of the story as complete, the only adequate reason for the grief would be God's rejection of Cain's offering.

What does it mean for God to reject our offering?

We come before the numinous, asking for an experience of Union, of reciprocity, and God says, *No*. '*Unto Cain and to his offering he had not respect.*'

With intent to move the story again into the realm of what we can more fully feel, I share the following observation: I have some experience with making an offering like Cain. I have some experience with making an offering that I believed to be sincere, and that God, whosoever and howsoever you would understand the Divine to be, rejected. What I can say in hindsight- with the clarity that comes from time, and grief, and loss, and suffering, and forgiveness- is that my offering, which I believed to be sincere, to be selfless, to be true, was in fact corrupt.

Was in fact arrogant. Was in fact ugly. Was in fact vain.

But what happened, when I made the offering, and it was rejected, was that I felt forsaken. It is one thing to feel forsaken by your peers. It is perhaps a suffering of a different order of magnitude to feel forsaken by your family. But to feel forsaken by the Lord? Well- this is painful beyond the endurance of most anyone I know. And in the face of it, we'd really rather feel anything at all. Lest you imagine it to be abstract, I want you to imagine yourself walking in that field, not to BE Cain, but to bear witness to him. I want you to understand the degree to which, in the moment when the Lord says *No* we find two brothers walking in a field, but only can we say that they are walking beside one another if we adopt the perspective of the field.

As the field, beholding two brothers walking, we see two men moving side-by-side. But move the narratorial viewpoint from omniscient closer to first-person in either of the brothers, and we see something like this, perspectives irreconcilable.

After the offerings, in a field, the brothers walking side-by-side:

From Abel's point of view:

Ah yes, for I can feel the beauty of Light dancing upon my skin, how it passes through and into me. And All That Is, moving in harmonious whole. Wheeling, in cosmic perfection, upon celestial axes: how the wheat of the field turns its cheek toward the light of the Sun, the wind himself speaking the name of the Creator, the call-and-response; how every creature has its place, its rootedness in the whole, and every cell says, Yes, there is but One, everything breathing together.

From Cain's point of view:

But. No. Wherefore even the Light is cold. The Sun remote. As if it was featureless, flavorless. How. Can it be? This field. Dead to me. Body as sudden winter. Light stripped of warmth. As though I were not in it, but behind it. Seeing it through a glass, coldly. As if from an inward distance. As though I were enclosed, life outside the room. Remote from myself. In here nothing but stale air. There is nothing here, not even life. I have been closed out. Erased from all tenderness and belonging.

It is this that Cain rises up against. This depth of feeling forsaken.

Thousands of years later, when the Europeans arriving in the New World encounter the Centro-American Indigenous cultures, they will recognize this, and call them 'En Dios', which is to say those still living in the Garden, e.g., in God. They will encounter, and many will recognize, that the people of the New World they are encountering are living, still, in that relating. Living, still, in the Original Garden. Eden.

15 - An Intrusive God

It aggrieves me that God does not give Cain a moment to reflect on what he has done. There is not a cosmic beat long enough for Cain *himself* to come to his senses and notice that he has acted from a fallen countenance, that he has become steam (war)– and to find the center of remorse within himself, such that he can begin inwardly to atone... In the same way that it aggrieves me that God intrudes here, comes searching for Abel, forcing Cain's attention outward to grapple with an angry Father when it should be inward, searching his own soul, I confess that the story of the Fall, this blaming of the turning away on a snake seems to me to let humans off the hook much too easily.

I lived a good part of my life in fear of an oblique, irascible, and unfathomable God: the notion of a Living Creator mysterious to the point of inscrutability. And I think the profound danger of this depiction, whether clothed in the body of Jesus, or the cloth of Michelangelo's Sistine Chapel depiction, this notion of a SkyGod, a ruler on High, is that it requires an antithesis. These western notions of God require the Devil. A Satanic force is the structuring recipe. If the ladder has a topmost rung, it must have a bottom rung.

Why is man alienated? Satan. Satan as a snake, whispering to the woman.

But what if, in the same way that God has intruded upon Cain, has taken his attention away from the possibility of genuine remorse by pulling it away from his inwardness, this notion of Satan is also a distraction?

What if both the pull of a SkyGod, and the pull of a demonic force are equal and opposite irrelevancies. Let's be clear, the Judeo-Christian vision is not the only cosmology ripe with Gods and demons. We are monotheists, so we consolidate the beneficence into a single being, and this requires that the malevolence consolidate as well, but the notion of benevolent and sinister cosmic forces is not merely Judeo-Christian. And I'm not for a moment saying evil doesn't exist. Just look at the dumb motherfuckers ruling the world. There is plenty of evil out there. I'm just saying that if our work is to overcome alienation, we need to be extremely prudent about where we place our attention.

And putting it on supplication to an inscrutable SkyGod or the warding off of a malevolent demon both collaborate with dissociation. What about the inward archeology required to touch the inward parts of ourselves that have turned to ice? What about the communal hearth, the fireplace at the center of the village, the possibility that we are part of a small band, that we are not alone with the agony of our alienation?

Because the thing missing from the story of Adam and Eve, the thing that tells it for the lie that it is, is that humans did not come into the world in a dyadic relationship. We did not originate as a married couple. This is a uniquely modern notion, and patently false. The human lineage comes from the small band. There is no first man, and no first woman. In the same way that the proper unit of human flourishing is a small band, the original human unit is the village. What of the first village? Where is the village in the Garden? Where is the fireplace and the circle of us around it? To succumb to the fable of there being a single man and a single woman is already to have accepted a falsehood at the origin of the tale.

16 - Always Digging it Out

I cannot help but feel, because I observe it in myself, that the taproot of supremacy is feeling alone. It comes from feeling abandoned by everything. Feeling abandoned, feeling cast out, we reserve some little part of the psyche of universe and call it self. We withdraw from relationship, and this contraction is ego.

I know something about this. My own seven-year-old self's balled-up fist. The root of supremacy breaks out from the fist, dropping straight down, this white tail. The bifurcation, the splitting that gives rise to the tree, is its mirror image extending in the opposite direction. The moment that we feel more-than, the moment supremacy takes hold, it births an anti-self. Inferiority. And from the sacred unity we split into this bivalent structure of better-than, worse-than. More-than, less-than. Good and evil, the knowledge of. Suddenly there is hierarchy everywhere. We are above, and we are below. A hall of mirrors, a world of ranked selves. We are in exile. Cast out.

I pick up with another origin story here, this one Greek. *The Odyssey* of Homer. The great Odysseus, that man skilled in all ways of contending, is marooned far from home, far from his native land, his steadfast wife, his beloved son. Taken for dead by the people, his hall has been over-run by suitors, whom his wife forestalls by weaving a tapestry, claiming that when it is finished she will marry one of them. Each night by candlelight she unweaves it, pulling the warp and weft apart. The governing yearning of this text is *nostos*, the Greek word that means longing for home.

We are a handful of millennia back now, three or so, by the time *The Odyssey* is authored. In this story, incandescent at its center, illuminating the entire arc of action, is this longing to come home.

At its inception modernity is already in exile upon exile. Cast out from home and hearth. No longer gathered around the original fire.

⊕

I didn't become conscious of social hierarchy until I had been taken from my people and from my place. At seven years old my family moves away from the small town where my sense of kinship to everything flourished. I experience this as a kind of kidnapping, of being abducted by those people who were supposed to take care of me. It shatters my trust in my parents. I go with them willingly at the time because I don't understand that we are leaving. Have you ever loved something so much that you didn't realize it could be taken away from you?

This is my own private experience of being cast out. As an outcast I become suddenly conscious of hierarchies. Of the status valence of different clothing brands, different makes of cars. Alienated, I suddenly adorn myself in symbols of worth, and I hierarchize others. Polo is better than Izod is better than JC Penny. Ferrari is better than Mercedes is better than Toyota is better than Ford. White is better than Asian is better than Indian is better than Black. The world becomes a ranking system. I only realize this because I no longer belong. My focus shifts from the feeling of kinship to the gaze of exile. In the Garden rank is meaningless. Outside of it, gazing back in, we seek to adorn ourselves with all manner of ornament, status, rank. We want proof that we are important because what we feel is empty.

⊕

There is a concept in biology that says ontogency recapitulates phylogeny. It means that the development of an individual organism expresses the evolutionary history of its entire lineage. Look at the development of a human embryo in utero, and you can see it passing through phases that resemble a lizard, a chicken, a monkey: all of our evolutionary forebears, before it starts to differentiate itself into something unmistakably human. Elements of the theory have been disproved, but the notion of this, the fractality, it holds up. Does the arc of an individual life also recapitulate the arc of cultural ancestry?

I know what it means to be cast out and not know why. The body wants to–needs to, perhaps–make up a story. Why were we thrown out of the Garden? Who writes the story? The priestly class? Let's blame it on the woman and the snake. My own grapplings with this give rise to supremacy.

Impotent in the face of what happened, unable to change it, unable to bear it, the grief too radioactive to name, the loss too white-hot to know, to feel, I cordon it off in parts of my psyche that are unreachable and the deepest most vital parts of my kinship with everything freeze. I become ice. Deeply deeply alone. Turning this alienation over and over in my mind, like a stone, I come to the conclusion that I am better-than. But as always with this formulation, its twin is also true. I come to the conclusion that I am worse-than as well, only this I refuse to know.

Thirty seven years it takes me to make my way home, back to this original self. My path there is circuitous, and it passes, in 2012, through psychiatric hospitalization when my mind cleaves around this birfurcated root. As a result of childhood trauma I had become someone with two acceleratingly opposed experiences of self: one seeking confirmation that I was superior, its manifestation in accumulating evidence of my own perfection. Things that provided evidence of specialness I adhered to this sense of self. Certain accomplishments. Degrees from elite institutions. Bulletpoints on a résumé. Things that contradicted it, and there were many, I refused to know, because I didn't have a structure of self that could accommodate them. If I was superior, then failure couldn't be part of me. And so if I failed there was then something wrong with the contest–I had to disqualify it. The parts of myself that felt grief, loss, absence, doubt, weakness...experiences of which I was ashamed, felt guilty, was embarrassed, or defeated–none of these had a place to live. They hovered, anchorless, tired birds with no place to roost on the tree of my superiority.

Ironically, neither of these stances–the stance looking down at, or the stance looking up at–have anything to do with relating. With feeling kinship. Both are brittle. Remember the woman in Iowa? We are in the domain of the hegemony of the eye. What is striking in her portrait is the gaze, and the place in consciousness it is coming from. The head is tilted off to the side and she is looking down at. Not at us only, but down at everything. Off to the side of the world, she looks down at it, at something beneath her. Something outside of her, unrelated. But what is beneath–the everything of it all–looks back at her and in moments of vertigo, of inversion, it is her beneath, looking up. The stance births its own opposite.

In my own life, in 2012, a series of increasingly stressful events took place that included the death of my grandmother, my parents moving toward divorce, me losing my job, and my wife leaving our spiritual community. I watched things break apart like a series of dominoes falling in slow motion. My ancestry, my family of origin, my livelihood, my community. Consumed by anxiety, I stopped being able to calm my autonomic nervous system, and I stopped being able to sleep. An internal edifice collapsed– I can remember it happening. It was as if all the things that were holding me together, all of the structures built on the stability of other people and parts of my identity, shook down in an earthquake. I didn't sleep for forty days, until I had completely lost control of my own mind. And what was revealed, plain as day when I could no longer in any way steer my own thoughts, was that I had cleaved in two. A taproot of supremacy, and a tree of inferiority. Everything went upside-down.

Supremacy is always schizophrenic. That's part of what I am here to tell you, the central point of this section. There is no such thing as superiority. It is always superiority and inferiority conjoined. They are coupled. The taproot and the tree it nourishes. The above and the below. It is always bi-valent, this forgetting. This is not something I read in a book somewhere. This is something I lived through.

I was plunged down into all of the parts of myself I had been unable to metabolize at all. A plunge beneath the surface, replete with terror. A hell realm.

But–and I feel that this is important to emphasize–while that place is real, as real as its ethereal opposite–what gives rise to it, the roadway that connects it to here, to this earthly plane, is this split structure of supremacy.

The evangelical fervor around sin, the pulpit hectoring about hell-fires and damnation, is a possible place to get sent only because, earlier in the sermon, the christians thought themselves to be superior; convinced themselves that heaven was their due. Thus the current pope's warning: *Never again can the Christian community allow itself to be infected by the idea that one culture is superior to others...* And yet. And yet- nearly all of the christian communities I've ever encountered do.

We think we are superior because we have been cast out. All of us. The entire lot.

We live in a supremacy engine. It is the fuel of this suicidal/

genocidal cult of death worship that passes for a culture.

And yet, neither superiority, or its anti-self, its twin of inferiority has anything to do with relationship. Both are contractions, balled-up fists, to avoid the pain of relating. Of how deeply uncomfortable it is to have contact-felt contact-with Self or Other. How much it hurts to touch and to be touched. How much contact pains us.

Whether we are above or below someone else doesn't matter. The point is that, in either case, we are not *with*. Neither one knows anything about kinship.

⊕

We are not superior to anything. But neither are we inferior. We cannot be either, for we are made of the same stuff as everything else.

I had to rebuild my mind.

It took me six years.

I would never wish the experience on anyone, yet neither would I trade it for anything. I was afforded the opportunity to perform an archeology of shadows, and what I excavated was not merely mine.

Yes, I had attached to it, and had made it my own, but much of it was inherited.

The reclamation of original self is something that we should probably all undertake. I remember the moment when my child-self came back online. I had gone to extreme measures to retrieve him. I've drunk ayahuasca hundreds of times, passed through the insane asylum, got spat out the backside of hell to rescue and resuscitate my original indigenous self.

When I re-united with him, after thirty-seven years, it was

about 5:30 in the morning and I was lying on the forest floor. I had just moved back to ten acres of pristine forest and was able, for the first time since being cast out of the forest of my childhood mind, to feel the grief of it without drowning– because I had returned to the forest.

I had been meditating on a cushion at the moment this happened, sitting before dawn in a circle of Douglas Fir trees, but when the grief came it enveloped me in a cloak as black as death and I couldn't hold my body up and I collapsed. The air itself became funereal.

I had met this child self before, in ceremonies, accompanied him back into vitality slowly, quietly, with simple presence over many years. But when he came back to me it was thermonuclear: there was nothing subtle about it.

From the deepest well of blackness, smothering in grief I crossed an internal threshold back into rage. An autonomic threshold. My body tensed as through encased in steel bands, and I felt a scream begin to organize beneath my body. I stood up.

It came up through me, slowly, yet whitehot, rising through my feet, into my calves, then my knees, my thighs, my hips. My throat began to organize as it moved up through my torso and I found myself gulping air, like some kind of fish.

When I screamed it knocked the roof off the valley.

A silence ensued, and then a cacophony of barking dogs followed.

17 - Prohibition on Lamentation

ἐκ γαίας βλαστὼν γαῖα πάλιν γέγονα
Peek1702.2

Having sprung from the earth, earth I have become once more.

Unangan (Aleut) Elder Kuuyux Ilarion Merculieff notes that a primary axis of the polycrisis of modernity is the imbalance between masculine and feminine energies. We have been seduced by the vertical, and therefrom suffered the splitting of Supremacy. Let us conceptualize this as the Original wound. We have then been seduced by patriarchy: male supremacy, a hierarchizing of the sexes. This second imbalance correlates well temporally with the establishment of city states, inheritance of property, and changes in the forms of governance. In exchange for promises of greater security from the state, we have traded parts of our sovereignty and constrained our expression. This compromise is more antique than many of us realize, and one of its archetypic formulations is in the legislative restrictions on lamentation that emerge in Greece in the 6th century BCE.

Among the earliest documentations of this legislation are the descriptions in Plutarch's *Life of Solon*. According to Cicero it was Kekrops, the legendary founder of Athens, who initiated the full pomp and ceremony of funerals there. The enormous circular *thóloi* and chamber tombs of the Mycenean period were large enough to house the entire clan, show traces of intricate burial customs, and were richly provisioned with gifts. It seems clear that the Myceneans engaged in funerary rites that were extensive and unconstrained, and that these rights were a central spiritual practice of the community.

Solonic law represented a significant departure from this earlier era, and was clearly enacted with political aims. The prohibitions on mourning were designed to counteract a culture of vendetta, as generational blood-feuds between aristocratic families had left a strong mark on Athenian culture, and were contemporaneous with its transition into a more democratic context. Yet the prohibitions fell asymmetrically on women, and removed agency from what had been a uniquely feminine ritual sphere. They seem also to have been particularly concerned with behavior that was regarded as out-of-control, yet that specifically involved the ritual and embodied transmutation of energies.

The laws tended to contain four explicit kinds of prohibition. There were prohibitions on extravagance, which limited the magnitude of expenditure on funerary rights. There were limitations of the right to mourn to immediate kin, a direct constraint on professional mourning, and an attempt to strictly delimit the number and degree of relatedness of those in attendance, which seems to have born on inheritance law. There was a ban on ritual likely to attract attention. And finally, and principally for our purposes, there was a ban 'forbidding everything disorderly and excessive in women's processions, funeral rites, and festivals,' as Plutarch puts it.

No woman was to go out with more than three garments, one obol's worth of food and drink, or a basket of more than one cubit's length. There was to be no procession by night except by lighted coach; also, no laceration of the flesh by mourners, no singing of set dirges and no wailing for other dead. Bull-sacrifice was similarly forbidden. No one was to walk about other people's graves unaccompanied.

-Plutarch, Life of Solon

Hellenic funerary rites were carried out in three stages. First,

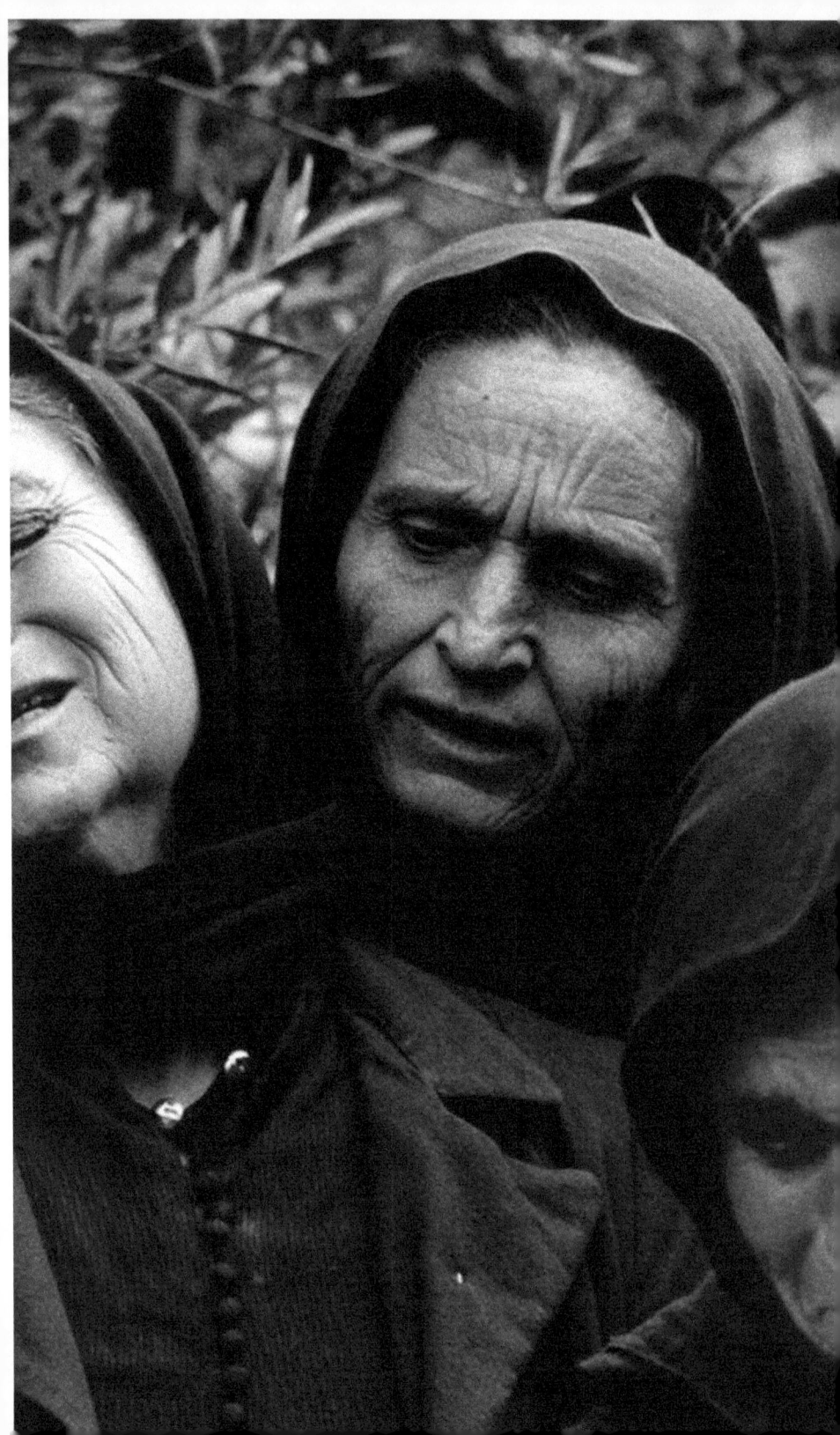

there was the *prothesis*, the laying out of the body. This was followed by the *ekphorá*: the funeral procession itself. And finally there was the internment of the body or cremated remains of the deceased. Regulations for the ekphorá are exact and strict in the Solonic legislation: the corpse must be closely veiled and carried in silence, and must not be laid down and wailed for at the turnings in the road or outside the deceased's house. The fact that this is spelled out points to how these processions had been conducted in the past. Previously the body had been moved slowly, lowered to the ground periodically, and wailed over. There were to be no dirges and no wailing at the tomb of 'those long dead'. In addition, the wake was to take place indoors, and 'be over by sunrise.'

We can feel the ways in which a ceremony that previously was designed to publicly transmute the grief of a community – a wailing procession that pauses at monuments in the road, turns and switchbacks, before the home of the deceased– that carries on through the night and into the next day, that gathers others, that stops to wail at the tombs of others fallen – attended by many members of the community, including professional mourners, and engaged in ritual acts of lamentation – *a true grief ritual* – is being legally constrained with precise and targeted prohibitions. *You may not do this in public, you may not do this outside, you may not do this with a large group. You may not let the energies of lamentation spread in the community.*

FACING PAGE: Professional mourners by a graveside in Mani, Greece, 1962.
© Constantine Manos

Women shriek. They tear their hair and clothing, scratch at their faces and beat their chests. They sway hypnotically and sometimes dance wildly, as if possessed. They scream out questions without answers, repeat themselves, call for vengeance. They will not be consoled. At times, their sobs, moans, and sighs compose themselves into song, into a searing melody or a mournful antiphony. They summon us to witness, but they seem mad. Unwashed and unadorned, they rub grime on their faces; they are alternately despondent and angry; they breathe unnaturally. They seem caught up in something both intensely sacred and dreadfully pagan, in an obscene exposure of women, their bodies, emotion: of the private in a public place. One is tempted to recoil, as if from contamination; one senses that the anguish will spread.

– Rebecca Saunders, *And the Women Wailed in Answer: The Lament Tradition*

Grief accumulates, does it not? It hides from us, sinks in, festers, builds. In the modern world we talk about stress, about allostatic load, as an accumulation. But mostly in our modern discussions of this we fail to recognize that there are two distinct kinds of stress. The kind that puts us into fight-or-flight: the high-intensity, hot, active, mobilized, jaw-clenching, tense, adrenalized stress that undergirds anxiety and aggression– and the kind that puts us into shutdown. This second kind, undergirded by different neurology: the subdiaphragmatic, the belly-based, and different neurochemistry- not adrenaline and cortisol but endogenous opioids that convey us into the realms of the dream-like, the landscapes of the surreal, is not hot but cool, sometimes freezing. It is subterranean, resides in the depths, shy, inaccessible. In pure form it contains no motion, no heat, no adrenaline. It is sober, cold, lifeless, without muscle tone: the tenor of collapse, the color of depression. Grief is of the latter camp and it requires different neuro and spiritual technologies to be alchemized; to move through us.

Grief is a deep belly affair: it touches us in our centers. Who were the women grieving, after all? Assuredly some of the funeral rites are for those who have died of old age, of natural causes. Yet 2,600 years ago, how many deaths are there that today are regularly avoided? How many women died in childbirth? How many newborns, toddlers, and children died? Today we have flu shots, homes with a thermostat that can be set to 72 degrees in winter. Twenty-five hundred years ago in Greece? To the baby arriving in September, what is the lethality of the common cold born in with the January damp? How many people pass away from diseases, infections, ailments for which there is then no cure? A cut that festers in a time before antibiotics? And how many are the dead from war? How many are the lamentations for husbands lost to campaigns, border skirmishes, violence between warring clans?

Unmetabolized grief, which moves us into shutdown, runs the risk of moving us deep into dissociation. Runs the risk of paralyzing the community: uprooting it. For in the grip of shutdown, when it takes over, there is not impetus for *doing*. There is no meaning in activity, and the necessaries of action: planting crops, tending livestock, harvesting...these require facility with action. A community plunged collectively into the dissociation of grief stops its tending of the inward and the outward realms. Fruit withers on the vine, weeds spring up. Babies go un-nursed, children unschooled.

Grief ritual is, therefore, a profound and necessary antidote to dissociation. It is a spiritual technology for transmuting the profound energies of grief. Grief is what we feel when we have loved and lost. It is not something unnatural, but simply the pain of love lost. We grieve in proportion to how much we love. The grief ritual is the obverse side of love: the same coin flipped over. If we are to love with abandon, to love unrestrainedly– and this is in large part why we are here– the twin of this love is grief when we lose someone dear.

⊕

There are no deeper mysteries than life and death. The funerary rites of a culture tell us a great deal about their cosmology.

μή μ' ἄκλαυτον ἄθαπτον ἰὼν ὄπιθεν
καταλείπειν,νοσφισθείς, μή τοί τι θεῶν μήνιμα γένωμαι.
Odysseus. 11.72-3

Don't abandon me, don't leave me behind, unwept and unburied, lest I become a visitation upon you from the gods.

In Homer's *Odyssey*, Odysseus voyages to the Underworld, where the first soul he encounters is Elpenor, who had been left unlamented and unburied in Circe's house after falling drunk from the roof. His warning words, *Don't abandon me, don't leave me behind* **unwept and unburied**, *lest I become a visitation upon you from the gods*...[emphasis mine] suggest that the funerary rites, both lamentation and burial, were required for a soul to transition safely to the Underworld. In Greek cosmology, funerary rites were foundational to the transit of the soul returning to the Underworld, and the manner in which ritual was conducted provided the necessary energies and inputs for this process to proceed smoothly. In this sense, the funerary rites are a way of assisting and honoring the soul of the dead. Yet, like lock and key, they form a symbiotic function for the living, allowing those of us who remain to release the dead.

There a crucial neurobiological and perhaps we could say alchemical role for the living in the lamentation. The funerary rites create a relational field where it is possible to alchemize this loss. The tearing of hair, the wailing, the alternation of feeling forsaken and enraged, the unnatural breathing: all of this viewed autonomically is the progress and process of the metabolizing of grief.

The soul's transit can be impeded by the soul not wanting to progress, yet also by the people who are left behind (the living) not wanting, or not being able to let go. The ritual context is a technology that creates a format for this metabolization process. We are digesting here (this is the reason that this is an autonomic act of the Grounding System) something nearly impossible. To become open to, and able to allow this experience of loss to fully move through us, we need the dilation and expanded consciousness of a ritual context.

A diaphragm must open between the worlds, threads of relating must de-tangle. A separation must occur, relationality must be parsed back into its parts. Some day our science will become nuanced enough, our understanding of quantum entanglement quantifiable enough to track the algebra of these ceremonies: their mystery in rendering the relating back into its component spheres. We talk in psychological circles about co-dependence, enmeshment, the way that people and psyches depend upon one another, become entangled across boundaries, and confuse. But there is something atomic and electronic happening here as well; something we moderns do not see clearly yet that ancestral peoples did and do. The San of the Kalahari speak of the energetic threads of relating that open between two beings engaged in the act of seeing one another. While this seeing can take place through the eyes, its meaning is not optical but of mutual accountability.

I am accountable to that with which I am in relation. To those with whom I tend the fires of relating, there are energetic ropes of relationship, and they are real, tangible. When these ropes are severed by the passing of someone from the earthly plane, it is necessary to tend to their re-knitting so that we are not permanently bereft. This is the province of grief ritual. In its deep contact with death, it is honoring the continuity of Life herself.

The early architects of democracy in Athens, men, do not understand the necessity of this ceremonial work, feel threatened by it, and fear its destabilizing effects without recognizing that it is an antidote to a different kind of inward destabilization.

An Indigenous shaman from Kalaallit Nunaat (Greenland) named Angaangaq Angakkorsuaq says "Only by Melting the Ice in the Heart of Man will man have a chance to change and begin using his knowledge wisely." Unmourned loss is in fact one of the primary origins of the ice in the heart of man to which Angaangaq refers.

The early architects of democracy, seeking to politically stabilize a larger population, which had now grown in size beyond the 150 reciprocal relationships that the human nervous system is hard-wired to organize, conclude that the outpouring of energies in funerary rites are too potent, too likely to stir up feelings in the population that cannot be controlled, too likely to make people 'irrational.'

Irrational here, however, really means sovereign. It really means feral and whole. It really means healed, re-knit, restored.

A people unable to mourn, a people who have lost intimacy with death, a people who are afraid of it– what else is the desire to live forever?– condemn themselves to a different kind of 'irrationality': the dissociated. This is a step on the civilizational progression of turning to ice: a moment in the history of western civilization where our constriction on ceremonial forms of lamentation begins to turn the people, at scale, into ice.

It bears directly upon our modern predicament today, and in this sense 6th century Athens is but yesterday: a direct antecedent of the moment we collectively find ourselves in.

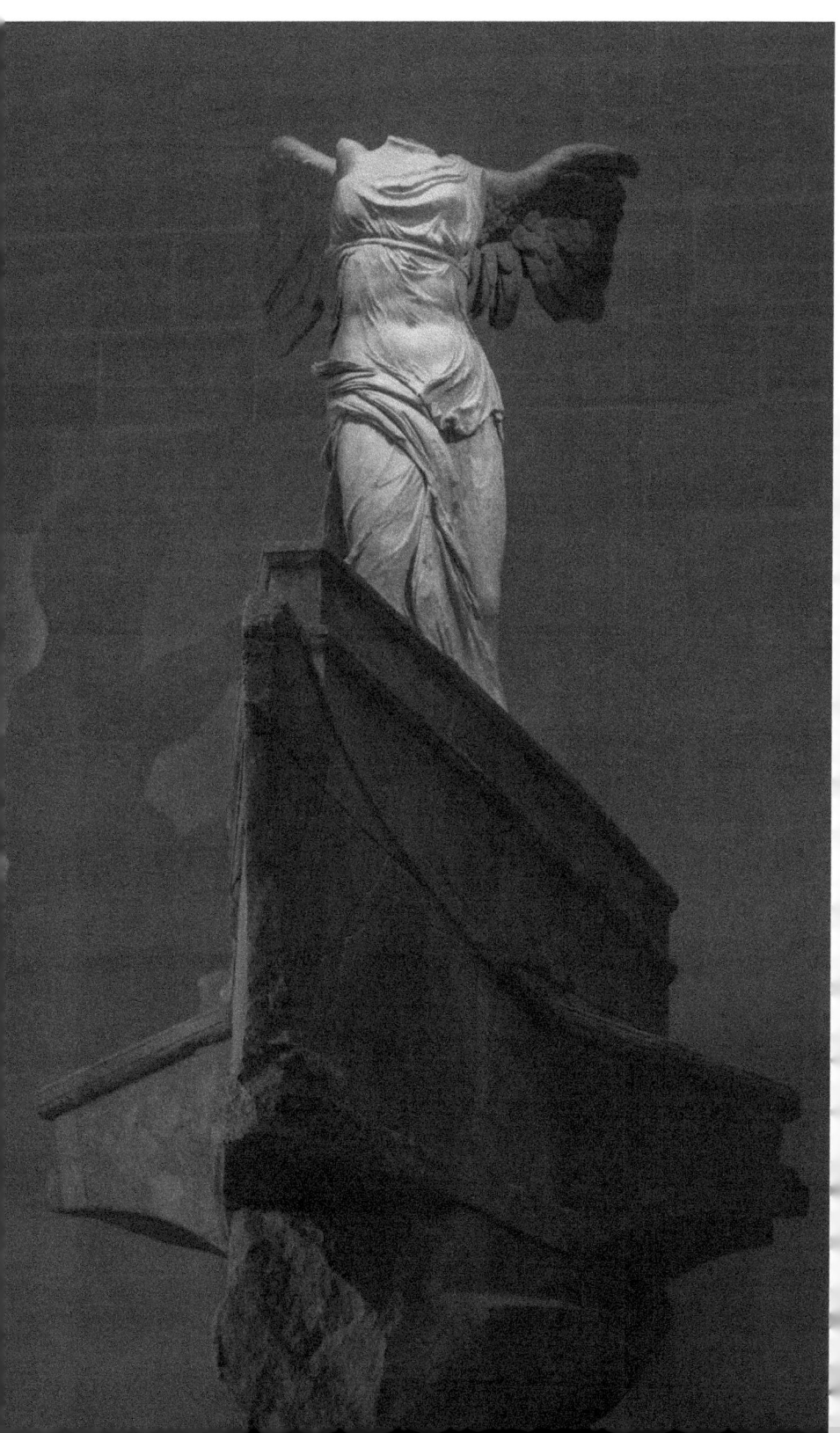

18 - The Nike of Samothrace

In the 6th century BC in Athens, the extent of ritual mourning was partly in response to the culture of blood fueds between aristocratic families: a culture of revenge. We would be remiss, it seems to me, in talking about cultures of mourning, if we failed to address at least some of the losses that people were grieving, and so we turn our attention here briefly to formulations of war as they relate to Supremacy mind.

In 168 BC, at the Battle of Pydna, during what would become known as the Third Macedonian War, the Roman legions, in flexible formation, moving over uneven ground, defeat the Macedonian phalanx, a more traditional war formation, ultimately routing the Macedonians, and sending their leader fleeing. The leader, Perseus of Macedon, is later captured from an island in the Aegean (Samothraki), where he had sought refuge in a temple (The Temple of the Greater Gods), which was under the guardianship of a Winged Goddess. Taken to Rome, he is paraded through the streets manacled, then expurgated to an underground dungeon in Alba Fucens in central Italy, where the Romans, who didn't believe in the Macedonian gods, but didn't disbelieve in them altogether, and were aware that Perseus was likely under the protection of forces they did not understand, demurred from killing him outright, yet did so eventually by depriving him of sleep.

The statue of the Winged Goddess was beheaded, as the Romans sought not merely to kill their enemies, but to kill the Divinities of their enemies. The Romans liked to kill people, but what they wanted to extinguish was a worldview, and worldviews are bound up in our comprehension of the Divine. Knowing that the Macedonians were animists, aware that the Goddess might come into the stone through the breath, they removed her head. I find myself wondering if this was done ceremonially, or at least ritualistically. Beheaded, and plundered from the Temple of which she was guardian, she might have been lost to history, except that you can visit her in the Louvre, in Paris, where she is known as the Nike of Samothrace.

Deprived of her gaze, her listening, her voice, it is hard for me to yet gender the statue female, though she undoubtedly is. Yet gaze upon her beauty. Gaze upon the sculpture, made of stone, the garments, which are rendered shear– and marvel at being able to see, somehow, her skin, as it were, through the fabric of the gown blown by the winds, knowing that she is in fact made of stone, and made several thousand years ago. The artistry!

It is, you will observe, a rather macabre statue at this point. I wonder what it says about us moderns, and our lack of sensitivity to the energies in objects, that we don't seem to notice this? The contrast between the regal beauty of the body and the absence of a head, which makes this notional aliveness a deeply vacated proposition, is not lost on anyone who understands that she did, at one time, possess a head. Imagine how beautiful and sovereign she must have been before she was beheaded by the Romans. If the artist could render the stone garments transparent, just imagine her gaze. But we are accustomed to statues without heads. We have seen Roman, Greek, and Egyptian statuary all deprived of limbs and heads. It seems normal to us. Its meaning fails to register.

The Roman Empire was nearly unmatched in its annihilatory glee. The Romans had a pure zeal for war engines, delighted in combat. They were whole-heartedly obsessed with what the Irish poet John O'Donohue refers to as our 'fatal attraction to aggression.' If we explore theories of war, which have been catalogued and outlined with precision since at least the time when Sun-Tzu authored the manifesto that is known to us as *The Art of War*, we can find two broad camps arrayed in terms of their understanding of what war is, and these camps are distinguished principally by whether or not the civilizations holding the beliefs are under the impression that Nature is above them, i.e., they are part of (or subservient to Nature) and Nature is superior, or whether they are superior to Nature, and Nature is subservient to them.

In my explanation here, I am referring explicitly to a body of teaching that I received from my friend and mentor Pete Jackson, an artist of reknown, and a soldier for peace. Pete is a master of the Afro-Brasilian martial art of Capoeira, and a profound student of the martial lineages. In my early years of friendship with him, I was confounded by his contention that the martial arts were a route to peace, until I began to understand what was required to master one's rage.

When a civilization is not alienated from the Source, and understands that culture is subservient to Life, with a capital L, war is understood to be a necessity at times, but it does not trump life. Civilizations with this view tend to precisely structure the rules of war, such that it accomplishes its objectives of dispute resolution, either vis-a-viz territory, dynastic succession, or conflict resolution, within prescribed limits. Pete taught me, for example, about warfare between African tribes where, when war was entered into, the warriors of the opposing tribes would line up, at a hundred yards distance, in parallel. In orderly fashion, moving down the line, a warrior from each side would hurl a spear at the warriors from the other side, until one was struck and killed. When the first warrior was killed, the opposing side was declared the victor. To necessarily complicate matters somewhat, the warrior who killed the warrior from the other side became responsible for the care of the dead warrior's family. This was war that made use of the martial and sovereign energies of self-protection, yet contained them. It recognized war, even killing, as a necessary part of life, but it held constraints upon it, and ended with the two sides bound together. War did not become total.

The fight response, activated hereby, aflame already, and in need of being mastered, was not fanned. No one poured gasoline on the rage.

This manner of war, in civilizations that understand themselves to be part of Nature, is in contrast to war practiced by civilizations that understand themselves to be superior to Nature. The Romans, believing that they were superior to Nature, elided all mention of the Earthly mother from the doctrine of Christianity when it became the official religion of the state, which happened in 380 AD, when the Emperor Theodosius I issued the Edict of Thessalonica, and which would have been no surprise to anyone who had seen how they conducted war. The Romans indulged their annihilatory glee. Drunk on domination, they exalted in it. When a civilization believes itself to be superior to Nature, it makes total war.

The streak of fear undergirding this total war, I believe, is the notion that if a single child of the 'enemy' so-called were to live, that child might carry in their hearts the seeds of rebellion. To this end, the civilization that believes itself superior to Nature seeks to annihilate all the seeds that might so one day turn. This story becomes the mythic fulcrum on which turn many stories of dynastic succession, war, rebellion, genocide, and attempts thereto.

The body I am wearing is Jewish, ancestrally. I grew up remote from the practice of this faith, with a spirituality I would call nature-based were I describing it now. When I was about nine years old, in St. Louis, Missouri, I visited a synagogue for the first time. It frightened me quite profoundly. I had trouble articulating this at the time, but from the moment I stepped inside, it felt like I was walking into a crypt. It felt cold as death. Decades later, as I would come to understand the multi-generational trauma of the Holocaust, and the way that it lives on in the bodies, hearts, and minds of Jewish people, I would come to understand that the synagogue felt like a crypt because it was the spiritual home of a people who had been through a genocide during the lives of my grandparents. It felt like a crypt because it *was* a crypt. Inside the synagogue I had premonitions and ancestral recollection of the gas chambers and killing fields I did not yet, at nine years of age, have conscious knowledge of.

The greatest tragedy of trauma may not be the trauma itself, but the automaticity of reaction that results therefrom. If we do not heal trauma, it repeats itself. We are drawn toward it, ineluctably, karmically, to rehash and repeat and resolve what we are stuck on. Moths, in orbit around a flame too incandescent with loss to allow us freedom of movement. Tethered in orbit to a dark star.

Perhaps the incandescent loss at the center of our modern civilization so-called is the first war, some 75,000 years ago I am told, though I believe it was older. What did it do, this first shedding of our brother's blood? I would propose that it turned us into automatons. Something that, when struck, strikes back. It robbed of us of the freedom of choice.

Why, oh why, do we seem drawn, gravitationally, to the opposite of what will restore us to Life? How have we become automatons orbiting loss?

It is little known that, at the dawn of the 20th century, there were two Jewish visions of the future. The vision that materialized after World War II, the Zionist vision, was the creation of a Jewish state. What is not well understood, by the general population, is that there was another group in the Jewish diaspora, another political movement that at the turn of the century had become very influential in Eastern Europe, and was known as the Bund. Central to the social democratic politics of the Bund, was the Yiddish notion of *doikayt*, or hereness. *"The concept of Doikayt (in Yiddish literally 'hereness'), was central to the Bundist ideology, expressing its focus on solving the challenges confronting Jews in the country in which they lived, versus the "thereness" of the Zionist movement, which posited the necessity of an independent Jewish polity in its ancestral homeland, i.e., the Land of Israel, to secure Jewish life."*

The Bundists pointed out what was factually obvious. The creation of the State of Israel would displace the people (Palestinians) who already lived there. Colonial displacement, of the sort practiced and prosecuted during the long reign of the church-sanctioned European fever dream that laid the colonial foundations of the modern world order, does not engender peace.

When Perseus of Macedon died, the Antogonid dynasty came to an end. Rome continued its territorial expansion for several centuries, until it too eventually fell. Yet the form of Imperial Christianity that Rome birthed has been more enduring, and continues. More than a thousand years after the fall of Rome, the thoughtforms of domination that gave rise to the logic of supremacy that caused the Romans to believe they were above the laws of Nature found expression in a series of papal bulls, including *Dum Diversas*, and *Romanus Pontifex*, which would lay the 'spiritual' (I use this word loosely and in quotes) and legal theories in place for the Doctrine of Discovery, based in Christian Supremacy, that created the 'justification' for enslavement and colonialism that has set the template for the modern world, leading to 500 years of colonial extraction of lives, labor, and land, and undergirds the polycrisis of modernity. The chthonic and earth-based peoples of Europe were again purged, as they had been in Perseus' time, this time in the name of religion, not Empire. The witches were burned.

Domination mind is never satisfied. It is a devouring beast, and it eats its young as well. The weight of history is so great right now. It is a burden. Christian Supremacy, Jewish Supremacy, Islamic Supremacy. All of them boil down to Supremacies, all of which boil down to this original deformation of reality, which is the recognition that we are not superior to

Nature. This is the form of the original deviation. Christian Supremacy, Jewish Supremacy, Islamic Supremacy, Male Supremacy, White Supremacy–*any* Supremacy gives birth, in the moment of its creation, to its opposite, carried like a dark twin in the formation of the notion, because when we exchange the horizontal plane for the vertical, the energy that lifts something up, through physics, pushes something else down. In the thoughtforms of the Dominator are the thoughtforms of the Dominated. The annihilated becomes the annilator: it is quite easy for them exchange places. This formulation is schizophrenic, always tethers us to its dark matter twin, always deprives us of freedom.

Supremacy births inferiority. The elevation of the SkyGod potentiates the demonic. This is basic psychic physics. If we do not understand it, we collaborate with our own dissociation. For people birthed into a civilization schizophrenic in this way, healing cannot be simply a movement up (celestial) and out (external). It must also be a movement down (chthonic) and in (internal).

If we want to awaken we have to go as far down as we go up, go as far in as we go out. And the doorway to this, for modern people, is reclaiming the feminine and the indigenous, because that is what has been defiled and exiled.

This is how we return to center.

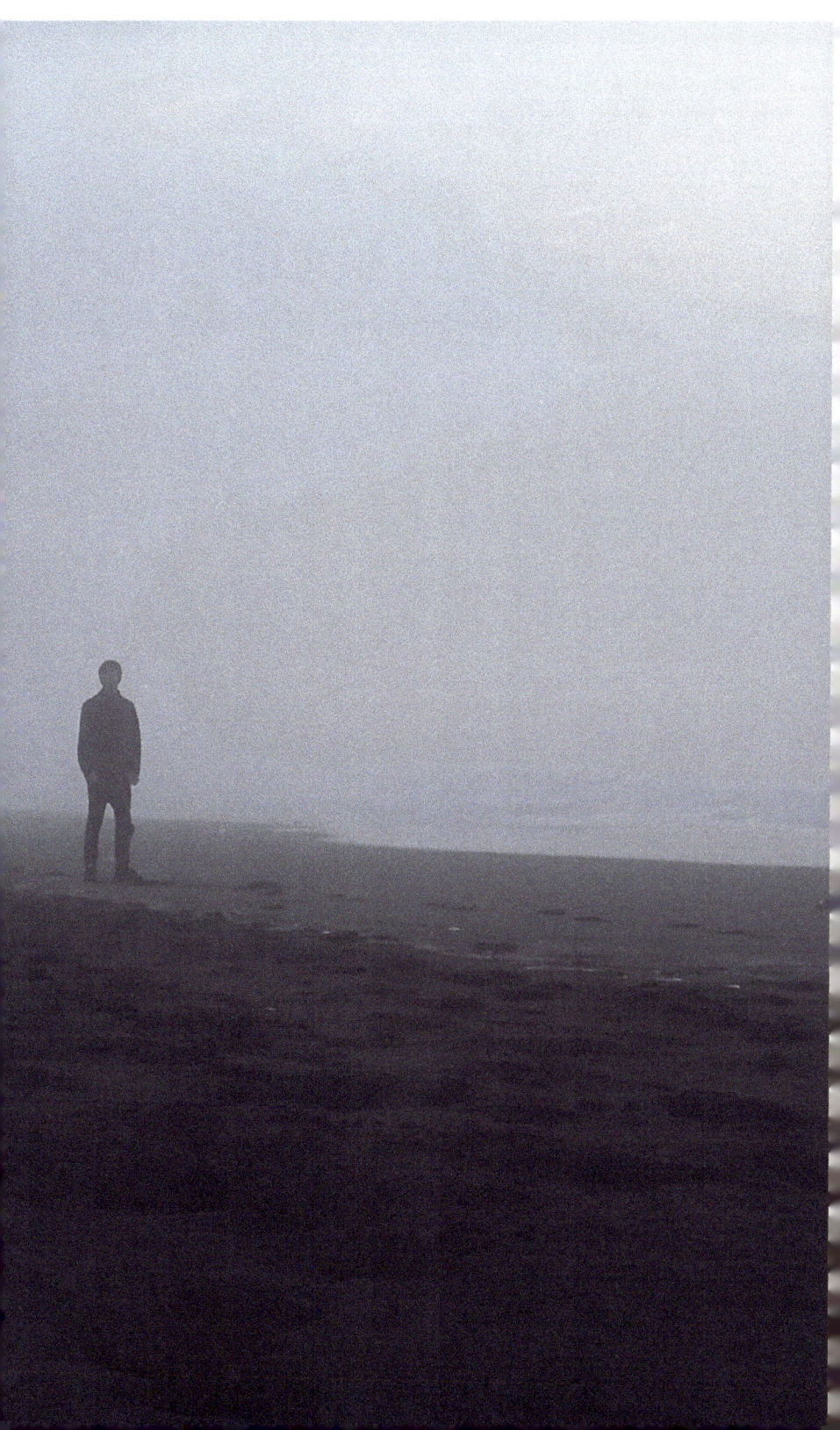

19 - Inverting the Logic of Enclosure

In *Post Capitalist Philanthropy*, Alnoor Ladha and Lynn Murphy propose that capitalism is a self-terminating algorithm based on socializing costs to the many while privatizing gains for the few. What does this mean? This lucid equation, which bears all the elegance of a formal mathematical proof, is the algorithm of capitalism. First, it notes that capitalism moves teleologically toward its own termination. This occurs when, functionally, someone owns everything. The end point of capitalism is when all of the commons (e.g., property, resources, labor, ideas, attention) have been enclosed and extracted by someone (namely owners), and their collective benefit has been transferred to those owners (the few).

Capitalism is an operating system. It is a kind of economic, political, and cultural software. The source code of this operating system is an extraction codex. To operate successfully in congruence with this operating system we must enact 'extraction mind' or 'domination mind'. This is how we advance within it. Since this system is a complex, adaptive, evolutionary system, and like all such systems wants to survive, it is self-perpetuating despite its self-termination logic. It preserves itself by drawing into positions of influence those people who best serve its purpose. As you climb, therefore, up the socio-economic ladder of capitalism, you find people who are increasingly adept functionaries of this system. Problematically this system is a death cult.

If the source code of capitalism is extraction, what context does it therefore make of the world? Capitalism, as operating system, turns the world into a mine. The capitalist gaze, intrinsic to its core logic, views the aggregation of material, energetic, metabolic, and psychic resources of the earth plane (e.g., the world) as a mine to be extracted. Extracting, within this mine, is virtuous, vis-a-viz the logic of this system. It is permissible to extract from our Mother Earth (notice that the evisceration of interiority in the English language abolishes the interiority of all beings), and we speak therefore of raw materials and natural resources rather than living stones and sovereign rivers.

It is permissible within this mining logic to extract elemental materials (e.g., metals, minerals, gases, etc.) and biotic materials. Language aligned with this project converts animate beings (i.e., trees) into inanimate objects (lumber). You will notice a linguistic alchemy whereby this system converts heinous acts, e.g., murder of animals, into palatable ones, e.g., pigs are not killed; pork is harvested. It is permissible and notionally virtuous in this system to extract labor from the bodies of the poor. That is the function and domain of corporations. It is permissible and notionally virtuous to extract ideas (intellectual property), i.e., white collar work. And it is permissible although possibly no longer considered notionally virtuous to extract attention (e.g., surveillance capitalism & the attention economy.)

Once extracted, all of these are permitted to be enclosed, i.e., productized. The gains of this process that converts common assets into enclosed forms are conferred to the owners of the respective mines that performed the extraction. These profits are cleansed, magically, by their magnitude, becoming virtuous by their enormity. Behold the extraction engine of the modern world.

⊕

I am interested in tracing, from the mists of deep time, and the silence before time, the birth and evolution of the denatured thoughtforms of modernity that are manifest in the death cult we are attempting to extricate ourselves from. I call it a death cult to point out what is at stake here, which is life on earth. Both a cause and an effect of the death cult is that most modern people's feet do not touch the ground.

The mine that capitalism understands the world to be is collapsing, because we have reached the terrestrial limits of the biosphere's capacity to be extracted without modifying its foundational climatological parameters (climate crisis). We have extracted so much that this mine is collapsing on top of us. Our collective response to this has, so far, been to extract more rapidly. Now that the mine is really falling in on our heads, there is an accelerating movement towards authoritarian regime, as if the consolidation of power and boundary fortification will save us. It will not.

We have, in parallel, extracted so much from our fellow humans (colonialism, racism, etc.) that our societies are collapsing. We are extracting so much from our own attention that our wellbeing is collapsing. The polycrisis of modernity is the perfectly logical consequence of this operating system. It is a feature of the operating system, not a bug. This is, in fact, exactly what this operating system is *designed* to do.

This operating system treats systemic death as perfectly acceptable collateral damage in service to its self-terminating end project. Unfortunately, only one person escapes this logic: the person who can exit the biosphere that has been destroyed. It is no accident that the richest white men on earth have become obsessed with leaving the planet.

For all the rest of us, those who do not want to live on Mars, or have the means to do so, this system is a complete disaster. No amount of material wealth on planet earth insulates us from the consequences of this.

With this as necessary preamble to what follows, in my tracking of the originating notions of capitalism, which are now expressed with such ruthless efficiency (or absurdity) by the current system, I bring our attention to the notion of enclosure: a foundational principle in this logic. If supremacy is its taproot, enclosure is the basement of the ossuary we have built.

⊕

Applied to property, the enclosure (or Inclosure) of the commons was the division or consolidation of communal fields, meadows, pastures, and other arable lands in western Europe into the carefully delineated (i.e., boundaried) and individually owned and managed farm plots of modern times.

This movement began in England in the 12th Century, and proceeded rapidly in the period from 1450-1640, when its purpose was to increase the full-time pasturage available to manorial lords. During a later period, from 1750 to 1860, it was done for the sake of agricultural efficiency. Between 1604 and 1915 over 5,200 enclosure Bills were enacted by the British Parliament which related to just over a fifth of the total area of England, some 6.8 million acres.

I am interested in the notion of enclosure as it relates to the psychic (i.e., interior) landscape, and specifically our notional sense of 'possessing' a self, i.e., the implications of an enclosure paradigm on our sense of interiority as a psychic space firmly delineated, boundaried, and enclosed.

⊕

I find the painting on the next pages very beautiful and a little bit strange because it speaks to a yearning with which I am in regular contact these days. What I find beautiful is the ripe abundance of the harvest, and the communitarian ethos of the farmers or peasants, or villagers, whomever they are, who have come together to eat lunch as the grain is being harvested. Through the lens of my own deep longing, I would like to imagine that this is a depiction of a village harvesting common land. I would like to believe that this harvest does

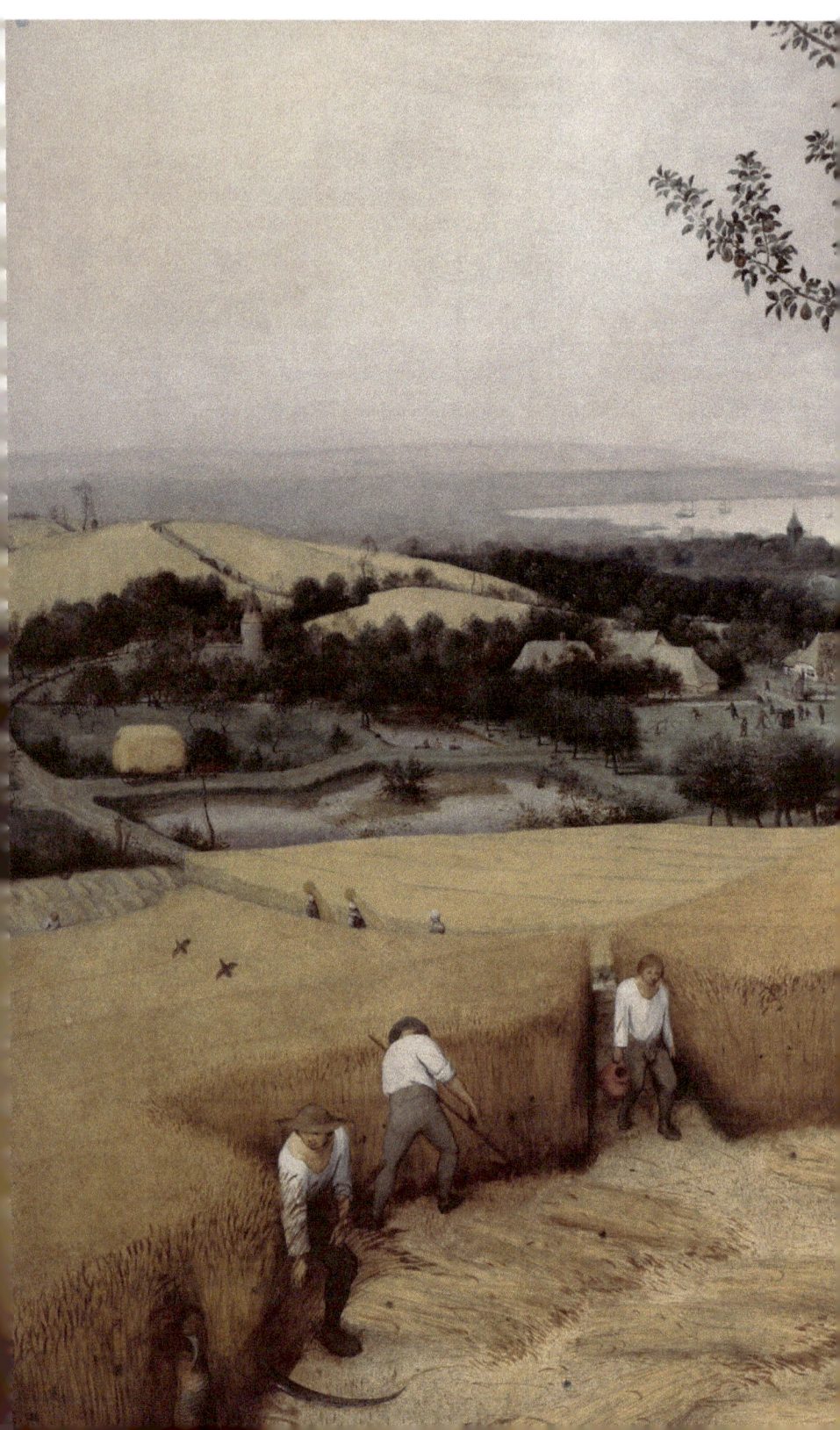

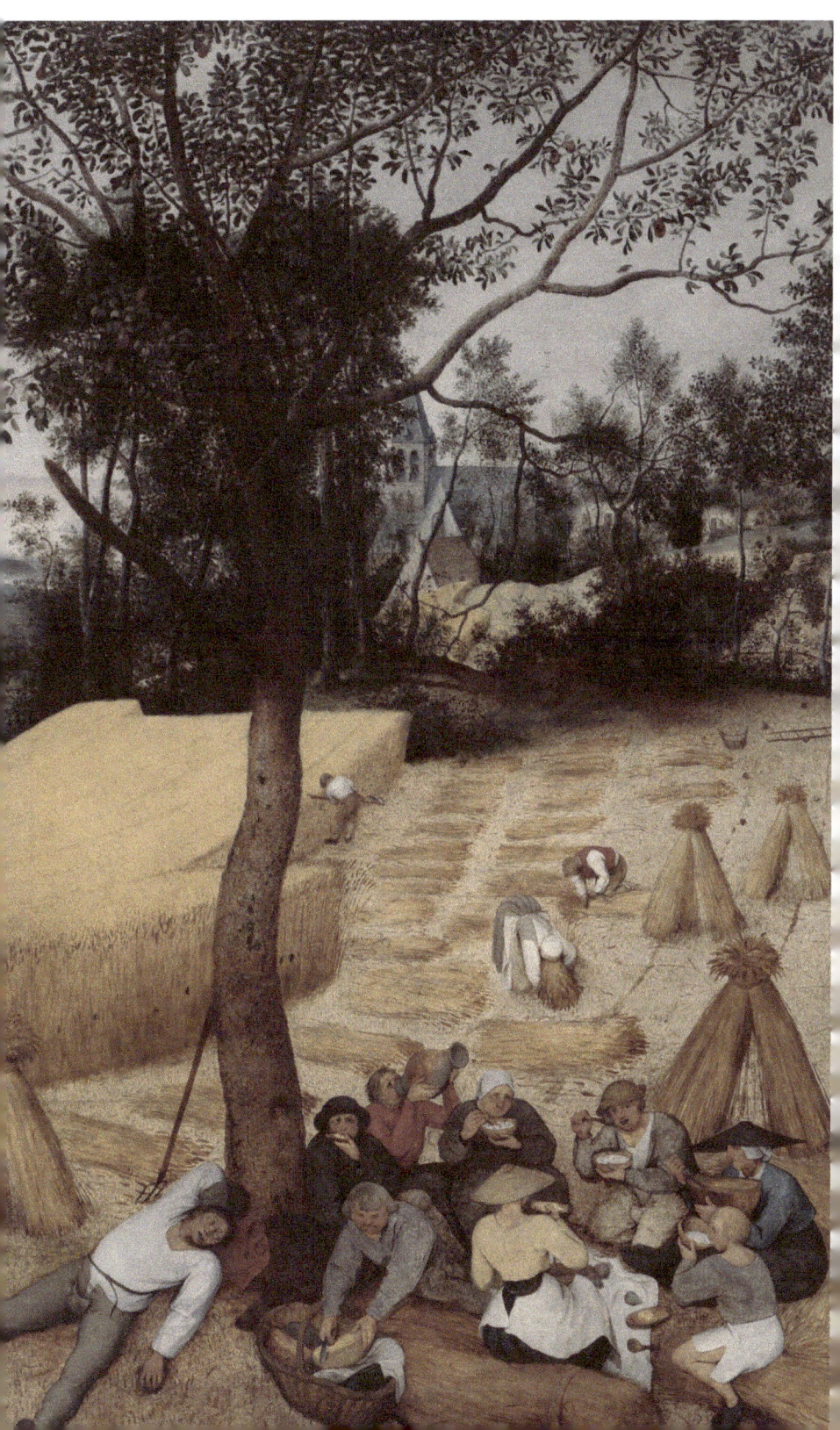

not belong to the lord of a manor who could not be bothered to come out and work in the fields, but that rather this is a collective enterprise of benefit to the village.

Look at how hard they work. The man at the left of the tree is exhausted and now fast asleep as a group of others takes their mid-day meal. The basket of bread represents the culmination of the harvest, and I love how everyone sits together on the ground in the shade of a tree that is intricately beautiful, and upon which the painter has rendered each and every leaf. This tree, strangely, occludes what I think is the church in the background, as if to say that the immediate spiritual life of the village is here in the field, not there, locked away in some building, but right before us with everyone seated in the shade, on the ground, together breaking bread. Here is the true communion, not indoors mediated by a professional.

I experience, in my interpretation of the painting thus, an image of the health of the village. To be honest, I'm not sure that this is really what is happening. I readily confess my yearning for a guild, for apprenticeship, for work of the hands, for community in these days of endstage capitalism.

This is Peter Bruegel the Elder's *The Harvesters*, from 1565. In an extraordinary reversal of previous representation, the peasants appear as dominant in the landscape. The curator of the Metropolitan Museum, where the painting resides, notes that if you look at the women bending over, putting together the sheaves of wheat, they have almost become them, so completely have their forms merged with the forms of the triangular sheaves. How beautiful.

Before the enclosures there is the experience, which cannot but be a psychic experience, of the commons of the village that dwarfs individual holdings. This notion of the commons fosters what Professor Darcia Narvaez calls 'the proper intuitions of relatedness.' In the commons we are part of something larger. We do not begin and end at or with ourselves, or our edges, for we are woven into a common tapestry of belonging, in which we find ourselves through sacred relatedness.

The commons is the terrain of becoming, the terrain of relating. When we have access to the commons, when we have both the opportunity and the concomitant responsibility to tend them for the common good, our private (e.g., familial) holdings are placed within a relational web (a mycelial, dare I say, network) of relations that constrains our sense of inflated self-importance while re-inforcing our (again dare I say it) sacred and necessary obligation to operate with a view toward the best interests of *the collective*.

Common lands were used for grazing, planting, hunting, fishing. These were collective resources stewarded on behalf of the community.

One of the astounding foundational errors of the European vision, arriving in the Americas, and due to the English colonizers having now been thoroughly acclimated to Enclosure because their own commons had been thieved from them, was their radical failure to understand the staggering beauty of the land they encountered as an expression of communitarian ethic of its Indigenous stewards, who wild-tended the garden/ forest / grasslands, etc., in which they resided.

The total European failure to recognize the flourishing of New World landscapes as the result of millenia of tending by Indigenous stewards (they literally could not *see* this)- their inability to recognize that they were looking at carefully and invisibly tended wild gardens of majesty, tended in ways that did not fit the European notion of gardening to create wild gardens that did not fit the European notion of what a garden is- led to the profoundly mistaken notion that the apex of natural beauty is nature undisturbed. On the contrary, this efflorescence of beauty is attained through stewardship uncontaminated by domination. Indigenous people were collaborating with elemental forces such as fire, and water, and wind, and also collaborating eco-systemically, helping shape the way that various herds interacted with and thereby moulded natural landscapes. Their communitarian vision extended far beyond the human inhabitants of place: they were and often still are master collaborators with the entire Living World: flora, fauna, elements, and super-natural forces.

Indigenous people had, for millennia, been stewarding a commons, and although would not use this language, because their cosmology had evolved along different lines, its implication is similar.

In each case, the familial life was set in the context of a community, a village, one of whose many functions was to steward common resource. *Within this commons grow the proper intuitions of relatedness.*

⊕

I am interested in the mental, the psychic contents of this moment, in the 12th century, in Britain, when the Enclosures begin. This is at a feudal moment in Britain, and there are manorial lords, but the villagers living there have certain rights on the land, including pasture, pannage, and estovers. Pasture is the right to graze livestock, pannage the right to graze pigs in the forest, and estovers an allowance of wood that a tenant is allowed to take from the commons for the implements of husbandry, hedges, fences, and firewood. (Etymology: from the French, *Estovoir*, "that which is necessary."

Manorial lordships were created following the Norman conquest of 1066. Let's back up a little. The Roman Empire abandons Britain at the beginning of the fifth century. Anglo-Saxon kingdoms are established in the 5th and 6th centuries: Northumbia, Mercia, East Anglia, Essex, Kent, Sussex, Wessex. These kingdoms are gradually unified during the 9th and 10th centuries, ending with the Norman conquest by William in 1066.

The origin of the manors was in the need for territorial

self-defense, in particular down the east coast of the country, against successive invasions by Germanic tribes and later the Vikings. William the Conqueror created 13,418 'manors' (areas of land administration), which the local 'Lord of the Manor' governed. The Lord of the Manor sublet this land to tenant farmers who paid the Lord rent (see our word 'landlord'.) In turn, the Lord paid taxes to the King. These manors were the pivot around which the feudal system swung.

Such a manor did not consist merely of the land. Rather, there were conveyed four distinct sets of rights. Beyond the land title, were the land rights (hunting, fishing, mining rights). Then the manorial documents. Finally the manorial title.

⊕

I want to see if I can place us here in the mindset of this moment.

I recently looked closely at an 800-year-old English manor, which was advertised for sale in *The New York Times*. 800 years takes us back, almost to this era. The manor, though immense, is dank and dark inside, the windows tiny. Roofs are strangely thatched. Stones worn into troughs down their centers through centuries of use. The sense of physical enclosure, of being totally indoors, walled off from nature, is the most powerful sense. We are deeply inside: the spaces, while often monumental, have the air of caverns.

We are long before the birth of nation states, and the villagers are gathered close together in towns. There are no proper sewer systems. No medicine. No electric lights. The most rapid conveyance is some remnant of a cart or chariot. There is no civic infrastructure. This movement to enclosure, a defensive movement, happens I believe for safety. To defend against the hostile onslaught.

Hostile neighbors. The ravages of winter. These are northern climes. Because materials technology at this time is not good enough to let in light but keep out cold the structures in which people live are totally enclosed. Only the rich have windows, really, and those are at best miniscule. Double-and triple-planed windows do not yet exist. Winter will kill you, as will the barbarians from the East...

And so a trade is made, the price of which will not be apparent for many generations to come. We give away some collective benefit in exchange for the promise of greater security. Sound familiar?

⊕

We say that the eyes are the windows to the soul. The mouth a doorway to the heart. A house is always a metaphor for the psyche. One dwelling where we live is a metaphor for another dwelling where we live. So what does it mean to live within an enclosure? What kinds of psyches develop inside of four walls, and how are they different than psyches that develop in the Living World? What is the price we pay inwardly for being boxed in?

Ask yourself. You know the answer. You were raised in a box. Ask a 3rd grader to cut through all of the political correctness, and name the archetype of European-derived modernity versus Indigeneity, and they will tell you: Europeans live indoors, Indigenous people live outside. Do you - *can you* - understand what this means? Do you – *can you* – understand what has been thieved from you?

If where we live cannot but be a metaphor for the psyche, what kind of psyche develops in people who live inside? I'll answer that: a closed psyche. Psyche as fortress. Psyche as defended perimeter. Psyche as contraction. This is another foundation layer, accreted beneath the known, in the basement of the psyches of the modern world. A taproot of supremacy and a basement of enclosure, which is the ego. A contraction into defense that pulls back from relationship.

The taproot gives rise to the schizophrenia of supremacy, the inability to have horizontal relations.

Enclosure fortifies the individual, reifies the individual ego as separate defended self, walls us away.

It migrates out of the house into the fields, where it eats the commons, partitions the land up. It draws cleanly delineated psychic boundaries across the fields, cuts up the eco-system with the same alacrity the butcher quarters the cow. What is lost in our seeing as this happens? What mycelial threads of relatedness are severed?

Suddenly the child is no longer permitted to go forth. Those woods, those wilds, they belong to someone else now. Robert Frost's *Stopping by Woods on a Snowing Evening* becomes impossible.

Whose woods these are I think I know.
His house is in the village though;
He will not see me stopping here
To watch his woods fill up with snow.

My little horse must think it queer
To stop without a farmhouse near
Between the woods and frozen lake
The darkest evening of the year.

He gives his harness bells a shake
To ask if there is some mistake.
The only other sound's the sweep
Of easy wind and downy flake.

The woods are lovely, dark and deep,

But I have promises to keep,
And miles to go before I sleep,
And miles to go before I sleep.

Today Frost does not stop. The woods are fenced in. They are privately owned, circumscribed by a wall. You could get shot for trespassing. And yet, not only have you lost the woods, you have lost the *imaginal terrain* of the woods. Not only have you lost the wilds, you have lost the *imaginal terrain* of the wilds. Both the place, and what it means psychically have been thieved from you with the deft legal swoop of enclosure.

Stay in the house! Stay in the yard! Stay in your proper place! How dare you venture into the unknown wilds! How dare you set foot in places that do not belong to you!

And so we have boxed ourselves in. Our psyches, our minds, our language, our thought forms derivative of enclosure. Like root bound plants, we moderns: domesticated animals, primed for impending slaughter.

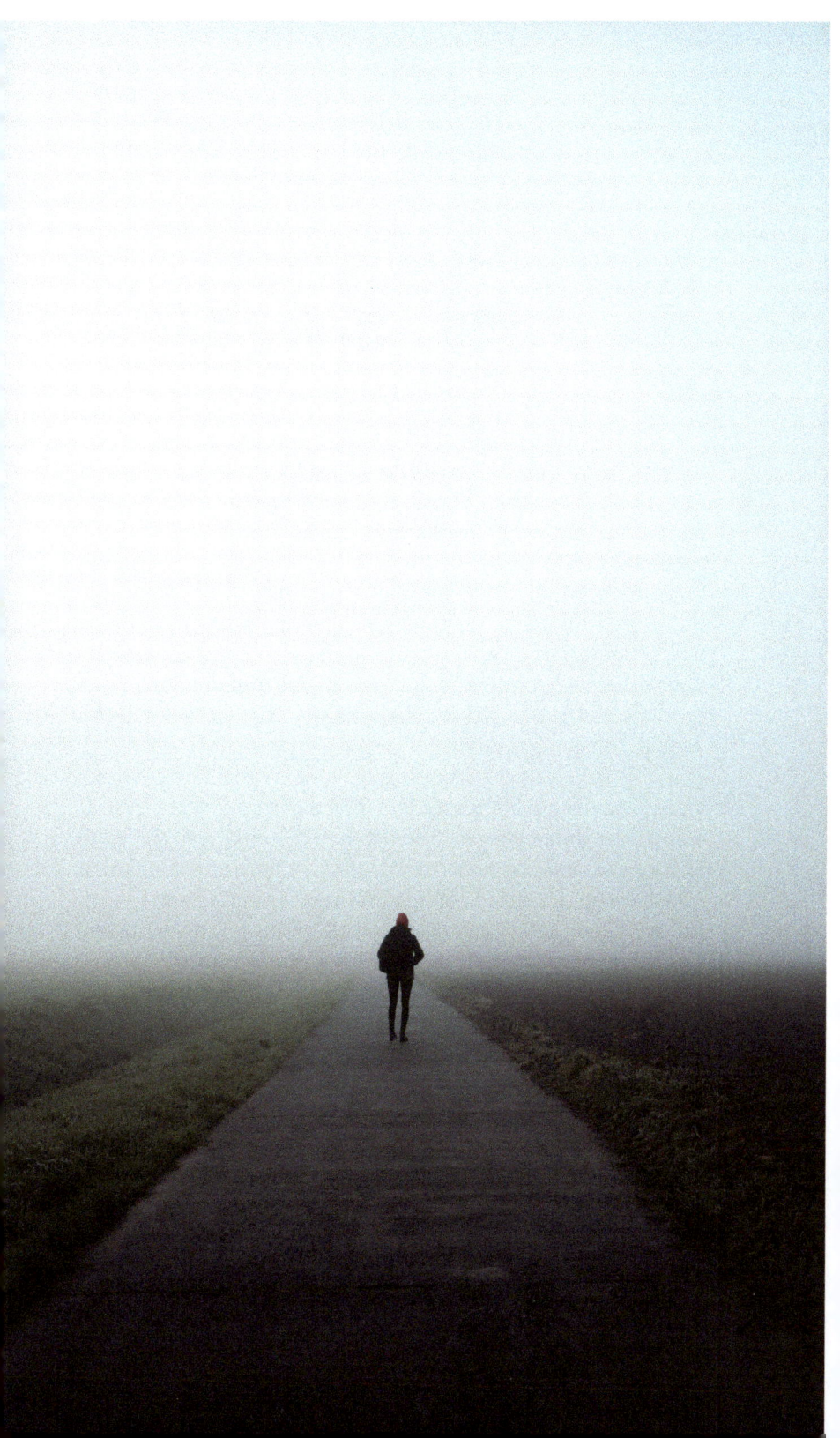

20 - Wrong Angles

In 1999 Stanford University acquired Buckminster Fuller's Dymaxion Chronofile. The idiosyncratic inventor, rebel mathematician, nature architect and cosmological inquirer had treated his entire life as an experiment, and never threw away a piece of paper after his early twenties. The Chronofile, Bucky's life in paper, was measured not in pages but in linear feet of material, of which there are 1421 if I recall correctly, and which were housed in horizontal files ordered numerically in a set of rooms off the main library that were not accessible to the general public.

I had been deeply impressed by Fuller since having entered, as a child, an immense geodesic dome of his design at the Saint Louis Botanical Gardens that housed a rainforest: a building unusual enough that it seemed to have been designed by, or for, an alien. Later, around the time when I dropped out of Yale, I had encountered his treatise on mathematics, *Synergetics*, which I liked to walk around with and pretend I was studying, but had difficulty making significant headway in. Synergetics, although a mathematics text, reads like a philosophical tome. I didn't make much technical headway reconciling it with my mathematics, but I understood what he was saying at a primal existential level, and found the book a great comfort. The premise of the book is elementary: nature designs in triangles and tetrahedrons. If mathematics is organized this way, it resolves the wave/particle duality at its origins, and we can calculate quantum effects using simple addition.

In 2002, while attending Stanford, I volunteered to work on the Chronofile, and was accepted onto the library's volunteer staff. I was assigned to the earliest section of documents, which included, memorably, a receipt from the general store in Penobscot Bay in Maine where the Fuller's owned a small island on which they had built a summer compound, and where young Bucky had charged a significant number of items to his mother's charge account, to her displeasure. This particular receipt was scrawled with her writing, and read: *Buckminster, do not charge items to my account without my permission, for I do not like it.* Ok, I thought. He was just like any other presumptuous kid.

But Fuller was not just like any other kid, and another story from his very early life makes this apparent, and perhaps lays out the groundwork for the manner in which he became an iconoclast. From a young age, Fuller had terrible eyesight. Before his vision had been tested, in kindergarten, he was given an assignment, with all of the other children, to construct a house or a bridge or some kind of structure out of toothpicks and peas. You can imagine this. The kids are sitting on the ground with trays in front of them: they have a pile of toothpicks, and a pile of green peas, and the teacher gives a demonstration and then encourages their creativity. Young Fuller couldn't see the demonstration that the teacher gave, and may not have cared about it anyway. He sits there with his toothpicks and his peas, and then makes a design decision that will shape the entire course of his life. While his classmates, emulating their teacher, as well as the design of their classroom, the angles at which the floor meets the walls, the ceiling meets the walls, the verticality of every building they have ever seen, the axis of horizontal and vertical, the entire received visual and architectural hegemony of every structure assembled in Europe since Rome, begin to build scaffolding and structure with right angles, young Fuller, who has been studying nature, decides that he is going to build with triangles and tetrahedrons. I say decide, but does he decide, or does this just happen? Is it trial and error as he is confronted with the raw challenge, or some assertion of intellect or intuition? I do not know.

The boy sitting on the floor, in his own private world, begins to assemble a structure composed of struts and braces where each pea is the cornerstone not of an assemblage of right angles, but of sixty degree increments. His creation gets progressively more and more unusual until the entire class is gathered around him, laughing. I cannot imagine that this is pleasant, but what happens next is even more interesting, because the teacher begins to berate him, telling him he is doing it wrong. The child is five years old. And yet, strangely, he resists. Persists in his design. And then, in an occurrence that will reverberate forward through his life, he insists on keeping his strange building, and using it in the contest to see which structures can best bear weight, and he wins. Flat out. Hands down. Definitively. Not even close.

All the other houses, with their dutiful right angles crumble. Fuller's structure does not fail. It possesses superior strength. How does this land with a child, this experience? This resistance to influence of peers and authority of elders, and the subsequent unequivocal triumph? Many decades later, when writing in *Synergetics*, he would explain that the close packing of spheres, twelve around one, is the strongest most stable structure in Universe. This structure he names a *vector equilibrium*. It is articulated through the centerpoints of twelve spheres of identical radius closest packed around a single center sphere. It is a mystical awareness, this. Twelve around one. The angles are triangles and tetrahedrons, the geometry he accidented onto as a five year old.

If Fuller's classmates and teachers had not laughed at him–if they had instead noted the brilliance of his creation and embraced it– would he have gone on to develop and articulate the vectorial energetic geometry of nature? Or did this need, this urge, this yearning arise in him particularly because of the rejection, and because he then could observe that he was right? This kind of experience seems to me the kind required

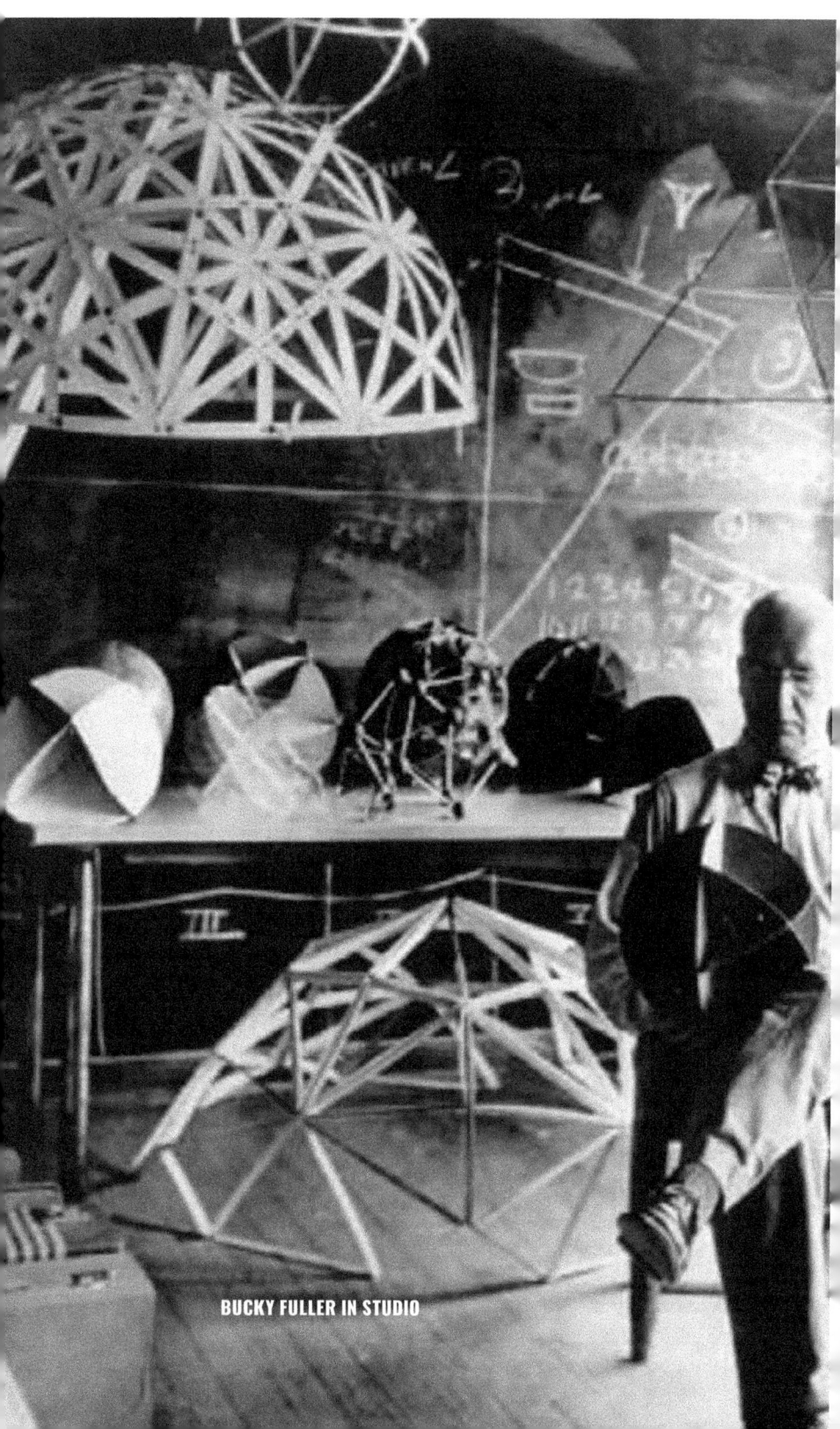

BUCKY FULLER IN STUDIO

to light an existential fire in someone. A five year old, in an act of pure creation, steps outside the fortress of four thousand years of received mathematics. Steps back into the geometry of nature, bio-mimicked, possibly accidentally: possibly in an act of pure intuition. That is what Fuller did. Synergetics are the mathematics of nature. Nature, Fuller would go on to say, would never use a strictly imaginary, awkward, and unrealistic coordinate system, by which he is speaking about our system of ninety degree axes, the horizontal and the vertical.

From Syngergetics: *The fact that 99 percent of humanity does not understand nature is the prime reason for humanity's failure to exercise its option to attain universally sustainable physical success on this planet. The prime barrier to humanity's discovery and comprehension of nature is **the obscurity of the mathematical language of science**.* [Emphasis mine.]

Drop the mic.

Stop for a moment and consider this. Have you ever seen a right angle in nature? How is it that every house, every room most people spend time in, every piece of lumber, which are the components of every house and every room, are pre-designed with right angles, when nothing in nature is made of right angles? Not a single thing.[1] Not any part of your body, not a single tree, flower, shell, fruit, mountain, river, planet, or star. Not an atom, a molecule, a cell, or an organ. Nothing in our actual lives, nothing in our lived experience that is not made by humans is comprised of right angles, except for some kinds of crystalline structures. Doesn't this seem odd to you? Who did this? Is it possible that right angles are the wrong angles?

That the fact that we have been trained to think in them is in

---

[1] My friend bio-acoustician Michael Stocker pointed out to me that some crystalline structures have 90 degree angles. I am hard-pressed to think of anything else.

fact denaturing us? Mathematics, as currently prosecuted, is one of many origins of the mindbody split. One of many origins of the man-nature split. Our math is a fountain of alienation because, like a funhouse mirror, it refuses to reflect the reality of our earthly world. So how did things get to be this way?

"Our current mathematics is one of the origins of the mindbody split."

Pythagoras (560-480 BCE), the Greek mathematician, was the first to prove, mathematically, the relationship between the sides of a right-angle triangle, e.g., a2 + b2 = c2. (a squared plus b squared equals c squared, where c is the hypotenuse.) But he did not discover it, as it was known to the ancient Babylonians for a thousand years before this.

We know this due to a fragment of cuneiform writing on an ancient tablet, which is known as Plimpton 322, and is from the ancient city of Larsa, which was located near Tell as-Senkereh in modern day Iraq. The tablet was written between 1822-1762 BCE. In 1945 the tablet was revealed to contain a complex sequence of Pythagorean triples. On the following page is a fragment. Beneath it the mathematical transcription of the fragment. This is the fundamental relationship that Pythagoras articulated nearly 1,000 years later, demonstrating that the ancient Babylonians already possessed a complex form of trigonometry. The Babylonians, who had a sexagesimal (base 60) system of calculation, rather than a decimal (base 10), had already articulated this relationship. But why?

Dr. Daniel Mansfield, a mathematician at the University of New South Wales (UNSW) in Australia with an interest in Babylonian mathematics, explains, based on a 3,700 year old cadastral survey, which sheds light on why there was a trigonometry table in ancient Babylon.

"With this new tablet [Si.427], we can actually see for the first time why they were interested in geometry: to lay down pre-

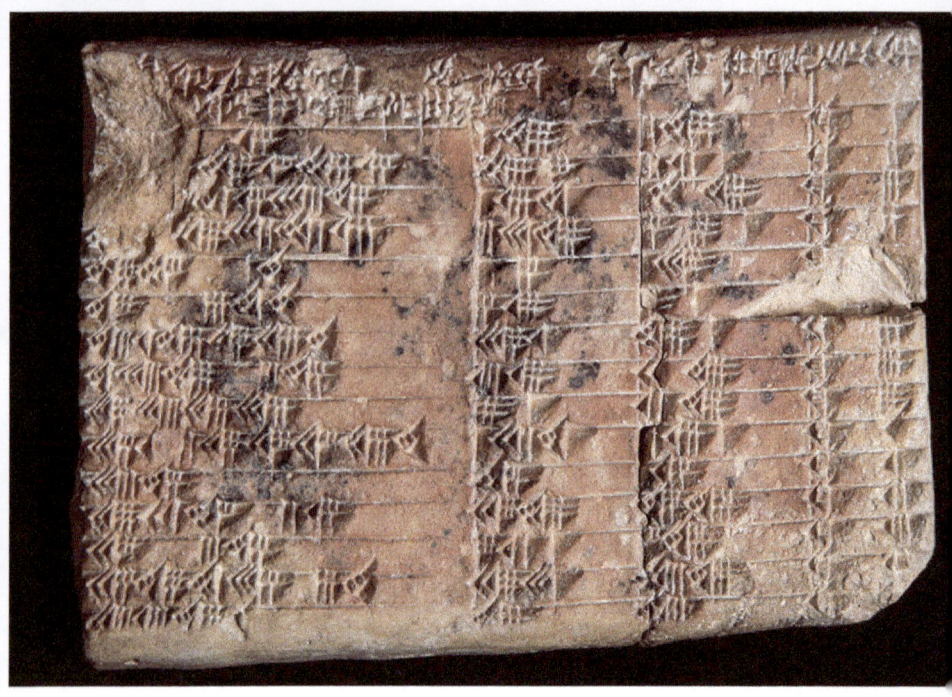

The Plimpton 322 tablet (above), and what is says (below).

obv	I'						II'		III'			IV'
1	ta-k]i - il- ti și - li - ip - tim						íb-si₈	sag	íb-si₈ și-li-ip-tim			mu-bi-im
2	ša 1 in] -na-as-sà-hu-ú-ma sag i-il-lu-ú											
3	1 59	15					1 59		2 49			ki
4	1 56	56	58	14	*56*	15	56 7		*3 12*	*1*		ki
5	1 55	7	41	15	33	45	1 16	41	1 50	49		ki
6	1 53	10	29	32	52	16	3 31	49	5 9	1		ki
7	1 48	54	1	40			1 5		1 37			ki
8	1 47	6	41	40			5 19		8 1			ki
9	1 43	11	56	28	26	40	38 11		59 1			ki
10	1 41	33	*59*	3	45		13 19		20 49			ki
11	1 38	33	36	36			*9* 1		12 49			ki
12	1 35	10	2	28	27	24 26 40	1 22	41	2 16	1		ki
13	1 33	45					45		1 15			ki
14	1 29	21	54	2	15		27 59		48 49			ki
15	1 27		3	45			*7 12*	*1*	4 49			ki
16	25	48	51	35	6	40	29 31		53 49			ki
17	1 23	13	46	40			56		53			ki

cise land boundaries," says Mansfield. "This is from a period where land is starting to become private—people started thinking about land in terms of 'my land and your land,' wanting to establish a proper boundary to have positive neighborly relationships."

Right angles emerge because humans have entered the epoch of ownership of the earth. Right angles are a byproduct of enclosure.

So tracking back here, to the origin of right angles, takes us back to the beginning of private land ownership, which is really the origin of enclosure. Between 1900 and 1600 BCE the nature of Babylonian land ownership changes, with smaller parcels being allotted to ordinary people. Prior to this, land belonged to the palace and the temple. Now, individuals begin to own lots. There is at this time, an increase in the number of surveyors. This is a poem, from the period, in which an older surveyor admonishes a younger.

Go to divide a plot, and you are not able to divide the plot; go to apportion a field, and you cannot even hold the tape and rod properly. The field pegs you are unable to place; you cannot figure out its shape, so that when wronged men have a quarrel you are not able to bring peace, but you allow brother to attack brother. Among the scribes, you (alone) are unfit for the clay.

The poem refers to the tape and the rod, which modern scholars state are references to the standard Babylonian surveying tools: the unit rod and measuring rope. Yet if we dig a bit deeper, we find that these items were not merely implements of surveyors, but rather implements of royalty, and beyond that actually of divinity. These were revered symbols of fairness and justice in ancient Babylon and were often seen in the hands of goddesses and kings. Now they are in the hands of the surveyors. Let's go deeper with this. (In the images on pages 142-143, on the Uruk cylinder seal (3500 to 3000 BCE), note the abundance of rods and rings.)

This rod of which the poem speaks is a surveyor's rod, but it is also a rod associated with kingship. So what does the rod do? What function does it have? We could say, at one level, that the rod is a unit of measurement, both actual and metaphorical. The rod is a standard unit of measure: the cubit rod. Anyone who has ever read, or heard the Bible read will have encountered this term– *the cubit*. Noah, for example, received specific dimensions about the ark he was supposed to build: 300 cubits long, 50 cubits wide, 30 cubits high. The cubit is a unit of measure in antiquity, and was derived bodily: the length from the elbow to the tip of the middle finger. *Cubitum*, in Latin, means 'elbow.' We can note that originally all units of measure were anthropometric. Our body, our nature itself, was the basis of the measurement.[2]

The ancient cubit was defined as this distance from the elbow to the outstretched tip of the middle finger, and was comprised of six palms of four fingers, ergo 24 digits, i.e., base 24. We were measured against ourselves. All ancient systems of measure were referenced, we should note, anthropometrically. Yet one can imagine, easily, that there might be some variation here, as people are of different sizes. Whose cubit are we talking about? The standard length of whose elbow to fingertip?

The rod, then, is a standardization of this measure. The ancient Egyptian royal cubit *(meh niswt)* depicted on the next page is the earliest attested standard measure, and dates back

---

2 I noted earlier in this chapter that an origin of the mindbody split was in the divorce of mathematics from nature. Another mindbody split is in the divorce of measurement from reference in our own bodies. You can see the ancient anthropometrism (to measure in terms of our own human bodies) in words we still use for measure. Horses are still measured as a number of 'hands' high. When our bodies are the source of measurement, we are measuring the world against ourselves, which preserves relationality. As measurement becomes standardized, this relationality is obscured. We gain precision, we lose connection.

to around 3000 BCE. But what do we measure? The gods who hold the rod measure the length of a human life. They are taking the measure of man. This symbol of divinity is held vertically.

In the Babylonian tradition, over several thousand years, we see these implements of divinity make their way into human hands. This happens gradually, and is depicted on stelae, cylinder seals, and tablets. In the earliest depictions, the rod and ring are held by Gods. Several thousand years later we see them in the hands of kings. This transition is marked by uncertainty. At first the kings revere the rod and ring, later they are holding them. I will assert here, speculatively, that by the time the surveyor poem is written, the rod and ring had moved into the hands of the surveyor, who were performing much the same function, e.g., taking the measure of heaven and earth, and who had become, *de facto*, the first lawyers. Let's dwell, for a moment, on perhaps the most famous depiction of the rod and ring, on what is now known as the Louvre stele (plundered, like the Nike of Samothrace), which depicts the Law Code of Hammurabi, in Akkadian and Cuneiform.

Here we have the Sun God Shamash seated on his throne (he wears a celestial crown that swirls about this head composed of four pairs of horns, holds a ring and staff, and has flames issuing from his shoulders) holding out the rod and ring, implements of divinity and sovereignty, toward Hammurabi. The laws? They are the rod and ring. Although Hammurabi is subservient he addresses the god directly. Even though he has his hand raised in reverence he shows that he has a personal relationship with the gods while mere mortals do not. Now take a very close look at the rod.

You will note that it is not symmetrical at both ends, but wider on the top, narrower at the bottom. It looks more, in fact, like a stake. A stake that would be pounded into the ground. The rod takes the measure of man, but it is also pounded into the ground to mark a boundary. The law code of Hammurabi, conveyed from the gods to the sovereign ruler, marks the

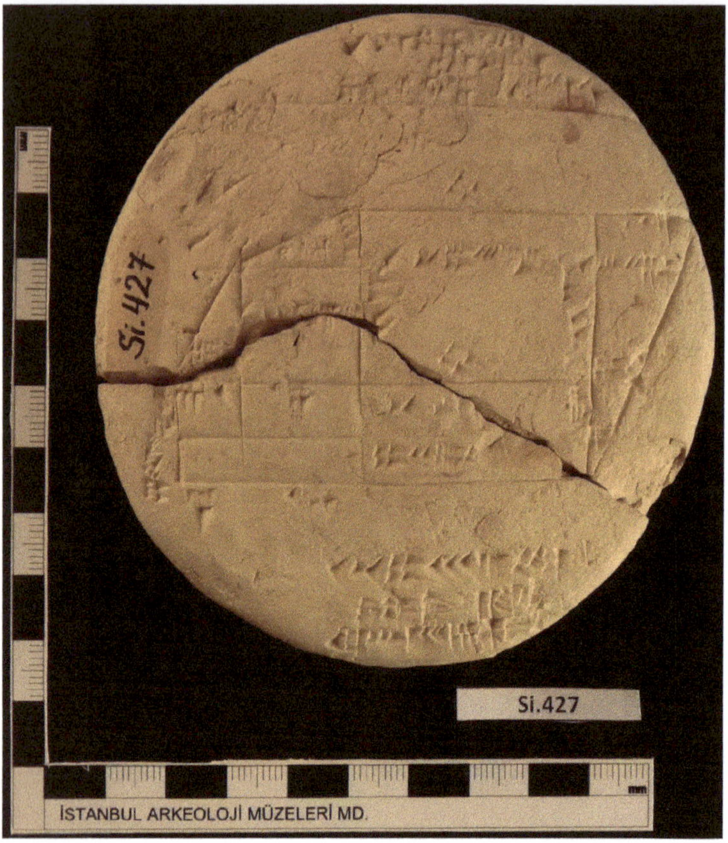

Si. 427 (above) – Cadastral survey on clay tablet. Right angles to demarcate land boundaries. Babylonian, 1700 BC

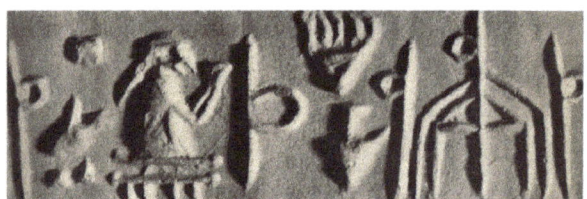

Illustration 3. Uruk Cylinder Seal, 3500–3000 B.C.E. As found in D. J. Wiseman and Werner Forman, Cylinder Seals of Western Asia *(London: Batchworth Press, 195-), 4.*

Uruk cylinder seal (above) – rods and rings

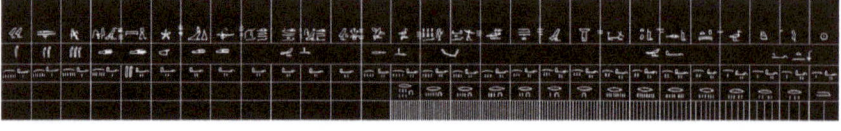

Egyptian royal cubit (neh niswt) (above) – a rod: the first yardstick

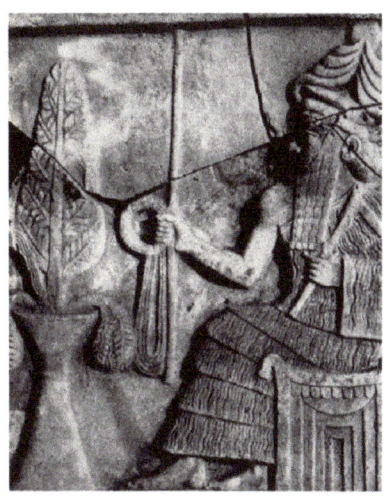

Two images of the Babylonian sun god Shamash holding rod and ring. On the stele below, The Law Code of Hammurabi, he hands these implements to the King. Notice that the bottom end of the rod is pointed, the top end is wider. It resembles a surveyor's stake.

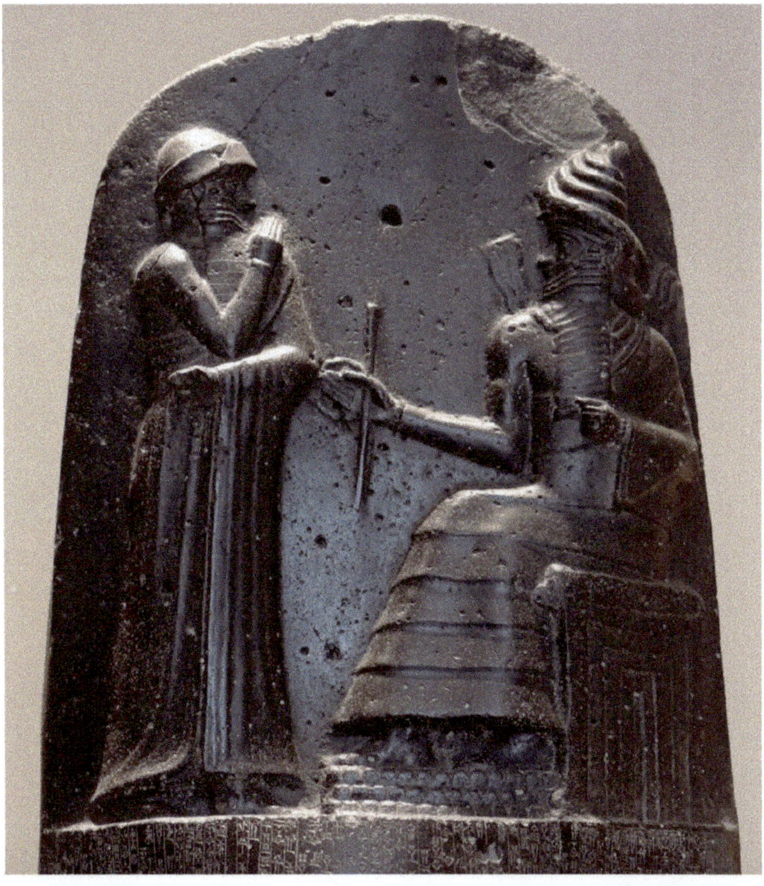

boundaries of the kingdom, both literally and metaphorically. The law is the boundary marker. Those who marked the boundary are therefore lawyers. To survey is to prosecute the law. It is the exercise of authority over the edge of the realm.

Let us dwell, for a moment, on the ring, which may also be a rope. There are no images of a rope other than a coil of rope, which is, you guessed it, a ring. You will perhaps remember from your own study of trigonometry that no two lines can pass through the same point in a plane. This is true in the actual physical world. A circle is essentially a flat coil. The symbols of divinity, held by the gods, are a rod, held vertically, and a circle, which while depicted in images is rotated such that we can perceive it is a circle, is actually held horizontally. Some say that the rod represents time, and the circle eternity. Some say the rod is linear time, and the circle cyclic. Some say the rod is masculine, the circle feminine. Yes to all of these interpretations.

The circle also represents horizontality. In the circle there is no above and no below. The rod is the implement of domination, of hierarchy. It is literally pounded into the ground. The circle is the implement of inclusion and relatedness. Divinity carries both implements. They are passed to sovereignty, gradually, where the sovereigns attended to the balance of the vertical and the horizontal, time and eternity. The edge (boundary marker) and the center (circle). The boundary of empire and the center of civic life.

The rod is a measurement of distance, but also of justice. The rod establishes a system of measurement. Vertically oriented, it connects the earth and the heavens. The cubit rod, unlike a staff, is too short to touch the ground if the divinity is standing, but it can touch the ground when the divinity is seated on the throne.

The rod's base rests on the ground, its tip points to the heavens. It depicts masculine authority, and is held in the right hand of sovereignty. The ring, born in the left hand, floats.

Held horizontally, it conveys notions of equality, and invokes the lunar, the feminine, the receptive. Imagine now, either the divinity or the sovereign aligning the two. The ring is slid over the rod, evoking the marriage of the earthly and the divine, the masculine and the feminine. An archetype of sexual congress. Viewed from the front we have a cross. A horizontal and a vertical axis. The intersections where they meet are at ninety degrees.

Yet something happens, psychically, of note, when these implements of the divine, which have become sovereign, make their way into the hands of ordinary men, the surveyors. The earth is now, on their cadastral tablets, being cut into right angle sections. Lest you imagine this being abstract, because these are farming plots, remember that an ancient Mesopotamian, standing on a ziggurat, the temples of the time, and looking out at the land, would have begun to see rectangles around them. The crops are planted to the edge of the property boundary. The Babylonians transform the world around them from a world of circles, spirals, waves: natural forms all, into a landscape of right angles. The rod begins to dominate. The ring recedes.

This is a concretized deviation from the ancestral baseline. This is the implementation of the imprint of the hand of man, inherited from divinity, passed through sovereignty, imprinting now on the landscape of nature. This looks natural to us because we are so accustomed to it. Yet it is very deeply strange.

Suddenly man – ordinary man – not the sovereign, is taking the measure of things. It is one thing when this measurement, of justice, of the human span, of distance is being done by the gods, another when it is transferred to the sovereign. Yet even the sovereign is still in league with the divine (this is the meaning and derivation of the 'divine right of kings'). When this measurement– of justice, of time, of distance– is handed to the surveyors, something changes. We move into the bureaucratic administration of empire. Justice (or its lack) is

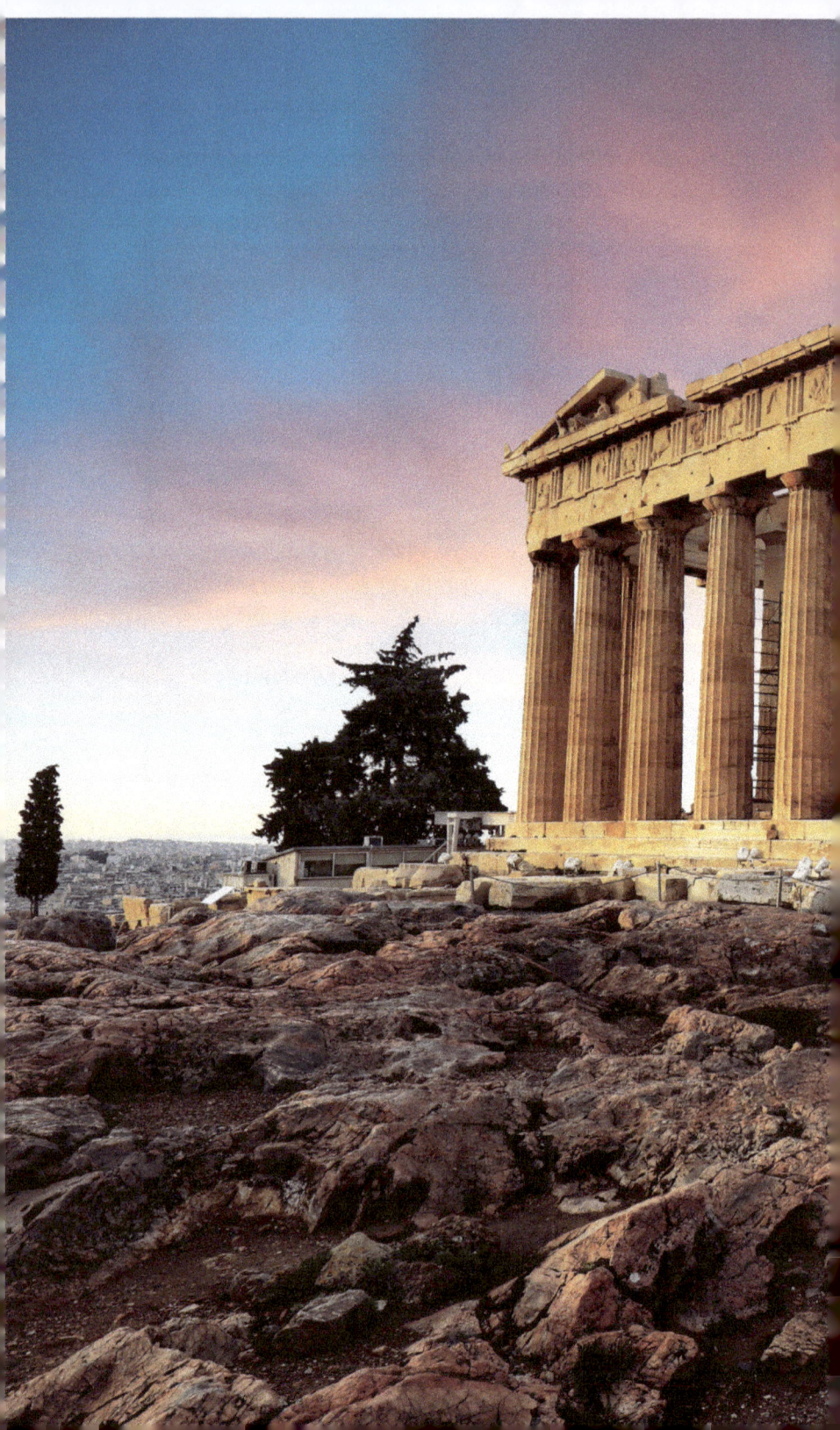

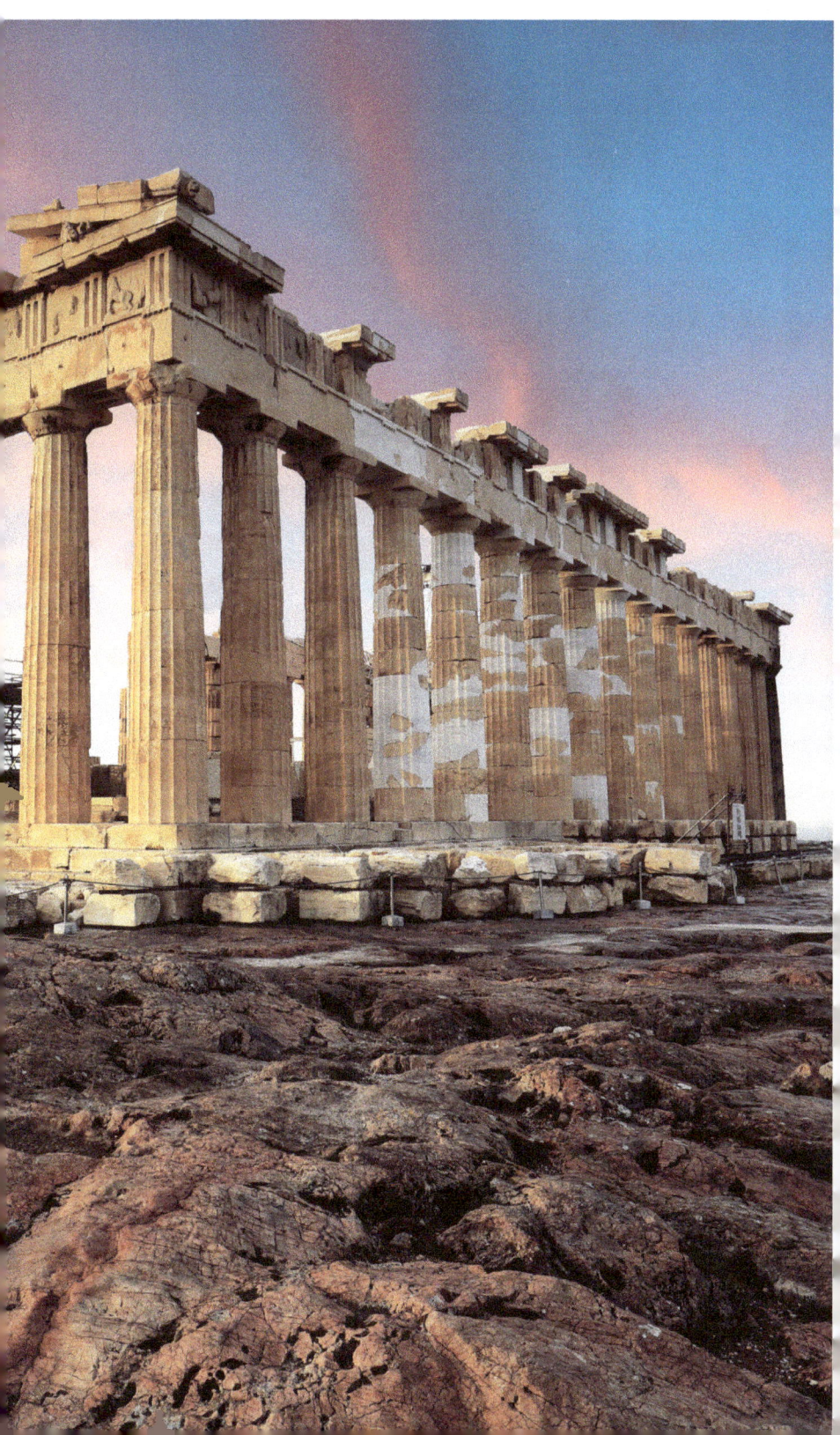

now meted out by functionaries.

Lest we forget, our ancestors knew there was something magical about building. The origin of masonry is in the guilds who built Solomon's temple. Building is congress between the celestial and the earthly. It leaves the imprint of the divine here on earth. And what were these builders, holding the rod and ring, these implements of royalty, these surveyors, building? They were building temples.

And now we can turn our attention to the familiar forms of temple architecture standing in the infancy of the Eurocentric hegemony we have inherited.

Here are the Greek forms. On the preceding pages is the Parthenon, built in the mid-5th century BCE and dedicated to the Greek goddess Athena Parthenos ("Athena the Virgin"), generally considered to be the culmination of the Doric order.

You can imagine the sudden order of this imposed on the landscape, its verticality, the way it marries heaven and earth. Exultant. This intersection of the vertical and the horizontal planes. Imagine it against its proper backdrop: a sea of organic forms (circles, spirals, rings). Imagine it for a moment as the root impulse of modernity, order against a sea of chaos. Man struggling to come into power in an elemental world of overpowering forces.

This is where my architecture education began, I don't know about yours. This is the reference thoughtform.

The temple architecture, at ninety degrees, expresses this intersection, this interface between the vertical and horizontal axis, the masculine and the feminine, the earthly and the celestial, in every angle.

And yet, at the time, it would have stood out, a singular structure in rectangles against a sea of natural forms. In its time it was the anomaly. In two millenia we have inverted this relationship, flipped it upside down. We are surrounded now by rectangles. Enboxed by them on all sides.

I have always promised myself that at some point, when I had more time, I would learn Fuller's energetic vectorial geometry. Starting with triangles and tetrahedrons, rather than squares and cubes, he develops a geometry that resolves the particle-wave duality. That can explain nuclear physics with simple addition. He teaches the mathematics that nature speaks. A mathematics of triangles, tetrahedrons, fractals, spirals, waves. A mathematics of flower petals, neurocardiology, the spiral arms of galaxies. It is the mathematics of the ancient divine ring. Not the rod.

We moderns, downstream of the wrong angle, cut adrift from anthropometric forms, a mathematics anchored in the reality of Nature, have lost our experience of relatedness through the language of mathematics, which is also the language of our 'modern' science, and like a noun-based language, no longer holds the imprint and vibration of the Living World.

We have been cut adrift from systems that foster the proper intuitions of relatedness. All around us the temple forms of an earlier era rise toward the skies, and we are lost.

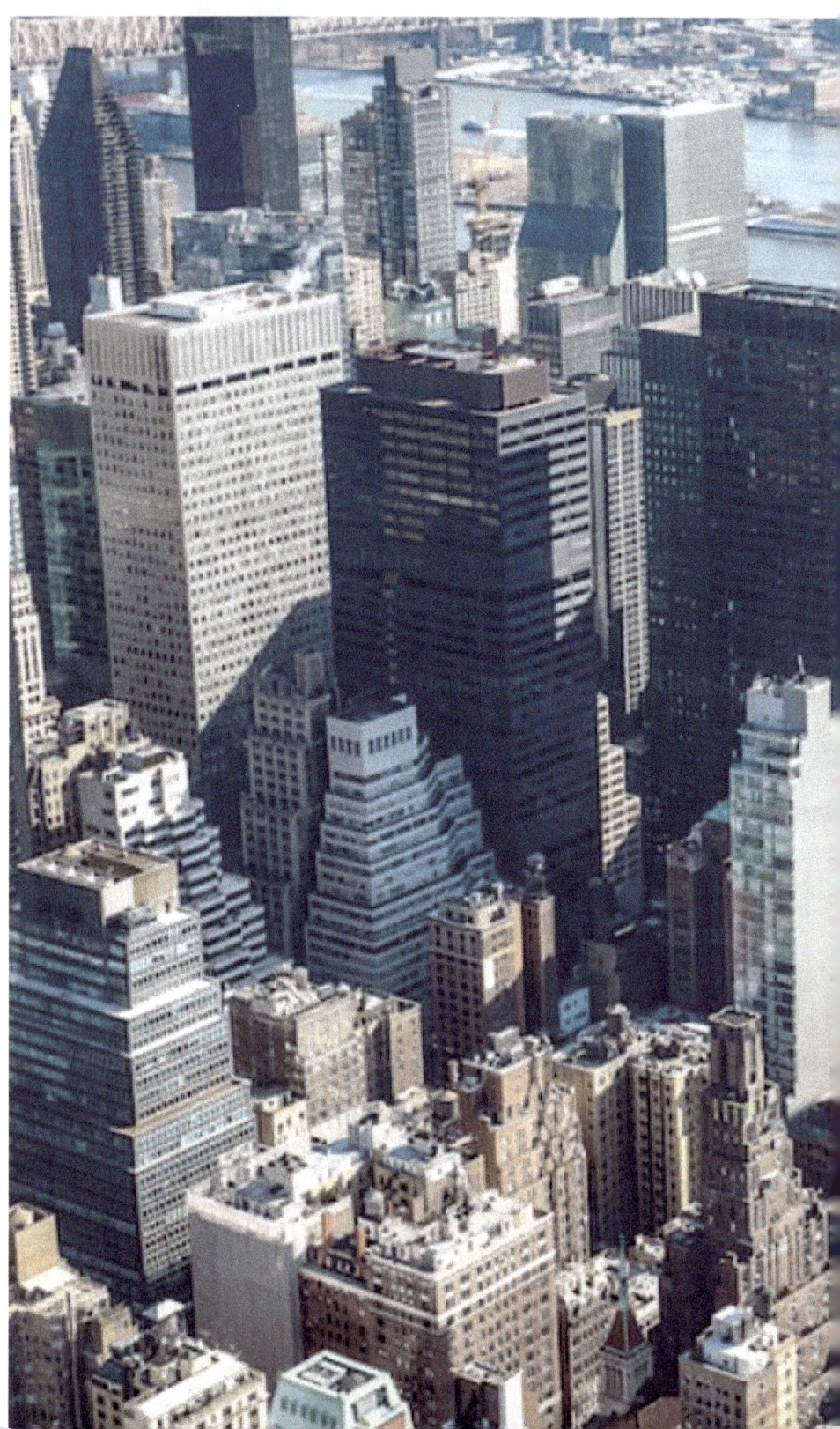

21 - At the origin of consciousness, a crime scene

I didn't get to meet Terrence McKenna while he was alive. I was, however, a grateful beneficiary of his writing, placing me squarely in the path of influence of his immense linguistic facility and playfulness, which was deployed in service to a vision of consciousness that was as deeply strange as it was plant-inflected. In the lineage of the great ethno-botanist Richard Evans Schultes, and like Shultes' student Wade Davis, McKenna made his way to the Amazon, in addition to other places around the world, to apprentice himself to plants. In 1992, in a book called *Food of the Gods*, he promulgated a theory, which became known as the Stoned Ape theory, that the deep origin of the human species, the transition from Homo Erectus to Sapiens, and the concomitant metamorphosis in consciousness that he proposed was of a cognitive nature, occurred as a result of earlier humans ingesting *Psilocybe cubensis*, a type of psilocybin-containing mushroom that likes to grow in cow dung. McKenna proposed that sometime around 100,000 years ago, when our Homo Erectus ancestors were following in the wake of herds across the savannah, we began eating the psychedelic mushrooms that grew in their dung. This, he proposes, is the origin of human consciousness.

We became cognitive giants by plucking psychedelic morsels out of piles of bullshit.

I didn't know McKenna personally, but I have friends who did. The stories I have been told about him, including a number of stories that he, as well as his brother Dennis wrote about, make numerous mentions of him taking what is probably an unfortunate choice of words to describe this activity, but is nonetheless known as taking 'heroic' doses of hallucinogens. A heroic dose, which I would propose to you that without proper guidance is more likely to be a 'foolish' dose of psychedelics, is one large enough, generally speaking, to dissolve the containment structure that has become known to most of us through therapy-speak as ego.

McKenna, by his own admission, had a propensity to take extraordinarily large doses of psychedelics without guidance. He was a self-described psychonaut, fearless probably to his own detriment. One of the problems, for someone who is deeply cerebral, in taking immense doses of hallucinogens outside of the context of a wisdom lineage, and without proper guidance, is that it is somewhat like getting into a rocket ship and blasting off, and we have a hard time not attributing significance to what passes by the window of such a cosmological transit despite the fact that we have almost no capacity to steer. You could end up literally anywhere in the universe on such a trip.

The structure of consciousness can be so altered, in these experiences– what we sense, feel, see, and interpret as a result of them so deeply otherwordly and potent– that we are likely to believe that what we have experienced is not merely real, but the fountain from which reality springs.

In 1980, in a book published by the anthropologist Michael Harner called *The Way of the Shaman*, the author speaks about a series of experiences he had drinking ayahuasca where he gradually became aware of more and more visions and information being presented to him by "giant reptilian creatures reposing sluggishly at the lowermost depths of the back of [his] brain". "I could only vaguely see them in what seemed to be gloomy, dark depths," he explained. He was given information reserved for the dying and the dead, he was told.

The "reptiles" projected a visual scene in front of Harner,

which showed the creation of life on earth. But first before that life there were hundreds of "large, shiny, black creatures with stubby pterodactyl-like wings and huge whale-like bodies" that dropped from the sky and landed on the barren landscape. Their heads were not visible. These beings were fleeing from enemies from outer space. They created life on earth "in order to hide within the multitudinous forms and thus disquise their presence."

Harner learned that "the dragon-like creatures were thus inside of all forms of life including man (almost like DNA, although at the time, 1961, Harner knew nothing of DNA). They were the true masters of humanity and the entire planet", the "dragon-like creatures" told Harner. He was caught up in a struggle between the aerial ship with the "bird" people taking his "soul" and the "dragon-like denizens of the depths." As he felt he was about to die Harner was able to cry out "medicine", whereupon in the real world the Indians frantically sent about making an antidote. A powerful being appeared before Harner to protect him from "the alien reptilian creatures".

Simultaneously the antidote to "the little death" drink [ayahuasca] was given, and the dragons and "the soul boat" disappeared. While the antidote eased his condition, Harner continued having "many additional visions of a more superficial nature... I made fabulous journeys at will through distant regions, even out into the galaxy; created incredible architecture; and employed sardonically grinning demons to realize my fantasies." He finally slept until waking surprisingly refreshed and peaceful the following morning.

Harner found that he could remember all of the experience except for "the communication from the dragon-like creatures". Eventually he was able to remember it. He was then seized by a fear that he should not know this material, that it seemed intended only for the dying. His remedy - he quickly told others, including local missionairies - who were startled by the similarities with parts of the Book of Revelations. This came as a surprise to Harner - an atheist.

Harner also sought advice on his "vision" from "the most supernaturally knowledgeable of the indians, a blind shaman who had made many excursions into the spirit world with the aid of the "ayahuasca" drink. The shaman said of Harner's "masters of the earth", *"Oh, they're always saying that. But they are only the Masters of Outer Darkness."*

The most vivid experience of Harner's life, it turns out, one with a coherent story, an internal logic, a felt depth, and a cosmological import, was, according to the most experienced guide to these realms he encountered, the byproduct of a conversation with beings who were lying to him. Put that in your pipe and smoke it.

What happens if there is no blind shaman around to point this out to him? What happens if, rather, Harner is in thrall to alien dragon beings who declare themselves Masters of the Universe, and are in fact demons?

Hey Elon? Hey Peter Thiel? Apocalypse merchants, you. You can't believe everything you think, or everything you are told. *I am the lizard king, I can do any thing.* No, in fact you are not. You are in thrall to Masters of Outer Darkness.

It is of critical importance to be very discerning in which thoughts we listen to. Not all of them, perhaps not that many of them, are true. Thinking, the way most of us do it, provides very tenuous access to truth.

McKenna was an extremely cerebral person. He identified with thinking. Thinking as being... He wouldn't take issue with Descartes' maxim, which I flatly reject. He encounters the plants, and they gift him an amplification of his own propensity for extraordinary hypothetical musings, which was quite keen to begin with. These they color with synesthetic vividness and character with insight. Is there some kernel of truth to them? Perhaps, I do not know. Is it possible that this happened? Certainly. Was our eating of mushrooms out of dung *the* catalytic event in the origin of a 'modern' consciousness? Was he encountering the origin of the species, or simply seeing himself? Each of us, the humans who I've spoken to, in an original encounter with the entheogens, has some version of this moment.

I had a moment like this the first time I smoked marijuana, which isn't even an order of magnitude approaching the psychic crisis that can be induced by a psychedelic. In some moment, you suddenly become conscious of your own mind as a structure, and you find yourself beholding it from some vantage that is not the same as how you ordinarily live within it. Is this the origin of consciousness? A shift in perspective from which you begin to observe the machinations of your own mind?

There is a disruption of the ordinary stream of self, and the dimension of awareness changes. We realize that we are not perceiving reality, we are filtering it through an interface that is mind. We cannot really recognize this until we step out of our ordinary mind. It is difficult to perceive the glasses you are looking through while you are wearing them. Is this the dawning of consciousness in the species? Or in Terrence McKenna? Is it ancestral memory or waking dream? Is it the mushroom that is important? Or is it the crisis it induces that is important?

Terrence McKenna died of brain cancer. My impression is that the brain, which likes to make thoughts and imagery, is not the most useful organ in which to center oneself when interacting with these forces: that the indole alkaloids, which are the chemical carriers in the plants that unlock such realms, are more usefully metabolized with our center of gravity in the heart and the deep belly. And yet that pushes against the western inclination to center the world in the seen (even be it inner seeing) rather than the felt.

Another theory of the origin of consciousness, one less hallucinogenic, yet no less brain-centric or vision-contingent, in its way, comes with Julian Jaynes, whose 1977 book *The Origin of Consciousness in the Breakdown of the Bicameral Mind*, suggests that the ability to introspect, which Jaynes' asserts as the origin of the uniquely human consciousness, is a byproduct of language and culture. He suggests that it arises specifically from metaphor, including metaphors of vision inwardly applied. Jaynes is concerned with introspective real estate: the origin of mind-space.

In both theories there is some catalyzing event that sparks the opening of a new inward horizon. There is a rupture in some plane of consciousness: the sudden arising of a new dimension, a relationship to a novel interior. We – our awareness – is conveyed, is birthed, discovers itself in a new space. We wonder: How did that happen?

And yet both of these theories are concerned with *mental* space. I find it interesting to notice that both of these theories, implicitly, build on the notion that consciousness is cognitive in nature. That its principal attribute has something to do with thinking, or the space in which thinking unfolds. I also find both theories impose a modern worldview invisible to the theorist onto a geography of ancestral consciousness that was in all likelihood unlike what either man was capable of imagining.

I find it unlikely that speciation was driven solely, or even primarily, by proto-hominids tripping balls, even if some of them undoubtedly did that. I find it unlikely that introspection is the advent of interiority.

I find myself wondering, personally, if the origin of consciousness, as it were, is not with introspection, but with *interoception*. Not with mind-space, but with felt-space. And yet, I will also propose to you, that in my own experience the origin of consciousness is a crime scene. I mean this archetypally, as it relates to the origin of consciousness in the species, as well as personally, which is an arena I feel more qualified to comment upon. But, for shits and giggles, let's start with the wide, the vast, the speculative, and then we'll come closer in.

I am a tracker. I have friends who track animals, and I have friends who track history. I track connection, and part of what I'm up to here in these chapters is tracking back into the mists of deep time to notice the source frequencies of kinship, and how we deviated from them, for we've erected edifices of nationhood, law, economy, and knowledge that are categorically deviated from Life. How we've come to be living in a death cult, which is what any sober analysis of our modern living program will tell you it is. I won't pretend to have certainty about any of this. I'm tracking background radiation emanating from behind the origin stories of our culture. What I'm listening with is not cognition at all.

I've spent a fair amount of time feeling into, and reflecting on the event described in the Bible as the Fall. This is not because I'm overtly interested in the Bible. It is because I lived the experience of falling out of harmony with All That Is at seven years old, and I recognized my own life in that story. I could have written the story of the Fall from personal experience—I just wouldn't have blamed it on a snake and a woman. In my case it was a recession, and a grandfather willing to rescue my mother and those attached to her (my father, her sons).

In 1982, when I was seven years old, the US economy entered a recession, my father lost his job, we packed our lives into boxes, and I got into a Ryder truck with him and drove out of the garden of Eden and into my life. I didn't know this is what happened until much later. My experience of the event, for most of my adult life, was that when I was seven years old I drowned. Some part of me—perhaps the best part of me—simply died. I didn't drown in water. My suffocation was being removed from my original context, uprooted, potted in emotional and cultural soil that couldn't nourish me, and being unable to grieve. That was what took away my oxygen. I was stunned by loss, a grief so immense that it froze me to the quick.

I didn't have language for any of this exile at the time. I was seven years old. I did not know how to express this, and no one in my family was able to intercede in a way that touched any part of what had happened. Part of me was dead, and not anyone in my world had the wherewithal to reflect this back to me. No one said, "Good morning Gabriel. I can't help but notice that today you seem to be hauling around some percentage of a corpse, whereas yesterday you were vibrantly alive." That would have been useful to me, I think. To have had someone notice this. Instead, it took me thirty-five years to figure out what happened, and to resuscitate the part of myself that was dead, which turned out not to be dead, only there is some mystery in this, because it was until it wasn't.

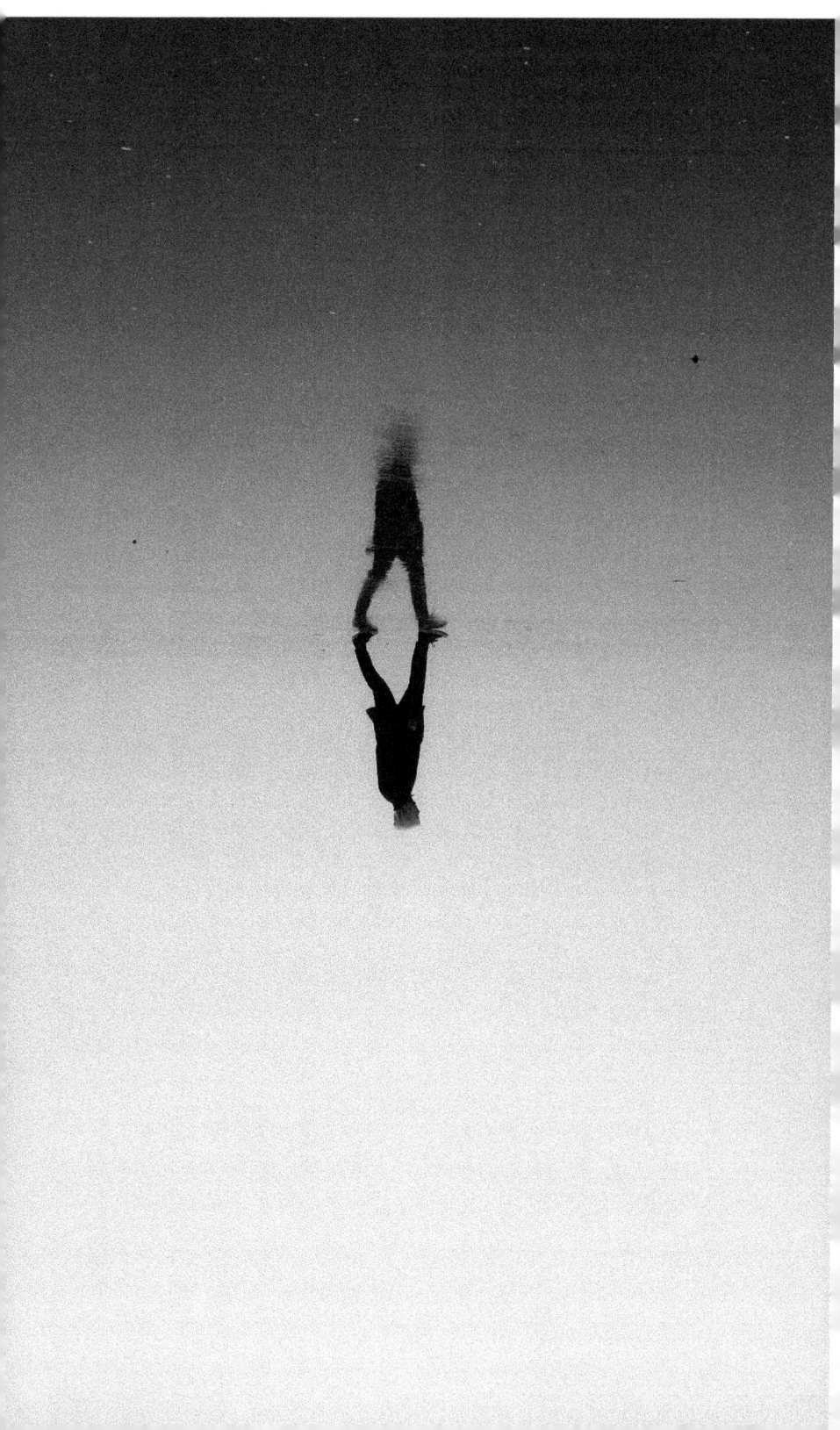

22 - Gate of Union

Neuroception is the moment-to-moment embodied detection of safety, danger, or lifethreat. Think about neuroception through the metaphor of water as a threshold that exists between primary existential states, between the liquid water, steam, and ice versions of ourselves. In water this threshold is temperature, across which elemental state changes. Molecules of liquid turn into gas or freeze into ice.

Different things happen at the boundary between safety and danger, versus danger and lifethreat. As we move from safety and connection into danger responses, our boundaries fortify. In connection there is no enemy; no *Us* versus *Them*. The movement into responding to danger is to create a boundary, an edge, a differentiation. I'm *here*, the threat is *there*. When people are arguing and put up a hand, palm open, as a visible wall between them and the other person this is a physicalization of the boundary-setting.

Yet something different happens to our boundaries in the movement from danger to life threat. Instead of becoming more solid, they dissolve. We refer to this gate as a gate of boundary-dissolution. We become permeable, porous.

Usually, if we are in a state of lifethreat, we crash into this gate under the full influence of rage or terror, and this impact vaults us out of the center of self as the boundary dissolves. It is, in other words, a terrifying dissociative experience. Part of the grace of this boundary dissolution, which is induced by the release of endogenous opioids, is to allow us to not have to be in the body that is being eaten by the saber-toothed tiger, or being beheaded by a Roman Centurion. The boundary of the body becomes porous, and we eject. It is fairly common for victims of sexual assault, for example, to report that they were watching their bodies from outside during a violation. This is not people speaking metaphorically. Self, spirit, identity, point of view– whatever you want to call it– steps out of the body.

Yet there are experiences in meditation, reported with frequency across diverse spiritual lineages, of boundary dissolution *without* displacement. In less formal contexts, the most everyday of these experiences, for many people, happens during sex. We are immobilized, yet without fear. It is called 'making love' because if this happens in a heart-centered way, through this boundary dissolution, we can unite with another. We merge. If this Other is *All That Is*, the universe entire, we are in the realm of spiritual experience. Union.

When we are in that Union, we can't use the word interoception, in its ordinary sense, because if we are connected with Source, there is not a boundary inside of which our feeling is constrained. We simply feel. This feeling harmonizes with the universal breath. The universe herself hums; she inhales, exhales. She expands and contracts. We are empty, in the way that the Zen Masters mean this: not void, not without awareness, but not constrained, not contained, not bounded. Self is pure verb: there is no object, no thing, no noun, no contraction, no boundary, no edge, no container.

In our day-to-day lives, most of us it would seem, cannot reside in such a state, and therefore exist within the sensing confines of a body, if we are not shut down interoceptively in such a way that we cannot feel ourselves from inside. This ability to feel ourselves from inside, this inward listening, as it were, this utilization of our body as a felt interior, as an apparatus of perception, an embodied field of awareness...interoception, in other words...this, I would propose to you *IS* consciousness. Not introspection, but interoception. This bottom-up, embodied, generally though not always co-terminous with the body, present-moment-centered feeling of electric vitality humming through a dimensional space. This *is* consciousness. Ego not required. Ego not even useful.

If this is our operating system, then ego, in the modern sense of identity-is not needed. My favorite definition of ego: a contraction to avoid relationship. (from Franklin Albert Jones, via Arthur Baker.) Ego is, dare I say it, the habit of contracting to shut out a hostile world. Ego is the boundary tightening we engage NOT to be in kinship. A boundary fortification reified through neurological habit and storied through narratives of identification with a particular point-of-view, and particular doings, into identity.

If the operating system we are running is interoceptive-the feeling of what is-and look: here is a magnificent autonomic neural architecture placed to support this, seventy percent afferent, uniting in the heart, upward-flowing, governing the brain- we don't need to be running an ego program. We can reside in the sensing. We can locate identity in the living embodied flux of feeling. The mind can fall silent and we are still here. This is why the Lakhota language has no word for 'I', 'me', or 'mine'.

Thinking, in the sense of cognition, rumination, a river of dialog, self-talk, turns on when we leave this location, or when we are forced out. Thinking turns on when we shift out of connection into defense.

Thinking turns on when we are not able to reside in the embodied feeling. When, in our autonomic analogy of water, liquid water turns to steam.

Thinking is what happens when we get kicked out of the body, when it doesn't feel good in here, when the neuroception shifts from safety to danger.

Slow down and examine your own experience, so that you can reference what I am saying in your own inward knowing. Thinking is a reaction to growing up unsafe. Do you understand the degree to which your experience of who you are is governed by lack of safety?

Most of us have firmly attached our sense of who we are to the inside of the cage we pulled back into because it wasn't safe to open our hearts out into the world. Most of who (and what) most of us hang our identity on is the residue of a habit of contraction forced upon us by exposure to environments-familial, social, cultural-where we cannot be who we actually are because it is not safe. If we cannot be who we actually are, then we do not know who we actually are.

"If we cannot be who we actually are, then we do not know who we actually are."

If we are not safe we pull back like snails, drawn inward. Ego is the sense-making and self-talk of the identity we experience pulled back inside our own defensive perimeter.

That contraction, my friends, is not who you are.

Yet we are in the habit of identifying with this contraction so completely that most of us are entirely identified with it, and if it stops running, even for a moment, we feel totally disoriented.

⊕

At the origin of consciousness: a crime scene. Something happens-some catastrophe. Some inciting incident; something goes horribly awry. There is a rupture. All of our ordinary ways of coping-everything we have learned thus far, are inadequate to respond. We enter a space of liminality where we no longer know the rules, where nothing is fixed, where nothing makes sense. A sort of between-the-worlds.

Mary Watkins and Helene Shulman, in *Toward Psychologies of Liberation*, remind us that Gloria Anzaldúa, in describing this, uses the Nahuatl word: *nepantla*.

Nepantla (nahuatl): the in-between-ness

This up-ending, be it the psychedelic experience of an early hominid ancestor on the plains, following in the wake of the herd, who pops a handful of small mushrooms in her mouth as she is walking, and some halfhour later discovers herself tilting into a novel perceptual landscape, a strange concatenation of sudden sensation, vividness, waves of color, variegated rainbow planes of luminescence undulating off living and elemental beings, the seeming solidity of the world melting down as if in a furnace, something entirely unknown arising, the mind grappling to steady itself...or be it the tear in the fabric of the non-dual, the sudden withdrawal into defense that grants an edge to the body...are related, these phenomena. Crime scenes. Moments when our worlds fall apart. WB Yeats marks the moment thusly:

Turning and turning in the widening gyre

The falcon cannot hear the falconer;

Things fall apart; the centre cannot hold;

Mere anarchy is loosed upon the world[1]

It is necessary. That's what I'm trying to tell you. This is how awareness is born. It's not the crime that is the awareness. The crime is the wound, the inciting incident, that makes it necessary to grow the awareness. Consciousness is the alteration of structure required to stanch the bleeding.

Awareness is not the mushroom. Awareness is the faculty required to not go crazy when the mushroom dissolves the world.

This is important. Because if it is the mushroom, you'll have

---

1 WB Yeats, *The Second Coming*, Collected Poems of WB Yeats

to keep eating the mushroom again and again and again. But if it is the faculty-you can grow the faculty. The faculty you can take with you. It is portable. Grow that faculty and life herself becomes the magical catalyst. You don't have to keep tripping balls to evolve. You just have to learn how to not go crazy when life dissolves your world.

My crime scene, seven years old, the Ryder truck, everything I love receding from view. The garden in the past, exile ahead. This is the inciting incident. This is the cross I will bear, my particular originating wound, what I will grapple with for 35 years, what will set the cardinal direction of my life's quest for meaning. The wound necessitates the awakening. It is initiatory. The traumatic injury is necessary foreground to the post-traumatic growth. The deepest teacher cuts you to the bone.

The crisis sets the banquet table. Yet can we eat it? Metabolize it without going mad? Let it make us mad and then grow a new self large enough to become sane again?

Is it not like this each time we grow into a bigger worldview? A wider field of awareness? I don't know anyone who does this willingly. Who would choose apocalypse? Who would choose to have their meaning-making system collapse? And yet, somehow, isn't it through the world ending that the new world begins?

Birth is a catastrophe with a marvelous outcome. The feotal ejection reflex-what pushes the baby out-is a massive dose of cortisol that creates a crisis we can't think our way out of. Creates a crisis that can only be overcome through utter transformation. A crisis so great that it gives birth not merely to the baby, but to the mother and the father. A crisis that breaks worlds open: one so great that it can only be overcome by love.

Another way of saying all of this: the crime scene is cortisol.

Is danger, is threat, is stress, is trauma. Who we are becoming is on the other side of that. Who we are becoming is the kind of love we have to grow to knit ourselves a broader version of ourselves; one large enough to include the wound from that crime scene. A version of Self broad enough to include the collapse, the breakdown, the apocalypse.

There are two verb-based flows here: a deathing and a birthing. Things fall apart, we have to overcome them in order to put ourselves back together.

This is initiatory terrain.

Transformation always holds the very real possibility of madness and death. If you are going to transform your mind, you could lose it. Psycho-pathology is, in part, those who have been incompletely or improperly initiated. Crime with no ensuing rebirth.

This is why the sages say—*don't resist the river.* The river is bigger than you are, it is stronger than you are. We are not in control. It is also why the sages say: *don't get your psychedelics in the mail.* It's not the mushroom. It's the faculty required to not go crazy. And when the stakes are that high—do you really want to go that alone? Or would it not be wiser to have an experienced community of support?

Is it possible to open to the inward apocalypse? It's a tall order, but if we recognize that the crime scene is the doorway?

And yet, study it we must. This particular wound that happens to each of us. What are its specific signatures. By what doorway did the apocalypse enter? What is its essence? What is the inciting incident? We must study it so keenly that we develop a new faculty of awareness: *the* faculty.

Anzaldúa again: *La faculdad: the ability to receive the depth of the world and soulfulness by breaking through habitual modes of relating to reality and perceiving consciousness.* La faculdad does not reside in reason but in the body. It is born not out of choice but out of the necessity to survive.

Can you knit a broader version of yourself large enough to include all the catastrophe without shutting down? Because western civilization, the death cult that has birthed this polycrisis? It was not able to do this.

The entire thing has gotten stuck on the threshold, like Christ on the cross. A crucifixion, a stillbirth, and here you have the world we have inherited, in all its agony. Frozen from the inside out, pinned though still alive like an insect to green felt. The body frozen, the greater part of us exiled, floating, detached, waiting for the proper ceremony to re-enter into the body which was, at one time, our home.

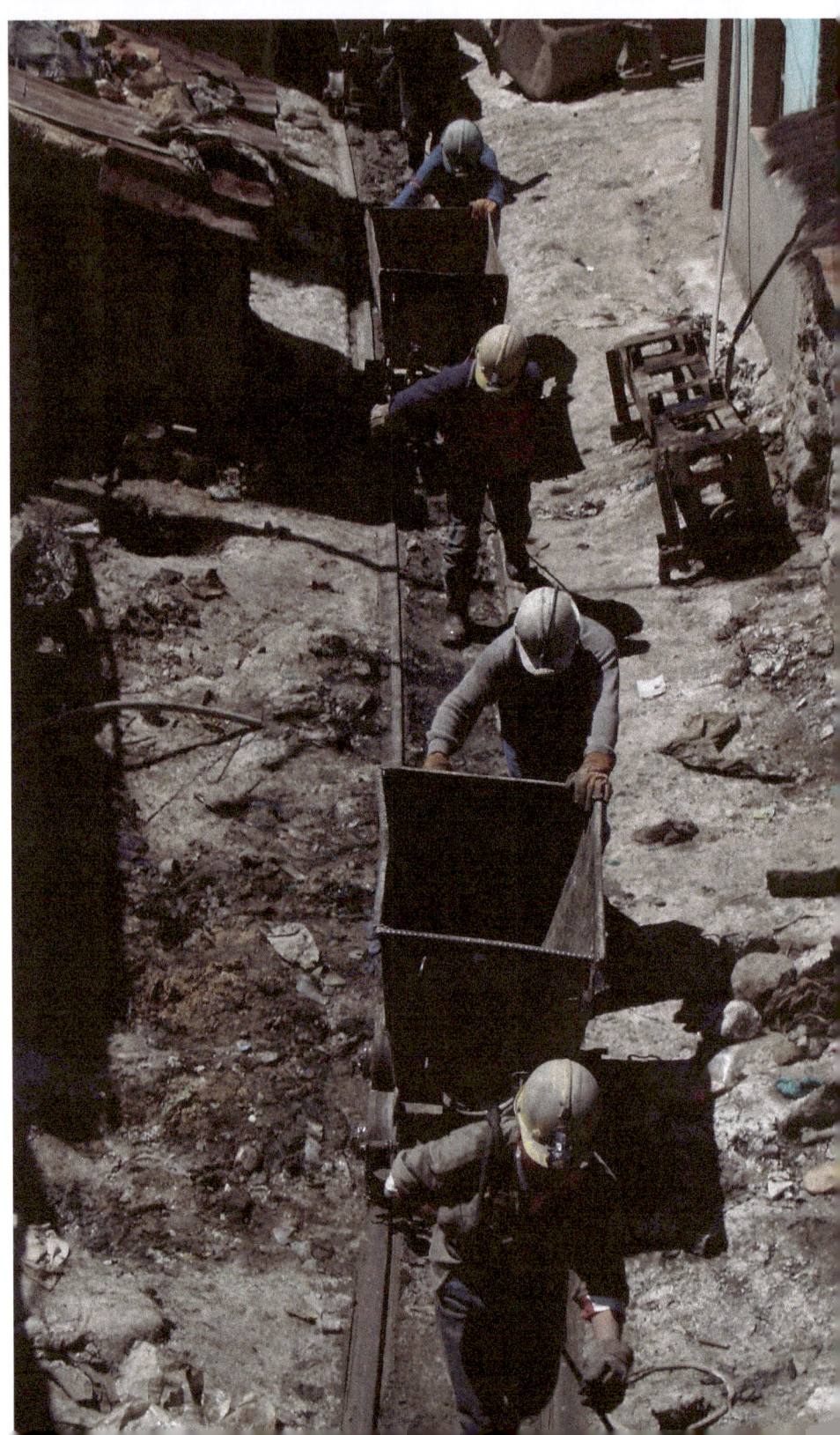

23 - Toiling in a Mine

For two thousand years, since Rome, everything has been oriented toward extraction. Domination, extraction, and enclosure, these have seeped into our thoughforms, poisoned deeply the well of language, the form of desire, the shape of our yearnings. We have become cloaked in the forms of death.

It begins with alienation, expulsion from the garden, fear, a sense of scarcity. The strip mine is the allegory for the age. A rape of the surface of the living earth, the female body– an act that can only be performed with impunity once we pull the roots of the Sacred out of the earth, which happens when Rome, in feverish annihilatory glee, kills off not only the chthonic (earth-based, earth-worshipping, Indigenous) people of the region, but dismembers their gods. A bloodlust to disembowel the Sacred. It is hard to comprehend the level of death worship here, unless we understand how drunk they were.

There are two philosophies of war, rising arightly from what our mentor Pete Jackson identifies as their root in worldview. One set of cultures, that believes itself to exist within Nature, uses war as a means to clarify boundaries, resolve conflicts, but there are rules for war and responsibilities, as prioritization is still of Life. Blood is not spilled wantonly.

That, as you may imagine, is not the lineage we come from. We (by which I mean the modern now globalized west) come from the lineage of annihilation. The lineage that declares that if even a single member of the enemy is left alive there are seeds of rebellion, which is perhaps not untrue. You crush rebellion, in this lineage of war, through genocide. You kill them all, down to the children. If the women are beautiful enough perhaps you secret them away as concubines, but this is not discussed, as it violates the dictum. This is the lineage that believes itself to be above nature, to have 'dominion over all the creatures of the earth.' (Genesis 1:26-28)

These are our grandparents, you and I. Ye who like me receive the unearned benefit of white skin privilege in this supremacy engine of a cult(ure). Remember though–white is not the color of your skin, but the mask that removes you from your indigenous self.

A trick of language, the association of heaven and sky, earth and hell. It seeped into the water in vessels made of lead, through drunken debauchery, moral corruption. Consolidation of power over, until those yielding authority were so far removed from the soil that their feet did not touch the earth, and they looked down on everything. The taproot of Supremacy is what I'm speaking about here.

One of the mechanisms of supremacy transmission is the adoption of Nicene Christianity as the official religion of Rome. From this christianity was expunged the earthly facet of Christ's teaching. Expunged were the angels of air, earth, and water: the elementals. Expunged was the great Mother herself. The prayer Our Father is inescapable. But did you know there was another prayer? A prayer to our Mother, which art the Earth? It was excised from the liturgy thousands of years ago.

Our attention in the polarity was shifted from dichotomies of benificence: the heavenly father and the earthly mother, to a polarity of antagonism: the heavenly father and the devil. How did that happen?

The answer, I would propose to you, once again, is very simple. When your connection system is online, you experience unity. There is no need for an enemy. It is all US in here, there is no THEM. Shift across the boundary line into defense, and suddenly the physiology is polarized. We require – it is a physiological necessity – to have someone to defend ourselves against. An enemy. THE enemy.

Here is a ground zero of psychic colonization. The space designed to hold the original polarity, that of the feminine and masculine, the earth and the sky, has been corrupted, denatured. Instead of the yin-yang, instead of the balance, there resides, in its place, antagonism.

I want you to stop and dwell here, studying this original wound. Studying this psychic massacre: this origin site of your own alienation. I want you to behold it inwardly and weep. Look at what has been done to us in the name of religion.

And as you study it, I want you to understand that it is a sort of structural fulcrum. That it is a force-bearing structure in the organization of your mind, this original wound.

It is also a palimpsest, written over and over with death story. A massacre site at the origin of western consciousness. I want you to feel the echoes pulsing within and beneath and around it.

This story is where the West begins: it is the ejection site from relationship with *All that Is*, when the civilization itself becomes unmoored from the physiology of connection. This is the story of Adam and Eve being expelled from the garden. Can you see it, how this is the same place in consciousness?

All the symbols are here. At the place where the good earth meets the sky there is a garden, and in that garden lived the original humans, speaking the original language. Until one day occurred an event. This is the moment after which the people's thoughts no longer dwell between heaven and earth.

Consider this. It is not that evil did not exist before this. That is not what the story says. This story is the replacement of one pole- the feminine, earth-based pole of consciousness- with evil.

It is the internalization of evil. What is the physiology of this? Defense. This is the moment in the western psyche where we leave a baseline in connection and relatedness, and retract into defense. With this retraction comes polarization.

Evil is internalized, and there is a *them* out there. We have moved from unity consciousness into Us versus Them.

The modern conception of evil, of a devil antagonistic to the skygod, is the reflection of a physiological shift from a baseline in safety and connection to a baseline in defense.

Lifeways do not say that evil does not exist. Jesus, himself, did not say that evil does not exist. But the Indigenous view doesn't dwell on evil. It is not fascinated by it. Neither was Jesus. He simply called it *unripeness*. They acknowledged and moved on. Neither clung to lurid depictions of it, summoning it for threat and condemnation. Neither of them organized a society baselined in physiological defense.

⊕

The story of Adam and Eve, in its particular contours, speaking of the first man, the first woman, a tree and a snake, is loaded with the potent elemental symbology of origins. But make no mistake: it is a death story. It tells of the death of relatedness with the Source. It is doctrinal in the death cult of modernity, a keystone bearing the weight of caternary arches, entire structures that configure reality.

We have a quadrumvirate of keystones in the ceiling of this death cathedral, which is properly an ossuary, a boneyard.

The taproot of supremacy, the transmogrification of the mother into the devil, then of darkness into evil, and the subsequent impulse to enclosure.

Look at the ceiling of the death structure thus assembled. It is made of bones. An architecture of death upholding the modern view. If the story of Adam and Eve is not true–and it is not true– you will need to rebuild the deep scaffolding of your awareness, because the shape of a world is architected by it, and it is the world we have inherited. The keystones holding up the caternary arches in the ceiling of this death cathedral? It is no temple at all. It is a mass grave in a mine. A mausoleum.

⊕

Despite all our apparent success, our 'elevated standard of living', all the attributes of convenience: our automobiles, endless purchasing power, access to exotic foodstuffs, can you not see the aching emptiness at the heart of things?

The origin story seeks to answer this question: why we toil in a mine and do not live in peace in a garden. At some time before, some time ancestral, wrapped in the mists of memory, we lived in a garden, the original garden. And we spoke a language, the original language. But now we find ourselves toiling in a mine. What is the mine?

The mine is the world after we have shifted into the fortress of defense. The fortress of defense is a contraction to avoid relationship. It is the pulling inward, a retraction. Causality is difficult to parse here, at the origin of the death cult. So many things have happened, an avalanche of consequence, and the techtonic plates have shifted. Millenia later, in the language of neurophysiology we will have a map to explain this. A map with the potency to unveil this transformation for what it is. We will be able to speak of the neuroception of danger, and the way that this creates boundary-fortification (the fortress of the ego, an US versus THEM), and then the neuroception of lifethreat, which creates boundary dissolution (the gateway to psychosis).

These sequential gates are the doorways that lead us first from the garden into purgatory, and then from purgatory into hell.

The mine is purgatory. In purgatory, we toil, the heartrate elevates, and there is the ever-present threat of danger. Of intrusion, invasion. Like Adam and Eve we are cast out of the garden. "By the sweat of your brow you will eat your food until you return to the ground, since from it you were taken; for dust you are and to dust you will return." (Genesis 3:19) At the perimeter of camp, darkness. Something lurking on the horizon. The dream landscape of danger. The blanket too short to cover our feet. This is where you wake up in the morning, fellow modern.

The purgatory of alienation is the mine we toil in.

24 - Archeology of Shadows

I write this for you, who are reading it, and I also write this for me, as an act of witness and an act of unwinding. I am writing it because finding this story, voicing it, is to bring up out of my body and into the light all of this stuff that my body knows, in joint and bone and muscle and sinew and memory, but that has not made its way up into words. It is to address lineage, and its occupation uninvited of the body. The act itself is an archeology of shadows, acts and histories that inhabit the margins.

It is my present self, my future self, descending, throwing a rope down to my child self, going back to retrieve him. It is Indiana Jones lowering himself, by rope, into the cavern filled with the living map of the ancient city, which it will shortly turn out is guarded by venomous snakes. It is act of self-love: a resuscitation.

Because what is down here, packed away in shutdown, the autonomic systems of lifethreat, are all things stuffed down that I knew and could not know, all the things we collectively know and yet cannot know. That our bodies know, and that our minds refuse to know. Things buried in the cellar.

There are bodies under the floorboards. Ancient dark things. Curses. Lamentations. The gnashing of teeth. It is not hell, do not be confused, but merely what we have endured. Things from which we have been taught to avert our gaze, things that are not discussed in polite company, things nice people do not talk about.

There are family secrets. Things no one wants to remember. Tragedies and crimes. Shameful things. Icky things. Yuck. Mess. Yet in order to clean the house out, and our psyche is a house, fool yourself not, we have to travel down here into the basement, the subterranean realms. We have to descend the stairs, find the source of that rattling. Find the precise nature of the haunting of the house. Find what we know that we don't know we know and claim it as our own. Bring it up into the living room, likely reeking of death, and scour it with clarity, until it becomes the bones of ancestors we can venerate. Until the ancestors line up behind us to open the way forward.

We cannot go forward without going back. We cannot ascend without descending. We should be aware of this, because we have been lied to about it.

And we should know, should be adequately forewarned, that the house is haunted, and that also it is not just our psyche, this house– because though we violently wish it to be so, have spent the last several hundred years in a fever dream of individuation– we are not islands, not isolated beings, not merely archipelagos, but the ocean floor through which they are linked. The place where the wave meets the ocean is us too. Not individual fingers only, but the hand they are connected to as well.

The house, this psyche, in its basement, connects all the way back and all the way down. To origins of life on earth. The first cell. Respiration. The vertebrate body plan. The origin of mammals. Seven million years back to bipedal ancestry descending from the trees. Seventy thousand years back to diasporas from Mother Africa. Seven thousand years back to the dawn of the agrarian. Seven hundred years back to the Middle Ages. They were not so long ago, in the span of our evolutionary history, these happenings we claim as ancestral.

We are witch burnings. We have been incinerated in ovens. Died many ghastly deaths. We know, in our bones, starvation. We have ordered people hanged. We have enslaved one another, buried one another alive. We have been shipwrecked off the coast, at some point, all of us. Someone has been raped. We have died making the crossing from there to here. There is incest, spoken or unspoken. Unspeakable crimes have been committed, unnatural and barbarous acts. Even if we have no immediate bodily experience of these things they are here.

Homo sum, humani nihil a me alienum puto, says Publius Terentius Afer, the African Roman poet, twenty-two hundred years ago. *I am human: nothing human is alien to me.*

In the basement are the desecrated bones of our ancestors, awaiting, sometimes impatiently, a proper burial.

Progress is another word for domination. An explanation for turning away from the look back, the look down, the look within. The seduction of Artificial Intelligence that will write all our essays for us, never-ending robot sex that asks nothing in return, autonomous driving to chauffeur us around the windswept city and visions of extra-planetary life on Mars.

Progress is another word for domination. We don't want to slow down, look down, descend. And yet, if we do not, we clammor into the jaws of death. For we have forgotten that, like it or not, often the origin of consciousness is a crime scene. And it is therefore a crime that has already happened. A crime that is in the past. Often the opening, the way forward, particularly in this demented era, requires a descent.

And so, an archeology of shadows for people seeking to unearth the demons, put the ghosts to rest, and properly bury the dead. Let us lower the ropes.

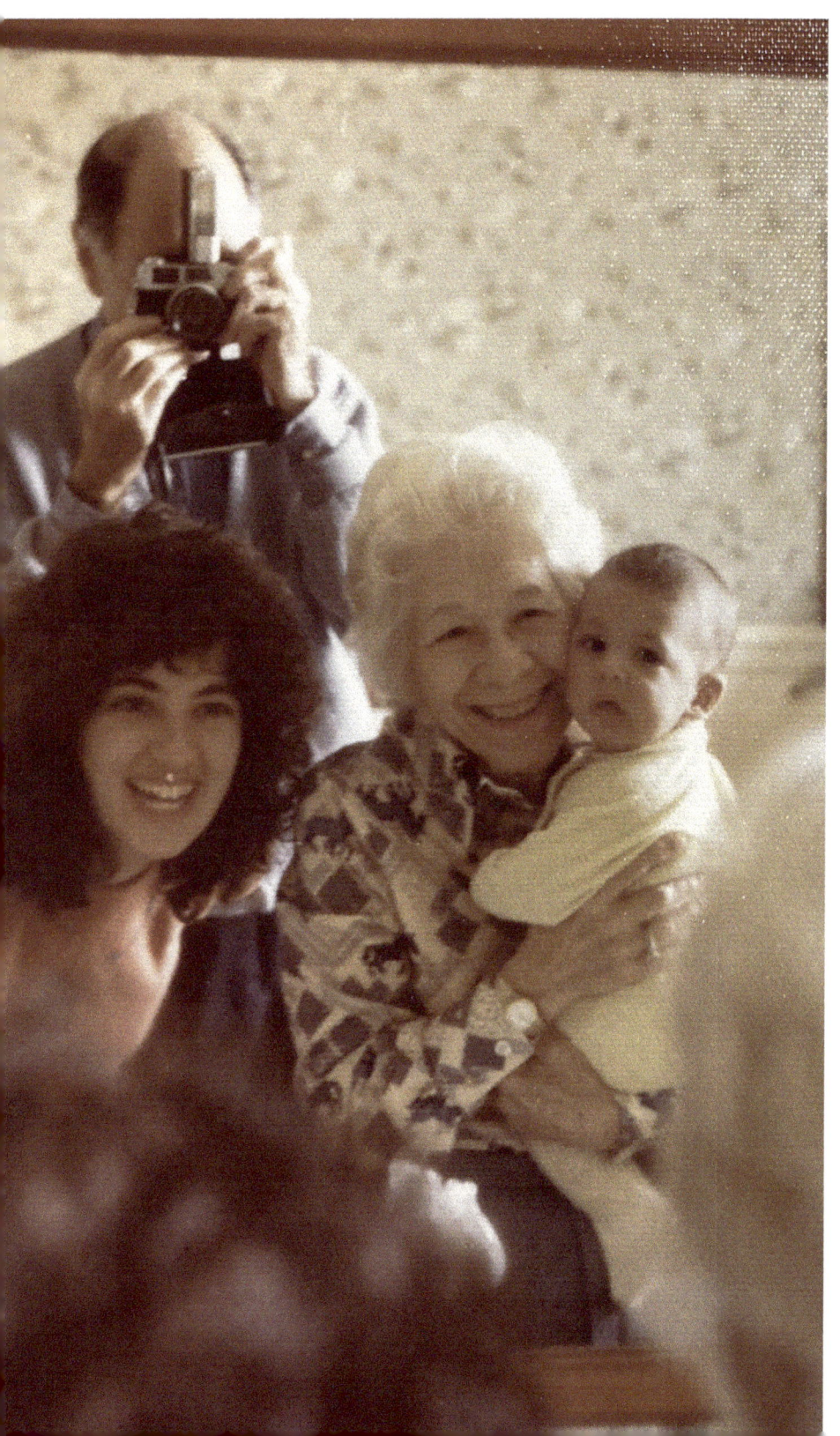

25 - Descent

The last time someone in the direct lineage of my family (e.g., parents, grandparents, great-grandparents) earned enough money to flourish was in 1969, six years before I was born. This was the year that my maternal great-grandfather took the company he had started in 1919, named at its inception the International Oil Heating Company, public as *Intertherm*. He had founded the company with two other people in 1919, and for 53 years he ran and grew it. They were in the business of building heating and cooling systems for manufactured homes. In the later years of the company his business ventures took him around the world, as far away as Japan.

In the home they lived in for over fifty years in suburban St. Louis was a formal entry with a slate floor, a case with tiny wooden dolls dressed in silk geisha outfits he had brought back from a visit to Tokyo, the fabric of which I can still vividly recall, rough and slippery at the same time, as we have nothing like it here. Nearby, a photograph of Mount Fuji. The ethos of the room both serene and severe, the stone floor making it feel nearly monastic, and the way it smelled would instantly remind me of them even today if I stood in their foyer. Their backyard was filled with antique roses. It is possible I have not thought of them for decades.

My great grandfather passed when I was a baby. I have a photograph of his wife, my great grandmother, holding me, as an infant, in front of a mirror with my mother. My great grandfather is farther back, his face obscured by the camera. I was less than six months old, alert, and a bit startled by him and the whole commotion it appears. I was old enough to hold myself upright, in that endearingly shaky way of babies at that age, but not old enough yet to walk. I'm wearing some kind of a onesie. My great grandmother is absolutely beaming, vibrant at nearly 80 years old as she holds my face to hers. My mother, her granddaughter, who was 26 at the time, is in the frame left. She is about half the age I am now. Behind them both is my grandfather, taking the picture. The photograph is reversed because it is shot into a mirror, an everyday familial moment transformed into art.

He was a very charismatic person, one of 13 children, generally considered a *mensch*. Fairly early in a successful career he bought farmland on a river in rural Missouri, about 90 minutes from the city, around which our extended family organized their summers for the next several generations. We called it *the river*, and everyone congregated there for half a century. When the company went public he added several hundred more acres to this landholding.

I never really thought about the reason that the primary dwelling at the river was a mobile home, at least when I entered the picture, but it is because they were in the business of designing heating and cooling systems for them. By the time I came around, this double-wide was so well-used that the linoleum floors bore familiar discolored divots in all the hallways, the indented curves of so many barefoot children and their parents who had walked and raced and crawled up and down them for generations. It was sprawling and dilapidated and cozy and filled with natural and cultural artifacts of various sorts: remnants of a hornet's nest that had come down in a winter storm, arrowheads unearthed from tilled fields nearby, raptor feathers. Several generations of us developed a strong enough bond with the Living World here that it would permanently shape the course of our lives.

In 1969, when the company went public, my great-grandfather passed its leadership to his son, my maternal grandfather. Although the title of CEO suited him, he did not have his father's leadership abilities or business wherewithal, and the decision was reached, during his tenure, to sell the company. My grandfather, who was yet young, retired wealthy.

It has been difficult, in my family, to get a straight answer about some of the economic trajectories here. When I was little I had the impression my grandparents were quite affluent, an aura that they did not wish to dissipate. This wealth was combined with a certain profound restraint that was never talked about directly, but rather translated into an implied expression of morality. They *could* have lived in a more palatial residence, but chose not to. They *could* have driven more ostentatious motorcars, but chose not to. Yet their home filled up during my adolescence with increasingly famous art, their gardens became botanical-grade and began to be photographed for magazines. My grandmother wore expensive jewelry and somewhat shapeless modernist garments that flowed and draped, and liked to take us to the St. Louis Fine Art Museum and then luncheon there. Sometimes they would take my family out to a restaurant in St. Louis, on special occasions, that was fancy enough men were not permitted to enter without a dinner jacket (they had spares on hand for boys), and the waiters all wore tuxedos. The menu was *prix fixé*, the food French, and what I remember most vividly was that if you took particular fancy to a course, they would bring you a second version of it, half-sized, and possibly even a third if you made it known that the dish was most extraordinary, and might it be possible on just this occasion to indulge just one more time? In this manner I recall feasting greatly on lobster baked into some kind of savory pastry at around the age of twelve. Absolutely delicious.

In most of the restaurants my grandfather frequented, at some point during the meal the chef would dutifully emerge and stand table-side, chatting with him. This was something of an event at the French restaurant because the chef wore a toque, and his movements through the dining room were not unremarked by patrons. The entire time I knew him, and especially when there was a large group gathered, as often happened on holidays, there was a moment when the check came, and he proffered a steady hand to the waiter for it, eyeing the other men in the group in what I came to understand later was an emasculation ritual. On one occasion a new uncle who had married into the family and was in actuality self-made took the hint and then the check and paid it himself in a buoyantly casual manner, but was I believe later roundly scolded in private for this come-uppance, and did not do it again. It didn't occur to me until much later in life that the reason I found myself staring at the check, as a small child-like, *who gives a shit about that when they are ten?*– was that my grandfather was conducting the entire attention of the table to his paternal beneficence.

My grandfather gave off the distinct impression of being a self-made man, a man with opinions formed in the furnace of action, prone to leaning back in his chair at dinner and holding forth about what rate of interest an investment should yield, what wines were worth drinking, Ralph Nader's work on consumer protection, the politics of the day, gun control, history-at-large, war, science, and God. My grandmother, who was the child of alcoholics, beautiful and remote, would parrot select bits of his pontification back to us, with him sitting there, like a faintly other-worldly transcription machine. Yet all of this command stance, this 'views forged as a man of the world' persona, was something of a facade. His father seems to have been the one who was successful: a man of the world. My grandfather simply inherited the windfall.

For purposes of simplicity, we'll call him the second generation of wealth. Not that he didn't make his own money, for he did. Later in life he became an expert witness, a consultant, and I am told he was quite good at it. Rather what I am saying is that the lifestyle my grandparents had was not one they could have afforded without inherited money. The Trova sculptures and Chihuly glass? Jewelry from Björn Weckström, the Finnish jewelry designer who made the necklace Princess Leia wore in Star Wars, purchased at the apex of his fame from his studio in Helsinki? The endless renovations and garden updates? The trips and travels and the gifting? The foundation of their wealth was not self-created, but a generational inheritance.

Looking back at your childhood with adult awareness is often complicating, because as a kid you just receive the world as it is. You feel things, and you make your best sense of what is going on, and you tend to, at least to a point, absorb the received narratives about why things are the way they are and just keep moving. Like many families, my family had a wealthy side (my mother's parents) and a not-wealthy side (my father's mother) and being downwind of money is more fun than being downwind of its lack.

I didn't overly dwell on my family's economic situation, except when my parent's stress about money boiled over. I never feared we would lose our house or not have enough to eat. The way I remember this tension primarily was that as a child, when we were out to dinner and my grandfather wasn't with us, which was infrequently, I would always look at a menu, find things that were priced in the lower middle-tier, and order those. I would have been mortified to order something that was the most expensive item on the menu, or to not know how much something on the menu cost. I looked at restaurant menus the way a stockbroker reads price-to-earnings ratios, pouring over them for the value stocks. The prohibition around ordering something expensive was so severe it didn't make my heart race, but was rather in the form of an immobilization. I literally could not have made my body do it. I would have experienced it as a direct betrayal of my father. I could not have spoken the words. As I contemplate it now, a residual artifact, I marvel at the severity of the internalized inhibition.

Not long ago, sitting with an older friend of mine at dinner, we were trading joking recollections of childhood. He said something along the lines of not remembering exactly what his father's face looked like at that time, except for the nose, but remembering his father's wallet perfectly, because what his father did all the time when they were together was take it out and pay for everything. I grew quiet and a sort of sedation came over my body at a cellular level: opioidal. I cannot easily recall a time in the whole of my growing up when my father took out his wallet to pay for something for someone other than himself. Maybe nachos at a Cardinal's game in Busch Stadium. I can however remember his wallet; a small bifold made out of brown eelskin, and that he carried a pale green American Express card.

If we went out to dinner with my grandparents I had to endure pontification, but at least I could order whatever I wanted. No one paid any attention to it at all. There were no ice-cold inhibitions on behavior freezing the table. No actions that might, undertaken, turn you to stone. At the time it seemed a worthwhile trade.

The thing that became pretty obvious, pretty fast in my nuclear family, when I started paying attention to these things, which was non-accidentally when we moved to St. Louis from the tiny town in New Hampshire where I was happy, and until this day, cannot remember ever having thought about, or even having seen money (can that be?) – was that my father was not having much success as a breadwinner, and so our family income was being supplemented, on the regular, by my mother's father. This was fraught for my father: a primary tension in their marriage.

In addition to monetary gifts, which we received each year up to the federal limits for a good part of my growing up, and were anticipated and relied upon and not supposed to be discussed, there was a regular procession of cars that we inherited. My grandparents would drive them for three years, and then pass them to us like clockwork, except for the odd interval when for purposes of filial fairness it seemed necessary to pass one of them to one of the other daughter's families. This was the basic cadence.

My grandparents helped my parents buy their house. They

helped my father start his chiropractic business, investing significantly in an enterprise that would start with a bang, and then shrink gradually over the years until it vanished and he changed careers. They also paid the tuition at the private school I attended in 7th through 12th grades, all six years.

It is not until this morning that it occurred to me to tabulate this. They helped buy my parent's house, which would have reduced the mortgage. Neither did my parents have car notes, since those were usually gifts. My sense is that they were receiving about 20K a year in gifts, and my tuition was paid from 1987 to 1993 when I graduated highschool. My great-grandparents had set up an educational trust, so my parents didn't pay college tuition when I first enrolled. When I dropped out of Yale, and later returned to Stanford I was no longer their dependent, and got a full scholarship. Those are a number of significant line item expenses. Many hundreds of thousands of dollars over the course of my childhood. I can tell you that if, in my own life, someone else was paying our cars, education expenses for my daughter, and kicking in 20K a year on top of that, my wife and I would be in a different position financially.

Yet my parents still struggled, to the extent that my mother went back to work full-time when I was about 12, and became first an art teacher, and eventually the Chair of the Art department in a private highschool, probably around the time I graduated. It was the first time in my life where they had seemed financially stable, possibly on the verge of prosperity. This gave my father a bit of a swagger: I remember this moment as a brief season of abundance, an indian summer in that season of their marriage.

That was the third generation of wealth. By that point my father's daily routine deposited him in a coffee shop with a buddhist or spiritual book from about 10 am to 1 pm each workday. Several years later, before they separated, he announced, *a propos* of nothing that I could discern, that he was retiring. My initial response, which I had enough sense not to speak out loud, was that someone had to be working in order to retire.

This was a fairly confusing milieu to grow up in, in the sense that my parents talked to me about the dangers of inherited wealth, how the third generation often blew it, things like this, while I looked around at our lives, the progression of used cars, our house as compared to the houses of other kids at the private school I attended due to my grandparent's largess- which was replete with students who were, in fact, affluent- the fact that we never took vacations as compared to the fact that about half the rest of my class decamped to Sanibel Island in Florida for spring break, and tried to figure out exactly what the fuck they were talking about.

My mother sent me books with titles like, *The Inheritor's Handbook*, and clipped and mailed to me articles from magazines with titles like, *The Three-Generation Curse of Wealth: Why Riches Don't Last*, which concludes with this bit of sage advice:

The three generation rule is a concept that explains why wealth tends to dissipate after three generations. The first generation, the builder, accumulates wealth through hard work and determination. The second generation, the maintainer, preserves the wealth created by the builder. However, the third generation, the squanderer, often wastes the wealth created by the previous generations. This cycle of wealth can be broken through financial education, philanthropy, investing in education, instilling strong family values and work ethic, and proper estate planning.

The thing I found strangest about all of this was that my mother didn't ever seem to realize that *she*, not I, was the third generation.

26 - Localized Shutdown

For the first decade that I studied autonomic physiology, I thought of the deep belly shutdown state as a full-body phenomenon. Only later, and in working with a series of skilled manual therapists, did I begin to understand the degree to which these response could be highly localized in the body. The way shutdown could reside in a joint, say. The knees. A hip. Some kind of localized deep-freeze. A pocket of numbness, or total immobility, the size of a coin, or the size of a baseball, where a parent's locked gaze had turned you to stone. A region devoid of feeling, sensation, warmth. Either totally slack (the muscles have zero tone; simply do not work) or totally rigid (completely locked with tension). Localized winter in the body. A sudden tundra.

As I write this I remember something from my childhood that is instructive, and that I had forgotten. This inhibition I felt, at the dinner table, this religiosity about not ordering anything expensive...I inquire in myself, where did that come from? How did I know that this was a redline I was not to cross? And why didn't I test it?

I search, in recollection, for a look my father would have given me, something that would have frozen me to the quick, and yet at first I cannot find it. Some severity which which he would have regarded me, and find it is not there. And then, quietly, I remember, first vaguely, hazily, something else. Something more disturbing. For it was not rage, not something hot, that I remember seeing in him. It was, rather, terror.

By this point, probably age ten, I had caught a glimpse of my father's terror. I had seen it gathering at the edges, like an enemy army encamped, massing vaguely and darkly on the horizon, indistinct. My father at this time wouldn't have turned to me stone-eyed or ferocious. That fever of anger had already burned out, more or less, in him by the time we returned to St. Louis. Had I ordered something at the expensive end of the menu, had I crossed that line, I would have, rather, conjured the animal terror in him. Caused him, possibly, to become entranced by it. Or at least I believed I might. He was already, by that point, in a precarious place. And that, as a ten year old boy, is not something you want to see in your dad, not something you want any part in inviting in.

My taunting adolescent self, the self that wanted to fight him, wanted to call the bluff, was years in the future. At ten years old, you need the small boat of your family intact. You don't want to play any part in tipping it over. You collaborate with its idiosyncracies, and wear them with pride. You know the unspoken rules of the tribe: what you can and cannot do, say, think.

I began writing this chapter having discovered, during a recent transit through studying lifethreat, a cyclic inquiry into the autonomics of the deepest defensive response of mammals, the localization of another profound pocket of shutdown in my body, this one related very specifically to a shutdown around money, related to the stories I have narrated above, the verbalization of which sets my body ashiver if I am truthful.

I think of our story about money- what it means to us, how we perceive it, whether we think there is enough of it or not, what we'll do to earn it, what it is- as being complexly socially constructed. We are acculturated to view money in a particular way, and this acculturation process is sociological. It is familial, experienced intimately in the sweaty grip of a nuclear family for most of us, in private interactions- *please don't order anything on the menu that is too expensive: it makes your fa-*

ther worry – some of which are then internalized. In the proximity of the challenging constraints– does anyone else at school know this sweater is a hand-me-down – or possibly unearned privileges (most 16 year olds with cars, or for that matter middle schoolers with iPhones, didn't purchase them with money they earned) it affords us daily. In relation to our extended families, where we might see our nuclear family's understanding of money confirmed (your uncle is a chip off the old block) or challenged (so-and-so's family is terrible with money).

And then we watch movies. I remember being deeply affected, at ten years old, by watching *The Karate Kid*. I look just enough like Ralph Macchio to have felt like I was watching a slightly older version of myself, and the story begins with displacement from where he grew up on the East Coast to California, a journey west I would later imitate, though not for the same reasons.

In the story Macchio's character is poor, not truly destitute but merely humble, surrounded by rich kids (again, I knew that story, or at least its relative emotional texture), and he gets trained by a mystic archetype, an old Japanese man who catches a fly with chopsticks and makes him wash a car until he can affirmatively kick ass with waxing motions.

We are in the terrain here of mythic archetypes, of the heroes journey, though I wouldn't know this for decades to come. This movie, I remember at the time, got inside of me, and started working on my psyche, something potent. It seemed to propose an escape route.

Something like: *If you can find a Japanese mystic to teaching you essential mystical arts, you're gonna be able to get away from your parents, buy a vintage car, kick a rich guy's ass, and get the girl.* In some strange way, that sequence *is* one of the stories of my life. Hero's journey implanted at ten years old, courtesy of Mr. Miyagi: *Man who catch fly with chopstick accomplish anything.*

Money is pervasive in modern culture, and so we are getting trained in what to think about it all the time. From cinema, to Instagram feeds, there is a cultural story about money that we have to navigate. We are surrounded by wealth porn. What I'm saying is that the terrain is complexly culturally constructed.

Yet this meaning-making about money– what it meant to me growing up, what it means now– lives in the body through the autonomic texture of what it felt like throughout our lives to be engaging with money. And what we receive, at this sensate level from the milieu in which we grow up. For me, both in my nuclear family, where my grandparents and parents both lived lifestyles that were based on inherited wealth that they did not earn, the felt experience of this was that economically my feet were never touching the ground.

Feet not touching the ground is a pretty specific image, if simply because this is something that happens with very young children. Your feet don't touch the ground when you are lying on the changing table, when you are being held by your mother, when you are sitting in a highchair.

And economically, feet not touching the ground is to be held away from the economic reality by someone else's money insulating you from the necessity to survive. I grew up in a closed economic system, with people whose feet had not been on the ground financially for generations. I grew up with people whose lobster dinners were paid for by the work of deceased entrepreneurs from previous generations. People buffered, by inherited wealth, from the realities of the economic present. People who could fail without economic consequence: feel poorly about themselves without going hungry or getting a job.

27 - Fishmonger

My father was the oldest of three children born to a fishmonger and his wife. Fishmonger is a word with antique overtones that bore no resemblance to the daily reality of the business he found himself in, my paternal grandfather, a business he hated, that by the time I met him, which was for a short duration, because he died when I was quite young, left him reeking of fish at night, grossly obese, tipped back in an easy chair eating a cavernous, and ultimately cadaverous, bowl of ice cream in front of the television.

Tell your Grandpa Bill goodnight. I could count the times I have thought about him in my life on two hands. I feel like I should end the previous sentence by saying, *I am embarrassed to say.* I could count the times I have thought about him in my life on two hands, I am embarrassed to say. But I am not. Embarrassed. I am not embarrassed to say.

I don't care.

The reason that I don't care is because even when I knew him, which was briefly, he was so long gone into defeat, so deeply collapsed inwardly into his own self-pitying woeful self-destruction, that he had no ability to connect with me at all. Not that he might not have attempted to, not that he might not have tried, though if he did I have no recollection of it whatsoever. By the time I knew him he was long gone, vacant. The only memories I have of him, and there is more than one, is of my kissing him goodnight, in the living room, with him tipped back and a bowl of ice cream, which was, I believe, laced with suicidal intent.

I remember how he smelled: fishy. I remember the flaccid stubble of his clammy cheek. I cannot actually remember him saying a single word. It was my grandmother telling me what to do. I cannot remember him getting up. I know that the reason he smelled like that was because he had been at the fish store, Kram Fish, but I never saw him get up from that chair that I can remember. That's where I leave him, with the vertically slatted blinds of the sliding glass door to their tiny concrete patio, the lights low, the television on, its blue-tinged shadows crawling the walls, licking up and down his face.

And so I don't care, because caring is predicated on connection, and we did not have connection between us, no vital spark, no mutual recognition. By the time I knew him he was a grossly fat old man eating ice cream in front of the television, in a living room in a house on the proverbial wrong side of the tracks in Olivette Missouri, circa 1980. And he was not available. There was nothing to connect to, even for a curious child such as myself.

The most I have ever felt connected to my grandfather Bill, my father's father, was during an artist residency I had in Brazil, on a small island off the coast of Bahia, called Itaparica. This was either before or after I attended a candomblé ceremony, in which I was a witness, not a participant, and before or after I drank ayahuasca there, in an Atlantic forest, but Brazil is a mysterious and spiritual place that bends the laws of space and time in ways that do not happen anywhere I frequent in the United States, and one day, near the beach, 26 years after his death, I saw my grandfather pedaling a bicycle and laughing.

Physics and time would suggest that it was impossible that this was my actual grandfather, but the fact that I had to do the calculations to prove this to myself, in the moment when it happened, may give you a sense of how strange and affecting the occurrence was. I knew it was not my grandfather for several reasons, including the deeply rational fact that this man, who appeared to be in his late sixties, would already have been alive when my grandfather died, and that if it was in fact my grandfather, and he was still alive and had simply gotten up from the easy chair and walked away from everything in his life, reappearing in Brazil to continue fishing on an island, he would now be too old to be the man I was watching.

In the moment that this happened, the man bicycling in front of me on the beach, he was probably fifty feet away, and I was too deeply startled, too discombobulated to do anything at all. But if I could slow time down, if I could rewind it to that moment, and re-insert myself, I would have gone up and talked to him, because I recognized him spiritually. I would have had a conversation with him, that would have been healing irrespective of what he said, because what happened in that moment was that it occurred to me that in some possible universe existed some version of my grandfather who was happy.

The event was so odd that it occasioned, on my return, a bit of genealogical research during which I discovered something even stranger. The people on my father's side, who had made their way from the environs of Cracow, Poland, around the turn of the century, eventually emigrating to the United States, most probably entering through Galveston Texas around 1903, had made their way from Europe not directly to the United States, but had traveled first to Brazil.

My great great grandfather, Louis Kram, who had eventually moved to St. Louis and established, in 1907, the eponymous fish business, had left Cracow at 19 years old and travelled to Brazil. The women in Brazil, not all of them of course, but many of them, are beautiful. It did occur to me that it was not impossible that my great great grandfather, at 19 years old, disembarking in Rio, might possibly have sought companionship, and the person I had resonated so deeply, momentarily, and strangely with, as though I was looking at someone from my own bloodline, was, in fact, from my own bloodline. It doesn't matter. The man on the beach was not my grandfather. I'll never find him to have a DNA test done to know if there is a long lost family line in Brazil. I recognized him, somehow, at a visceral sensate spiritual level, and in seeing the possibility of my grandfather as a happy person, the depth of his sadness became dimensional, rather than simply flat, as it had felt to me knowing him.

And in that moment, he became both more real, and more unreal, than he had been to me in life.

28 - Fathers of Fathers

This same person who could not find his way out of the labyrinth of himself to notice his first grandson (me) was the person who raised my father. When I use the word raised here, I use it not in the traditional sense in which it is used in the realm of parenting, but more agriculturally, as in raising corn, or more euphemistically, as in raising Cain. For to be raised by someone who cannot find their way out of the labyrinth of themselves, as I know from experience, is not really to be raised. In my particular case, there were a series of crises required to finish the job, the very real possibility that the entire project would collapse under its own weight and end in suicide through self-destruction, and then a vast series of functional men, surrogate uncles, if you will, required to salvage it. But my paternal grandfather, I am told, was not always this way. He was not always defeated. That began, I am told, with the death of his mother.

⊕

We grow up ensphered by nested contexts. We are wearing a body that resides within a family, that resides within a society that resides within an ecology and a civilization. Our body is loomed inside the womb of our mother, and we are surrounded by her. And likewise, when we leave the womb, when we are born, we remain enwombed by the vectorial energetic geometries of the ensphering contexts.

We are not as solid as we seem, quantum mechanically. We are spiritual beings having a human experience, not the other way around. And this means that we are energy beings. And energy beings organize in energy contexts.

A family is an energy constellation with gravity and mass. Children are brilliant, many of us until this original seeing and feeling is down-regulated by failures to have our intuitions validated, and educational systems that stuff us full of sedating information in environments of sensory and felt deprivation with adults who don't know how to connect. We arrive, parbaked at birth, fresh from Union, with skylights in our skulls, feeling everything.

We are in orbit around our parents and the family members in close proximity, the cultures in which we reside. In ancestral and indigenous cultures, where we are held against the body of an attuned caregiver for the first nine months, our feet do not touch the ground at all.

Yet consider this. If you are, at this age, transparent- permeable in the extreme to the energy contexts around you- and you are carried on the chest, the back, the hip of your caregivers- you inherit their energy contexts. You absorb them autonomically. You resonate with them. The way they wear their experiences, how this lives in their bodies, architected through their autonomic physiology, its experience of safety or threat, its residence in connection, or, rather, appeasing, fight, flight, fawn, shutdown, or collapse, is entrained into our physiology, encoded into our breathing patterns through each inhalation, in waking and sleep.

We tend to think of inheritance as being genetic, and epi-genetic, but this is because our culture is materialist at heart, because despite the new physics, despite Newtonian mechanics having been shown to be insufficient to describe reality a hundred and some odd years ago, we still culturally fail to understand what it means. And so we anchor our thinking in the material, the concrete. But it is not genetic, uniquely, the inheritance. It is also autonomic. And autonomic is *energetic*. Our inheritance from family is therefore epi-autonomic in addition to (and possibly more than) it is epigenetic.

We inherit the autonomic contexts we are born into. We are molded by context. Your Autonomic Nervous System is the altar of your spirit. Your nervous system is, broadly, the mediator between interiors and exteriors, and your Autonomic Nervous system in particular is the energy grid that governs how you metabolize safety and threat into a body loomed by the Universe that you are wearing. It is the setting the levels on the energy processing templates that govern your interface with your experiences.

What you know as your body, *the way it feels to be you*, is the habitual structuring of the flow of attention through energy gradients sculpted around the fundamental calculus of whether your feel safe or in danger.

When we really start to understand the Autonomic Nervous System, we begin to see it as a kind of sound engineer dynamically working a set of master control sliders that adjust the physiological parameters of the body with each breath, tuning them to optimize the conservation of energy in every present moment.

If we are born into a context of deficient relating– and all modern people are born into a context of deficient relating: that is part of what is means to be modern– your ANS structures a contraction designed to help you avoid relationship. This is what Freud called 'ego'. The thing, the entity, the awareness around which most people accrete a sense of self is actually a tightening. A clenched fist, metaphorically speaking. The habitual felt flowthrough of energy and attention through biology contracted to avoid a threat.

What most people understand to be their identity is the feeling texture wrapped around a threat response.

Think about the harmonics of this. We are designed to relate, endowed with a connection architecture that unites, at birth, the neural regulation of the face, voice, eyes, ears, turning of the head and neck, with the breathing and the heartbeat. This physiological social engagement system is the only myelinated voluntary musculature in the newborn's body: the physiological mechanism undergirding attachment.

We come here to fall in love, to be revered by a village, our arrival to be celebrated, to be held up to the Sunlight and blessed like the tiny Simba in *The Lion King*. This is our innate biological expectation.

We come to crawl up the mother's belly, attach to the breast, coordinate the flow of breathing with sucking and swallowing, and dissolve once again into the ensphering context of unconditional love pouring into the windows of our eyes from our Mother, who is all mothers really, the Mother Earth herself. Only at this moment of birth no longer in a physical womb inside the mother, but moving into a womb-with-a-view, the formation period of the first 18 months outside the mother's body.

But– *do you know anyone who arrives like that?*

Were you blessed by such an ancestral context or set of greeting customs? The photograph of me in the mirror with my mother, great grandmother, and great grandfather, which was sent out that year by my great grandparents as a holiday card, with the caption – *Our newest great-grandson, Gabriel Ethan Kram, being photographed and trying to figure out what it is all about*, is about as close as it comes. But most of us? We get Grandpa Bill.

Most of us get taken from our mothers immediately, who have been heavily sedated in a hospital, given an injection, blasted with eyedrops, put on a scale, wrapped in burlap (it's not burlap really, but you've spent nine months in velvet jelly, what do you think it feels like?), and so on. And then we get handed to parents who are trying to upload our photos to Instagram and ask the nurse to hold the baby because they themselves have been raised in contexts deficient of relating, and are transfixed in a narcotics-grade haze of narcissism and dissociation and want to turn the event into a performance that can be consumed by others, like most of modern culture.

What the actual fuck?

At some point in the not-distant future, we are collectively going to look back at the childbearing context of the 20th and 21st century, the way that we have been raising our children, and realize that our entire civilization has failed in its most basic duty to create the conditions where it is possible to become a real human being.

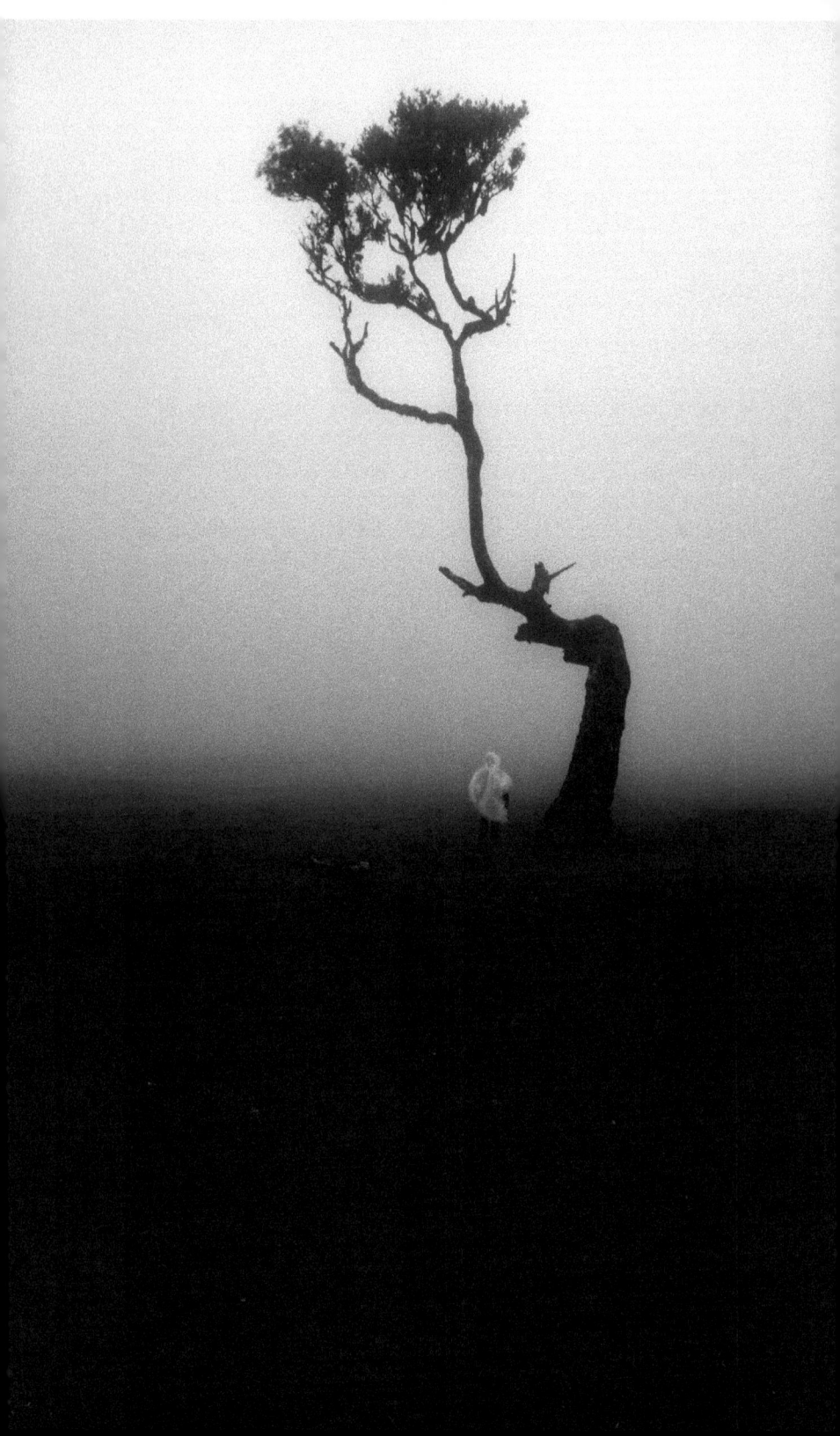

29 - Feet Not Touching the Ground

When I realize, nearing the age of fifty, that my feet are not touching the ground economically, it is in part because I have grown up in a multi-generational energetic context where no one's feet are touching the ground. And since my feet touching the ground is not primarily a question of the physical location of the foot, not a question of gravity and proprioception, not weight and balance, but a question of the energetic pattern inside the body that connects the root chakra to the ground, it is (it was) very hard for me to learn how to touch the ground economically inside the context of my family. *How would I know what it felt like if no one raising me knew what it felt like?*

Some people want to get into the family business, some people want to stay close to home, but as soon as I got my bearings I found myself torn, because even though I was still, by late adolescence, deeply enmeshed with my family, I desperately needed to get away from them. I needed to put some distance between us so I could start to figure out what stuff was theirs and what stuff was mine. Start to sort the boundary line and evaluate what they had installed in me that didn't actually belong to me.

I think part of the reason that we have become as a culture so fixated on individuation is because we know, as we start coming to our senses, that our families are full of sick animals, and we want to get as far away from them as possible.

Yet the problem, the paradox, is that we have been raised by sick animals, and these sick animals have installed their sicknesses in us.

We could put it like this: *How come your parents are so good at pushing your buttons?* To which the response is, *Because they installed them.*

Yet what does that mean? It means that when you were permeable, which all little ones are, you absorbed, through your original non-cognitive brilliance, the context in which you were raised. You organized the way you feel yourself by pushing into it. Either by merging with it, or resisting it. These are the only two ways you can come to feel yourself. Either you inhaled it, or exhaled it. This is the dance of relating. Every small child is occupied with the dance of relating, whether those who are raising us are likewise engaged or not. Or sometimes, they are way too engaged. And so we organize, or dis-organize, in the context of this relating, and in the context of what it is providing or not. In the present moment, either needs get met, or they do not. The caregiver notices baby is crying, brings attention, problem-solves, checks the diaper, makes sure baby is fed, is warm enough, burps the baby, holds the baby, comforts the baby, or does not. Baby cannot tell the caregivers what she needs, because she cannot talk, but she has been endowed by Nature with this marvelous social engagement physiology, a set of literal doorways into her felt interior, so caregivers who are paying attention can read what is happening inside.

First time parents are generally not that good at this, and so we require, to thrive, the village. We need aunties and uncles and grandmas and Elders of all kinds who are carrying the wisdom of the village and vibrating in their whole intact energetic embodiments to train the parents in how to create the contexts to nurture a real human being. The proper unit of human flourishing is not the nuclear family: it is the village. A village with Elders connected to the spiritual Source. The nuclear family is rather a nightmare for most people: a constellation of alienation.

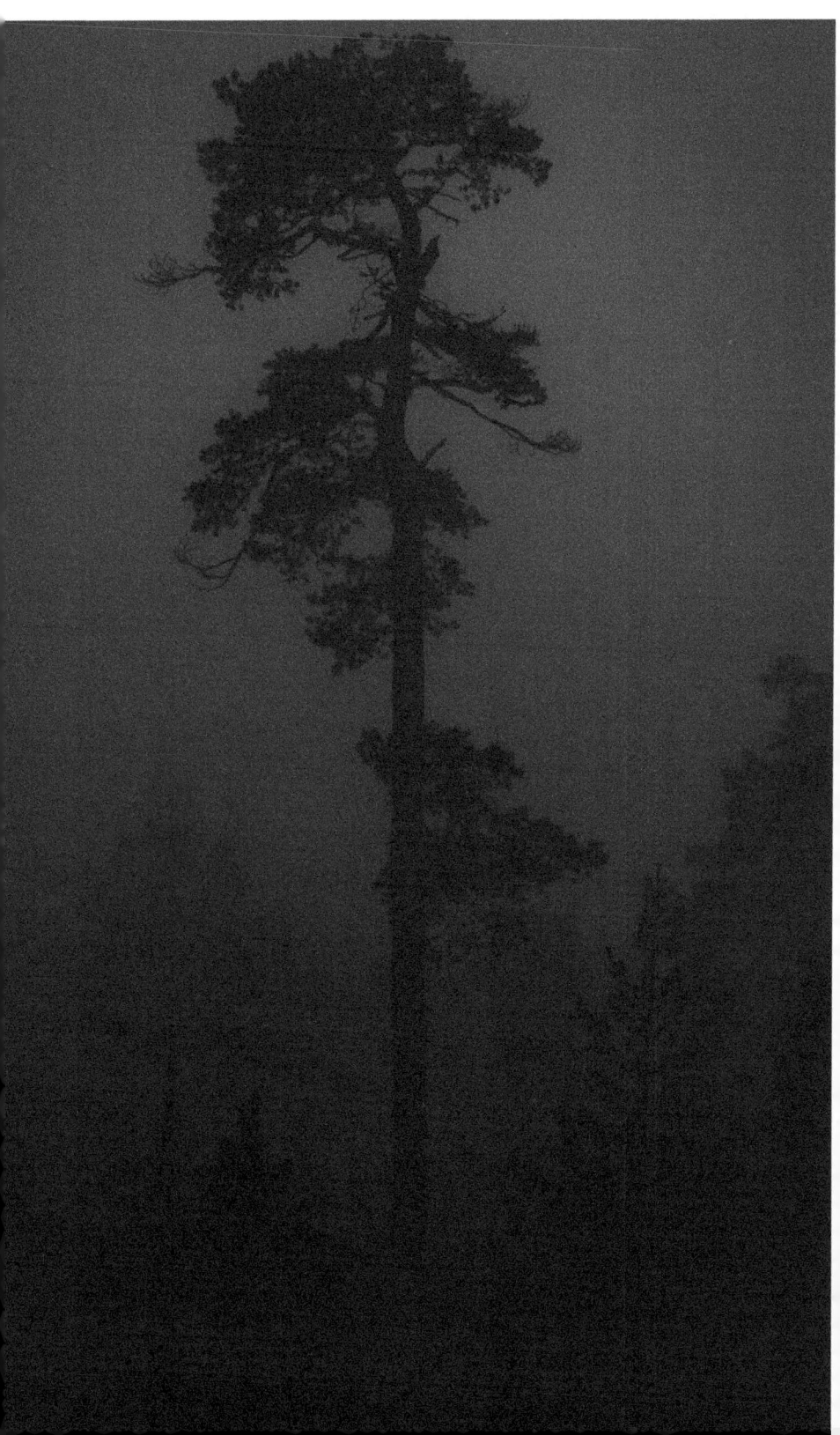

30 - Clear Seeing

Many people reading this will at some point have heard the word *clairvoyance*, which is a French word whose etymology is 'clear sight', and which refers to the faculty of discerning matters beyond ordinary perception. The word harks back to this notion of *seeing through*, a gaze that penetrates surfaces, exteriors, illusions, and this notion of clear seeing is also at the root of the name that the Huichols of Mexico give to their shamans, who are known in the Indigenous dialect as *marakames*. A *marakame* is 'one who sees'.

Shamans are the ones with clear seeing, the ones who see through. In most Indigenous traditions, the way that you get to be a shaman is through ordeals. Generally, if the culture is intact, children with aptitude are identified fairly young, but then they have to be trained. Generally this training takes a very long time. Clear seeing is not developed casually, and developing it is generally not very comfortable or all that much fun. Shamanic initiations that are not successful generally end in madness or death of the initiate. But those who do pass through the initiatory ordeals develop this penetrating sight.

The closer you get to the source cultures of the world- the deepest, oldest, most antique of our surviving human lineages- the more democratic the cultures tend to become, and in the oldest of these cultures, all of the children are trained to be shamans, although they do not use that word. In the San culture of the Kalahari (small band hunter gatherer bands that are the genetic origin of all modern European peoples) they do not have leaders because they do not need them. The San simply train every child to be a leader. They are all trackers, all shamans. Clear seeing is developed as a matter of necessity, because it is required to survive in the Kalahari, which is an extremely dangerous place. Faculties of penetrative awareness are required to keep you alive in a source (aboriginal) context.

Anecdotally, when westerners (ecologists, biologists, etc.) travel to the Kalahari to study its flora and fauna they hire San people to accompany them. If they have the temerity not to do this they do not complete their studies because they die. The Kalahari kills them off, generally quickly, and their corpses get picked apart by carrion until the bones are clean, and then gnawed by rodents for calcium. Their skeletal remains are scattered and bleached white by the scorching sun: little piles of osseous arrogance. A scatter of teeth too hard for rats to chew, some vertebral segments that look like alien mouthparts: that's all that remains. Those who survive do so because their San guides keep saving their lives and their asses– again and again and again. From poisonous snakes, apex predators, storms that swirl up out of nothingness, heatstroke, getting lost and disoriented, running out of water, losing the animals they are tracking in their studies. This is true– you can go look it up.

In a small band hunter gatherer band, where you are living outside in the elements, following the seasonal migration routes of animals, if you do not have clear seeing you die. It is pretty simple. In modern western cultures, where we have climate-control boxes to live in, work in, and travel between boxes in, and climate control boxes to hold slices of the animals we purchase at the deli counter (all we have to find is the deli counter, not the animals themselves), this faculty can lapse (it has lapsed) with apparently little adverse consequence, except that our civilization is destroying the only biosphere in the known universe and is unable to stop this despite being perfectly aware of it. In the Kalahari, if you do not have clear seeing, you fucking die. In the West, almost no one has clear seeing, and the externality of this is that we are killing the world herself.

Lest I digress here, part of the reason that we do not have clear seeing is because we are unable to successfully train our gazes on our families. We are not able to look back, with clarity, at the families that we come from, because we are structurally incentivized not to see them clearly.

A primary way we are incentivized not to see them clearly is the multi-generational transmission of wealth. This is because, to put it bluntly, if you tell your maternal grandfather to go fuck himself, he writes you out of the will. Yet the price we often pay for inheriting is that we inherit not just money, if our family has accumulated that- we inherit the stories, the blindness, and the bias of the family. We inherit the *not seeing*. We acculturate to a tacit agreement not to overturn the apple cart. And this *not seeing* of the family is generalizable into not seeing much of what surrounds us, much of what we are enmeshed within.

Yet we choose not seeing because in order to not disrupt the family system, in order to maintain contact, congress, and reciprocity with the family, we don't generally dig up the cellar and throw the rotting bones from the basement onto the family dining table and ask, *What exactly are these unmetabolized fragments of death?* If we do this it is generally not well received. So we elect not to see clearly. Often we don't even realize we are doing this. This is how indoctrinated we can get into the cult of the family.

And you know what happens when we do not see clearly? Of course you do. We get sick. Trauma is transmitted multi-generationally because we are sick animals raised by sick animals who were raised by sick animals. If you want to track back to where this started, you have to go back really far. Not just a few generations.

Realize that if you immigrated to the United States, or Canada, at some point in the last several hundred years, the decision your people made was to get on a boat for months that was as likely to splinter in the middle of the Atlantic as to make the crossing, in order to start a new life from nothing in a place you had never seen and knew nothing about apart from stories. In order to do this, things had be pretty bad wherever your people started, otherwise this whole enterprise would have seemed batshit crazy. I mean think about it– *Would you take those odds? Leave everything you know, and everything you have to embark on an uncertain venture that could end in disaster and from which there is no return?*

My point: if you elect clear seeing you are in for an ordeal. The bones in the basement? These are some really old bones. Some rat-gnawed bones. Some ancestors that have been reduced to a few teeth. Vertebral fragments like alien mouthparts in the Kalahari– only these are dirty.

31 - How the Wound is Passed

My second year at University was the year I started to get an inkling that not all in my family of origin was well. That there was something about the way that they were relating, in which I was tangled up, that was not healthy. It took me awhile to get clear about this (decades) because my principal task, and this took me about twenty years to figure out, was to identify the source of my primary childhood trauma, and to tend to that wound deeply enough that I could focus on anything else.

The chaos of this process I have documented in other books, and I will not dwell on it here, beyond noticing that in my experience some things have hurt us so deeply that it is not until we have gone a long way down the road of healing them that we can begin to grieve the loss. All of this is to say that it took me a pretty long time to be able train my attention steadily on the family itself, that particular context, and not my reaction to it.

At a certain point, I began to realize that I had inherited a broad number of patterns of relating that were pathological. I want to normalize this for a moment by saying not that this is normal, in any absolute sense, but that it is quite common. In the same way that early childhood adversity is not normal, but it is pervasive, pathological patterns of relating are not normal, yet they are pervasive.

My mother, whose boundaries were serially violated by her father, could not differentiate, for most of my life, the difference between emotional connection, merging, and intimacy. Places where she should have had an edge there was no edge. She has been crippled by chronic auto-immune disease for the past 15 years, I will note. Auto-immune illness is, in its most essential form, a breakdown in the body's ability to differentiate self from other. A middle child, an appeaser, someone who wanted to keep the peace at all costs, she was expert at pouring herself around people and merging with them, and understood this to be love. She and my father, who married young, had fused together into a sort of codependent amalgam by the time I had the wherewithal to begin seeing their relationship as something that existed beyond its impacts on me.

My father, whose own father succumbed energetically to defeat long before his body failed him, was so repeatedly and consistently crushed by the world, and then my mother's father, his father-in-law, that he retreated into a spiritual bypassing that was funded by my mother's inherited wealth, and simply withdrew from the world and stopped working at the age of fifty-five in the wake of a third or fourth bout of severe depression, with no savings whatsoever. He was only able to do this by living as a financial dependent of my mother. He moved to Colorado, joined a Tibetan Buddhist sangha, and devoted himself to the dharma, living off an allowance.

If I set down judgement, and observe these patterns in clear light, I can simply notice that I did not and do not want to be like either of these people. And yet they were the ones who raised me. They were the ones who taught me to relate. And this teaching was not in words, and pictures. It was not scholastic. It was embodied, and energetic, and it happened before my cognition was formed. They left an energetic imprint upon me, as loving and imbalanced as they were and are. The stamp parents leave on their children, etched into the lacelines of the nerves. This is the multi-generational imprint of autonomic patterning. It is how trauma is passed from one generation to the next.

When I interviewed Dr. Vincent Felitti, the Co-Principal Investigator of the Adverse Childhood Experiences study, one of the things he said that impressed me most deeply, was that the protocol he gave physicians at Kaiser Permanente in Southern California, where he was Chief of Preventive Medicine, when one of their patients came into the office with identified ACES, was to ask them if there was anything they wanted to share with the doctor so that the doctor could better support their wellbeing. The patient had completed an adult health questionnaire of some length, in which were sprinkled the ACES questions, ten of them, which were then separately tabulated and turned into a score. A patient might have an ACES score of three, or zero. If the score was anything more than zero, the physician would bring it up in the next office visit. First, they would normalize this, explaining that 67% of their adult patient population had an ACE. Then they would say, *If there is anything you would like me to know about what happened to you so that I can better help you, I would be happy to listen.* The hardest thing, Felitti said, was getting the doctors to actually listen.

The things that are in the basement, the things that are rotting in the root cellar, are things that we know and that we don't know. We know them down in our bodies. Down here where we feel things, we know them. But epistemological questions arise. *How do we know them?* Some of it isn't rational. What does it mean that *the body* knows them? And then questions of loyalty arise. *If I know this, what does it actually mean about the people who raised me? Who loved me? Who said they loved me? Who said they would take care of me? Keep me safe?*

The deeper question of loyalty is often the following: *can we know what we know and not tell ourselves it was our fault?* Because this knowing/ not knowing? It is generally protecting the status quo. It is protecting the elites, the patriarch, the powers-that-be. These are not things nice people talk about. It is thanking the patriarch for fancy dinners, and not confronting him about the endless litany of extramarital affairs, the emotional havoc his boundary violations have wreaked, the possibility that he is a sociopath.

I was sitting in a conference with Dr. Nadine Burke Harris, the former First Surgeon General of California, as she spoke about this. She said, "I have patients in Pacific Heights [a very wealthy San Francisco neighborhood, primarily white] and in the Bayview/ Hunter's Point [a very poor San Francisco neighborhood, mostly black]. The only difference," she said, "Is that in Hunter's Point, *everybody knows* who the molesting uncle is."

The origin of consciousness is often a crime scene. Something happens that shatters our world. A fissure, a rupture. But this wound, the healing of which can be, might just be the doorway to our transformation, can only be walked through if it is known. And it can only be known if we dig it up, if we allow it to come to the surface where it can be transmuted by air and light and water. Scoured clean. Down in the basement it festers. And so Felitti's admonishment to the physicians. *Listen.* You don't have to do anything, you don't have to fix it. If they dredge it up into the light of day, into conscious awareness, that act, in itself, is healing.

What do you know that you cannot know? What do you know, what are you holding, that you have not spoken? Who, at this point, are you protecting by this? And what price have you paid?

My maternal great grandfather, who is generally considered a mensch, also sent his wife and my grandfather and great aunt, his two children, to the river every summer for a couple of months so that he could go whoring.

My great grandmother knew this, and she could not know it. He sent her out to the river with her two children, and she could not swim. Until the day she died, she could not swim.

My grandfather, his son, simply knew this.

My great uncles, they knew this. Did they tell her, my great grandmother, this secret, that she knew and didn't know? Knew and could not know?

My grandfather, my mother's father, was also a serial philanderer. Yet not merely this. He had a particular lover somewhere, I do not know where she was, with whom he maintained a 30-year relationship. My grandmother, herself the children of alcoholics, knew this, and she could not know it. My mother knew it. My mother, from the time she was a teenager, was the keeper of this poisonous secret. How did she know this? Because her father told her. Made her the guardian of this betrayal of her own mother.

Things we know and don't know. I had a memorable dream in my early twenties. In the dream, my grandfather, who was about six foot two, probably close to two hundred pounds, comes running at me. He is large, and the way he is moving is like a zombie, like a freight train. His eyes are open, but they are not seeing, they are blank, he is asleep. His movement is inertial. There is spittle in the corner of his mouth. This is the whole focus of the dream: him bearing down on me, frothing, absent, running mechanically, with great force. In the dream I square myself, root down into the earth and hit him in the face so hard his entire body collapses, crumples to the ground. I hit him with my left hand, I can feel it now as I write this. The strike is so clean, so hard there is a cracking sound, like a baseball bat connecting. It feels so good it makes my entire body hum, every hair in my skin shiver, both in the dream and in the re-telling now.

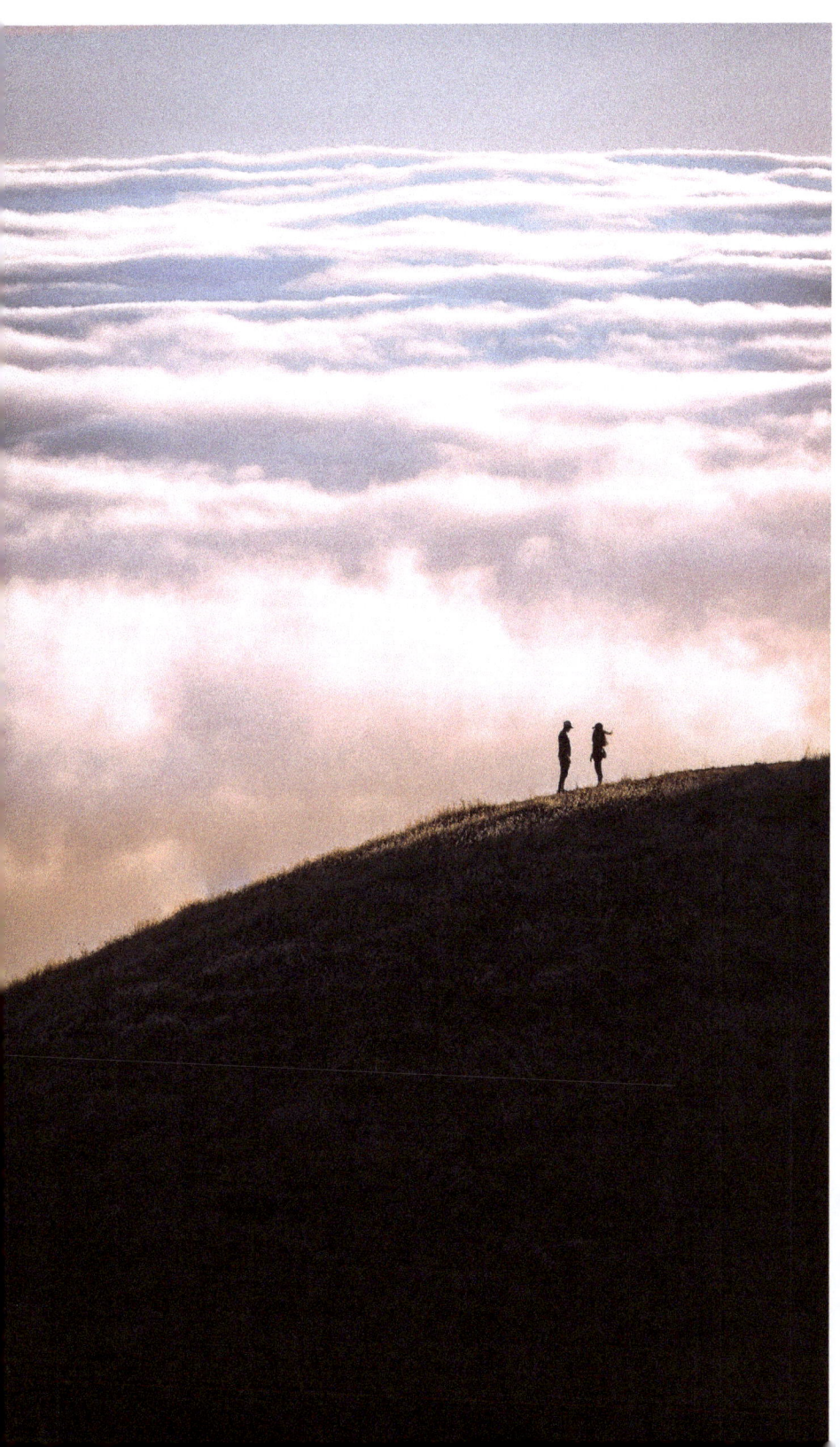

32 - Variants of Shutdown

When we think about the shutdown aspect of the unmyelinated deep belly vagal system, the Grounding System, which is understood broadly as our autonomic lifethreat response system, it feels important to go back to its origins in embryology. The earliest version of you is organized flat, before it begins folding back on itself. In these earliest embryonic stages, before you have a spinal cord, inner organs, a heart, or a brain, the cells are simply organized in two layers: an endoderm (inner skin) and an ectoderm (outer skin).[1] Neural development begins with a cord that starts to invaginate (fold in on itself), and the subsequent genesis of a layer between the endo- and ectoderm that will give birth to the heart and the blood system and blood and the visceral organs (the mesoderm). As the embryo continues to fold in upon itself, the endoderm becomes the inner tunnel of you (the mouth connecting to the esophagus connecting to the digestive tract connecting to the anus), while the ectoderm becomes your skin. It is not wrong to think of your guts and intestines as your inward-facing skin.

We are in touch with the outer world on the outside, clearly, through our skin. Yet it is helpful to remember that we are in touch with the outer world on our insides as well, through digestion. We open our mouths– this hole at the top end of our organism– and we insert things from the outside world into it, chew them up, and swallow them. Digestion then distinguishes what we can use from the outer world from what

---

1 This is called the blastula.

must be discarded, and the discards exit the other end of the tube.

I'm simplifying, for the purpose of reminding you that this inner tunnel, your inmost layer, is also both a barrier, and a sensate feeling organ, touching the world outside. It is so deep within us, so profoundly inward, and yet it is in direct contact with the world around us, because we put stuff from the world around us into the tube every day: this is called eating and drinking.

Clearly we digest food. Yet I will also propose to you, and this is not my idea, it originates in the dawns of time, that *we are digesting our experiences*. Our enteric system digests not merely proteins and carbohydrates, but what happens. Most of what happens we don't need to digest. Or said a bit differently, it doesn't hit us deeply enough that we need to digest it in our guts. But sometimes something happens that is so profound we feel it in our center in the deep belly. The level of knowing it activates is what is called, in Yiddish, *kishkes*: the knowing that comes from the guts.

And this is crucial for our understanding of the Grounding System in general, and shutdown in particular, which is its configuration in lifethreat, because sometimes something happens that we cannot digest.

Digestion is to break something down so that we can use it. We separate what will enter us through the intestinal wall, and become resource for our system, from what is chaff, garbage, toxin, and needs to pass through. The intestines are responsible for this discernment, an embodied filtration intelligence. It is a chemical and biological and immunological intelligence, in the specific sense of knowing what nutrients and chemistry to invite into the body, yet it is also a more subtle intelligence that determines what can be used from what must be removed. What can become part of us, from what must not.

The intestinal lining itself, the lattice of endothelial cells, has differential porosity depending on our stress state. And sometimes something presents itself inside the field of the body (our experience) that our intestines do not know how to digest. We cannot figure out what it is. We cannot figure out what parts, if any, we should allow to come in, and we cannot figure out how to excrete what we cannot use. And then we have a problem, because stuck there, this undigestible experience can literally bleed across the mucosal barrier of the guts and into our inward ocean.

From the deep belly center, on the lifethreat side, there are several variants. While I think all of them share a *what-just-happened?* kind of quality, all of them can be experienced as a social death, all of them take away our breath, and all of them shift us into stillness (immobilization, technically), collapsing us inward and altering the texture of our experience of reality, placing it into a liminal or between-realm that can gradate into the surreal or the dream-like (all make use of the chemistry of endogenous opioids), the contour of these shutdowns are different.

The first variants are pure shutdowns, and can arise in response to grief in all its flavors, of which I am told there are at least five. The second is lifethreat-level shock, which often moves us into freeze responses, the casual name for the state of tonic immobility: rigid and immobilized like a deer in headlights. A third is the kind of appeasing that happens when we exhibit sociality over the shutting down of our bodies, something we might do in the face of violence or overwhelming power: placating. These are primary ways that people enter shutdown, and it is important to distinguish them, I believe, because the paths out of them are different. My best educated guess is that how we come out of shutdown has to do with the state that just preceded our entrance into it.

⊕

Many of us, most of us, have not grieved enough. And we do

not do so because it was forbidden us by law, and we have forgotten how, and now we are afraid of drowning in it. And because we are afraid of drowning in it this grip of grief grows stronger in people. We used to tear out our hair, gnash our teeth, keen, ululate, wail. We used to give grief her due, which is, if you really stop to feel into it, to give love its due. We grieve because of how deeply we love. They are the same, really. The grief – the tearing of our hair, the beating of our chests, the wailing– is to honor what has been taken from us. The bodies of whom we love, which are also part of us. We don't end at the edges of our skin. We, who we actually are, is woven of the spaces between us, and when we lose someone we love, the space between us that is the relating is altered. We don't lose their spirits, because spirit is everywhen. But the touchability of them, the embodiedness, the hand holding us back. This is why we grieve. And Empire, selfish for the lifeforce, selfish to extract it from people, forbade these demonstrations of grief, because they move energy through and preserve sovereignty, and Empire desires that energy for its own uses, desires that labor to work the mines.

You have been acculturated by millenia of Empire to stuff your grief, and to hold it alone, and this is killing you. The Dagara people of Burkina Faso, in a gesture of extraordinary generosity, have taught some outside the tribe their grief rituals. They are rituals done in community, with altars to the ancestors, with the accompaniment of the drum. Rituals to restore grief to its proper place and to bring it back into community, where it belongs. We can apprentice to grief. We can honor her as the necessary companion to love, the *as below* to her above. She is a teacher of descent and renewal: the twin elements of which we moderns are sorely in need. Through apprenticeship to grief we can see the proximity of shutdown and connection, see how there are pathways from shutdown straight back to connection.

Let us speak here of the second category of shutdown: shock trauma. These are often shutdowns where what preceded the movement into lifethreat was an extremely high-energy fight-or-flight state. These are the shutdowns more generally understood as traumatic. These are shutdowns entered under threat. These are the lifethreats of being screamed at, abused, raped, nearly killed: the lifethreats of violence, of war, accidents, natural disasters. Of surviving something we didn't think we would. I know some small thing about these shutdowns as well, and these, which are entered by passing through the roof of the fight-or-flight-entered through the doorways of terror, most typically (sometimes rage)- these are different shutdowns, and the exits from them are different as well.

When shutdown is entered through flight-or-flight, the high-voltage charge of the mobilization causes the boundary dissolution characteristic of shutdown to eject consciousness, often from the body. This particular transit into shutdown is what is often reported by victims of abuse who speak about watching their bodies from above, or being stuck outside of themselves. This is the dissociative aspect of shutdown.

The repair and recovery of these shutdowns is different from the shutdowns of grief, and what we can say categorically, I believe, is that if we enter shutdown by going through the roof of fight-or-flight, when we exit shutdown we will move back across the threshold of dissolution (we will re-consolidate) and into the fight-or-flight state that preceded the exit. This is important to understand, because post-event, the experience of shutdown, unintegrated, exists along a continuum of dissociation. People feel numb, depressed, or dream-like.

These states are typically characterized by a low level of embodiment, interoceptive deficit, and dissociation. When people begin to heal from shutdown, when it resolves, what happens very often is that they shift back across the threshold into fight-or-flight states, and suddenly find themselves experiencing very acute fear or rage. To someone who has become homeostatically accustomed to living in a shutdown state- we can endure with our neuroceptive center of gravity in one of these states indefinitely (this is commonly called

PTSD but most modern people are walking around with significant unmetabolized shutdown)– these heightened and seemingly inexplicable surges of anger and fear can be profoundly distressing, and make someone feel like they are getting worse. *Good God*, we think. *Before I was just numb, but now I'm freaked out by everything. What is wrong with me? I must be getting worse.*

Being numb in a culture that is replete with numbness– staring at an iPhone for hours is dissociative and yet also considered normal– doesn't make you feel out of synch with the state of the world. You look around and everyone is doing it. On the subway, in the café, everyone who can afford to is tucked into their own private sensory island. To go from being numb, comfortably, to being freaked out, to being enraged? There must be something wrong with me. Only, there is not.

The neuro-circuitry of shutdown comes from a 500-million-year-old diving reflex, where animals held their breath, immobilized, and dropped their metabolic rate.

Acute defensive autonomic states, because they are concerned with survival, are given biological priority. Both fear and anger are on a continuum, and as we approach the end of the continuum that precedes the transition into shutdown, time slows down until its forward movement functionally ceases. At the threshold of pure shutdown time has stopped moving forward. Put slightly differently, the gates of eternity yawn open. The experience of being present in an experience that takes you through the roof of the sympathetic nervous system is marked by time dilation. When we almost die, we experience these moments as lasting forever. This happens as a matter of course, although it is nearly impossible to describe in ordinary language, or to someone who has not experienced this.

When people have been in a car accident, or been nearly blown up by ordinance, or survived a tornado, or almost been murdered, or been abducted, there is a consistent story that is told about the way that time slows down. People talking about a car accident, in the final micro-seconds before impact, will describe the way time congeals, the way sensory phenomena granulate, the way a weird calm descends (the endogenous opioids of shutdown). Our subjective experience of time is calibrated by arousal and sensory input. When an experience contorts the ordinary limits on our arousal thresholds, when it takes us to the heights of fear or rage required to conduct us across the threshold into shutdown, time begins to bend and dilate in characteristic yet non-ordinary ways.

When we then come down out of shutdown, back into the fight-or-flight range, we alight on these mountain tops. They are so much higher than ordinary arousal states as to be unrecognizable. Surfers understand intuitively that a wave that is twice as high is more than twice as powerful. As the height of the wave doubles, its power multiplies exponentially. So a wave that is twice as tall is four times more powerful; a wave that is three times as tall is nine times as powerful.

Looking down from the peaks of high-intensity arousal, the everyday waves of anger and fear are mere foothills. Up here in the vertiginous peaks, the contour of these waves is totally different. Their violence is astounding.

Our subjective experience of time is related to our ability to metabolize incoming sensory and interoceptive information. Ordinary time flows at ordinary arousal levels and ordinary amounts of sensory inputs incoming. Time becomes progressively subjectively non-ordinary as arousal levels rise or amounts of sensory inputs increase. (Entheogens, which dilate the senses, change the subjective experience of time by massively dilating our sensory and interoceptive inputs.) The topographies we are describing here occur at acute levels of arousal with extraordinary levels of sensory input, which often cannot be assembled in the moment because the parts of the brain involved in memory consolidation drop offline at these levels of arousal.

When a wave of this magnitude engulfs us, we will simply be taken by it. If we do not have skillful help outflowing its energy, it will simply carry us.

As we come out of shutdown, back to fight-or-flight, we need healing modalities that help us metabolize these extremely labile ultra-high energy states, and continue to ground and integrate them through the physiology.

Hakomi method, Somatic Experiencing, and Sensori-Motor psycho-therapy can all be very useful in this terrain. As can trauma-informed yoga, dance, movement practices, and grounding exercises. Shutdown is a hurricane trapped in a bottle. The threshold just beneath it is the hurricane unleashed. To come back down to connection we need to unwind that hurricane.

By the time that you are an adult, and most of you reading this are, you have organized a sense of self whose deepest primal layers are a set of neuroceptive setpoints, centers of gravity, if you will, around which you have organized your visceral experience of identity. These neuroceptive set points are the deepest layers of your embodied organization in relationship to safety and threat. Because neuroception is triphasic, with three parts: safety, danger, and lifethreat, you can think of this as a triangle.

By the time we are grown, most of us have a fairly stable and enduring set of neuroceptive centers of gravity. These can be altered by experiences of either intense or enduring danger, or lifethreat, or safety, for that matter, but typically, our neuroceptive center of gravity has organized our visceral sense of how it feels to live in the body that we are wearing, this embodied visceral landscape has shaped the envelope of the emotional terrain in which we feel like ourselves, this emotional terrain has sculpted the kind of thoughts that move through our cognitive territory, and these have all together shaped how we perceive the world around us, and how we therefore behave. (They also accrete our ordinary sense of self.)

To undertake, or to undergo a profound healing process, as an adult, is to shift these neuroceptive centers of gravity. Think of a building, that is, in this case, six stories tall, with the foundation laid in neuroception, then the first floor as visceral state, the second flood as sense of identity, the third floor as emotional terrain, the fourth floor as cognitive territory, the fifth floor as perception of the world around you, and the sixth floor as behavior.

To shift the neuroceptive center of gravity in your system is to do foundation work on a fully-erected building that is six stories tall. You can imagine that this psychic structure, which is also an embodied physical structure, has a certain mass, a certain weight, a certain inertia, and is used to dealing with incoming forces by moving them along continuous load pathways. In San Francisco, where I lived for many years, people would sometimes add a garage underneath their Victorian house, which required the house to be jacked up and stabilized by enormous support beams. You are a six-story Victorian, to extend this analogy, and if we are working on your neuroceptive center of gravity, we are going to have to jack up six stories and hold them stable. This is why I don't recommend working directly on neuroceptive set points.

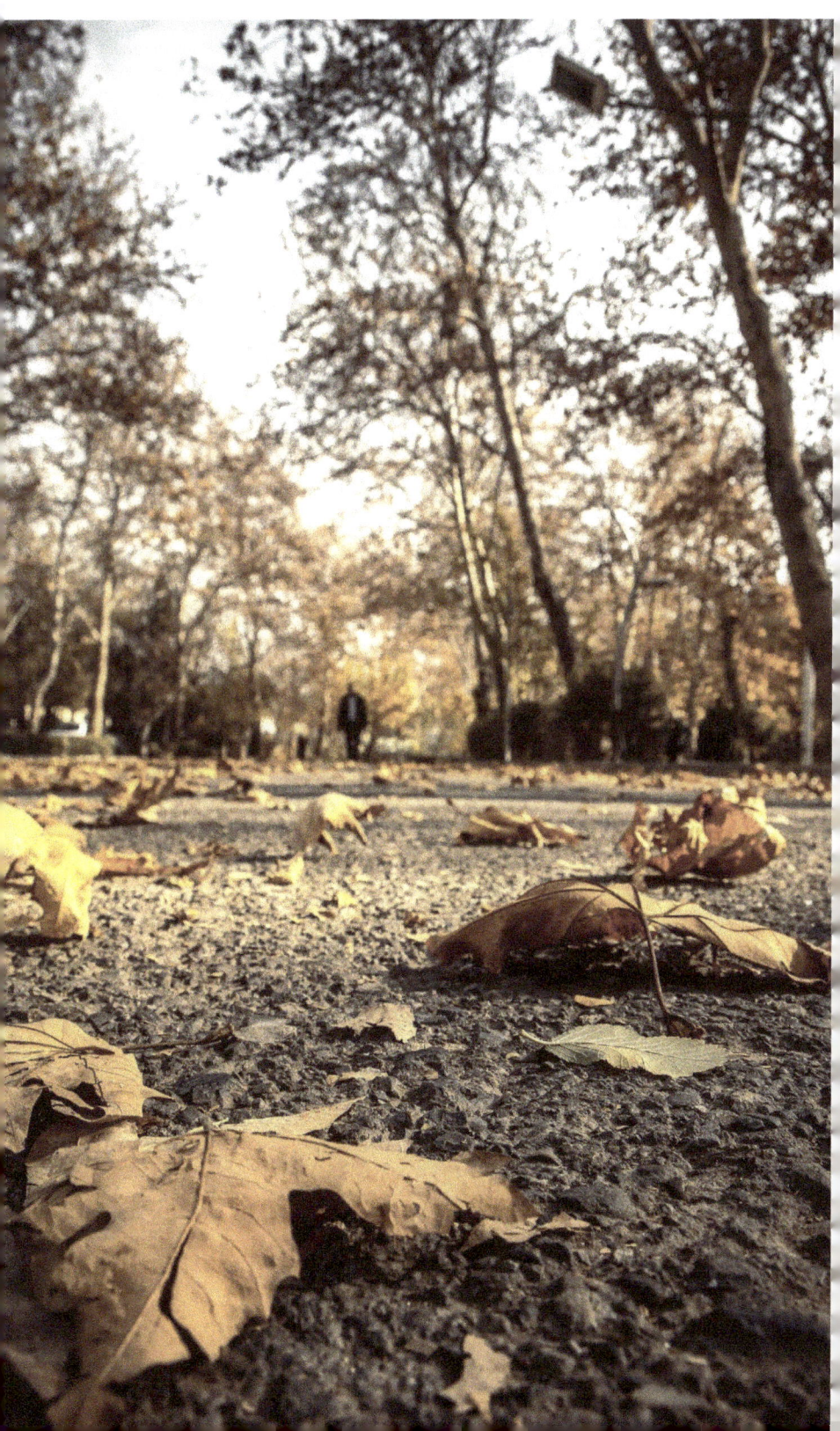

33 - Everyday Powerlessness

And thus I bow to what leaves me bereft.

The word power, in Latin, is *poder*. We can talk about the *power* of the Emperor, the *power* of the state, the *power* of money. But all of these speak of power in its *thingness*, as a noun. Poder, in Latin, is also a verb. It means- *to be able to*. To have the ability. This translates into everyday usage in the verb 'can' in English. *Can I leave?* means, do I have the power to leave? Do I have the ability? In Portuguese, which is the closest modern language to Latin, we would say, *Posso sair? Do I have the power to leave? Can I go?*

Power is ability. And when the ability is taken from us, we experience its lack. Power is an action word, autonomically-speaking. Ability is *to act*. To do. To make happen. And this doing, this making happen, is generally speaking, a mobilized affair. It involves movement. Ability is agentic. And because of this it is important for us to explore the particular shutdown that is a result of having our agency removed.

Powerlessness is shutdown when we cannot act. All shutdowns, by definition, are the removal of agency, so in a way all shutdowns are forms of powerlessness. Shutdown is captured in the phrase: *I couldn't fight back.*

Yet the traumatic shutdowns of removal of agency-the traumas of sexual violation, abuse, the being overwhelmed by forces of nature let loose, these shutdowns of powerlessness, must be contextualized also against the everyday shutdowns of powerlessness (I can't get my iPhone to work, I can't get this document to print, I can't get traffic to move) and the civilizational shutdowns of powerlessness (I can't get outside of capitalism, AI is taking over, there are demons running the government.)

My point here, with shutdowns of powerlessness, perhaps with autonomic state writ large, is that associative memory is clustered together by feeling tone, and when we come into more stable contact with our feeling bodies, those things that have the same tenor of vibration, whether seemingly everyday and minor, or existential, vibrate the same chord. What this means practically, is that the everyday powerlessness of not being able to get my iPhone to work- my experience of being powerless to do anything about this- resonates with my other experiences of powerlessness. Having been moved away from my home and hearth and people and place at age seven. The ancestral powerlessness of my parents and grandparents' people to stop the genocide against the Jews. My powerlessness to get outside of capitalism or stem the flood of AI garbage taking over the world. Without awareness I don't realize that the iPhone is making me bonkers because it is resonating with all of the other times I have been powerless. Without awareness I don't understand why I have vivid fantasies of smashing the shit out of it with a hammer. Of throwing it as hard as I can against concrete. Of annihilating the iPhone.

I'd like to here surface and differentiate three layers of defensive autonomic response: the everyday, the developmental, and the traumatic. Most of our attention these days in the healing arts goes to the traumatic. Some of it goes to the developmental, very little goes to the everyday.

Yet the place where our archived history meets the present moment is the place that we have a window into what is moving beneath the surface. And often, as in *most days*, there is something that makes me feel powerless.

I feel powerless to get my teenage daughter to hurry up in the bathroom. I feel powerless to accelerate the line at the coffeeshop. I feel powerless when the bank charges an overdraft fee, or when wi-fi doesn't work. I feel powerless when the very cogent email I wrote was mis-interpreted.

I detest feeling powerless. And so you know what I do instead? I get indignant. Indignation is the fight-or-flight suit I dress powerless up in so that I have something to push against. *Can you believe how slow this line is? Are you kidding me with this freaking wi-fi? What on earth are you doing in the bathroom?*

I love my daughter beyond imagining, and I almost said to her today, out loud: *Look, I know we've had a lot of rain this winter, and the reservoirs are full again, but that doesn't mean you need to use it up on ONE F*CKING SHOWER.*

That's the level of indignation I had to tamp down, but you know what? Underneath it is the shutdown of powerlessness that I do not want to feel. Underneath is the defeat of not having the energy to cajole, plead, and wrestle with her to hurry up.

This everyday level of activation- in this case my powerlessness around the shower- is the place in my life today where I can feel and be present with shutdown. If I hold myself with enough grace I can recognize that pretty much any time I am getting indignant about something what is underneath it is this feeling of powerlessness, and that somewhere along the line in the recovery of my agency and in the healing of my child self I decided that I would rather fight against than feel that.

That somewhere in my inability to get my daughter to shower faster was my 7-year old self utterly incapable of stopping my parents from moving away, forever, from everything and everyone dearest to me. And it is here where the everyday touches the depths of everything we have survived in order to arrive at this moment.

In this way, at the same time, the everyday is a portal to working on my deepest healing. As we live in each moment, so we live our lives. Can I find it within myself to simply acknowledge that this everyday moment makes me feel powerless, and to feel that and not like it and still not shut down? Can I weep with my inability to get my daughter out of the shower, knowing that I am also weeping for my powerless 7-year old self?

34 - Archeology again

My mother thought her father was her husband, and my father thought his wife was his mother. Of course, *thought* is not the right word, but there is no correct word in English. The thought was acted out, embodied, lived, behaved, and beneath the threshold of conscious awareness.

I think I did know this as a small child, the parent thing. I think I knew this, and could not know it. If I had known I knew it, I wouldn't have known how to say it, because I didn't mean that they thought this in their minds, in words and pictures, I meant that they behaved this in their bodies. It was how they acted.

Why else was my grandfather the breadwinner? Why did he pay for our house, give us cars, pay for my tennis lessons and my school tuition? And why else did my mother pay my father's bills?

Why was my father responsible for paying for things for himself, and my mother responsible for paying for things for everyone else? Why was my mother's car the family car and my father's car was my father's car?

And then- the emotional nourishment, the closeness she was seeking from her husband, but that he was incapable of giving her, she looked for from her boys: myself, and then my brother and I. Again, we know and we don't know. I didn't have a word for this. It wasn't a concept, it was a feeling. The motoric expression of which was, *Back up. You are standing way too close to me.* There was, at a neurophysiological level, almost nothing personal about this. It had nothing to do with who my mother was at an identity level. It had to do with the reality that there was this large animal standing emotionally too close to me, too involved, too inside my perimeter, crowding in. That I couldn't feel myself clearly, because she was looming.

For years her lament was, *You are pushing me away.* And I was like, *That's because you are standing way too close to me.* But again, feelings, not words. We know and we don't know. And so I spent a good part of my adolescence, teaching her, knowing and not knowing what I was doing, to back up.

Tolstoy opens Anna Karenina with the observation that, "All happy families are alike; every unhappy family is unhappy in its own way." Because we don't have language for this autonomic layer, this felt sense of the vocabularies of safety and threat, of boundary and edge, of the contours of energy vampirism, why we feel intruded upon or unmet, clarity about how to untangle ourselves, people's intuition gets all twisted up.

Because we don't have Elders to lean into, to push against, Elders to validate, *Yeah, your parents are kind of a mess*, we take it personally, we grow enraged, we grow disgusted. In reality, most people's parents are kind of a mess. They are a mess in their own particular way, which is what Tolstoy is telling us, but the problem isn't simply that this is happening, it is that there is no trusted Elder, no aunt, no uncle, no one in the village pulling us aside, staring deep into our eyes, and going – *You're not crazy. You are correct. You are clear seeing.*

If I had had just a little bit of that as a teenager, just a tiny bit younger, it would have gone a long way, and I might have avoided the intensity of self-destruction I rode for several years that culminated in my tripping LSD with a gang member who took me out late at night in downtown St. Louis on a summer night in 1997 and tried to get me to murder someone.

I might not have had to go all the way to that perilous edge to find my limits. I might not have had to go that far to teach my mother that she couldn't keep me safe. That she didn't have that power. That my life belonged to me. That I would make my own decisions.

We don't need to be fixed. We need to be accompanied. We need to be witnessed. We need to have what we know, in parts of ourselves that don't know how we know it, validated. Such that the yearnings enchanting us are not coming up from the decaying bones of the improperly buried ancestors in the root cellar. So that we are not seduced by death. In late adolescence and my early twenties, I was under the potent sway of darkness, because I had no language or maps for drawing up the corpses from the depths, no notion of what was required to scour them clean. Rather, their subterranean gravity called to me, in cadaverous ways, inviting me to join them in the land of the dead. I almost did.

The origin of consciousness, a crime scene. And at that crime scene there is a knife. If there is a crime scene, and a knife, the question is who is holding it, and at whom is it pointed?

Down here, in the basement, the knife generally gets pointed in one of two directions: at ourselves, which is how it happened with me, and this is called *suicidality*. Or at others, which is what happens for those inclined towards harming others, and this is called *homicidality*. Same force, same pain, pointed inward or out.

Yet what we really need to do? Learn how to jam that knife, to its hilt, into the GROUND. There are uncomposted ancestors and their ancient autonomic traumas here. And they are arguing over whether you should stab yourself, or those people over there, because they are trying to work out their unmetabolized ghost karma through your living body. This shit doesn't all belong to us.

By the time we have gotten to this point, and I have dialed

down deep into the socket of the hip, on the inside, where the psoas muscle joins into the interior, the basement of the hip, I'm in pretty deep dialogical discourse with the knowing in my body. I began this archeology as a project of interoceptive tracking, with the disovery of a pocket of numbness in the interior of my right leg where I simply could not feel myself.

Tracking this awareness, from its edges, led me to the great-grandparents and the grandparents, both sides of the family. This whole thing about my mother and father, and who each one acted like the other one was, came up out of my embodied knowing, packed down into that joint, in a way that astonished my conscious mind. This is the nature of the knowings that we carry in the body. They can be sitting in there, latent, for decades, waiting to be noticed and known, felt and understood. Deciphered and unwound. Decoded.

I have spent the last several days systematically unpacking the material that has lodged itself as awareness deep into the fulcrum of my right leg, and this after thirty-plus years of archeology: work on myself, and in myself, to find my way home.

The place in the body that awareness resides, the place it gets trapped, bound up, frozen, stuck, does not seem to be to me particularly accidental. This part of my body, right at the juncture of the torso, and the leg, is the junction from which I would begin to walk. The junction an infant makes from being held, to walking under their own power. First crawling, and then standing upright, the orthogonal shift made by our ancestors seven million years ago in deeptime.

And walking is a sort of forward motion that requires us to have our feet on the ground. How, with my family of origin, insulated by multi-generational autonomic dissociation, am I supposed to walk forward in my life? This has been the question.

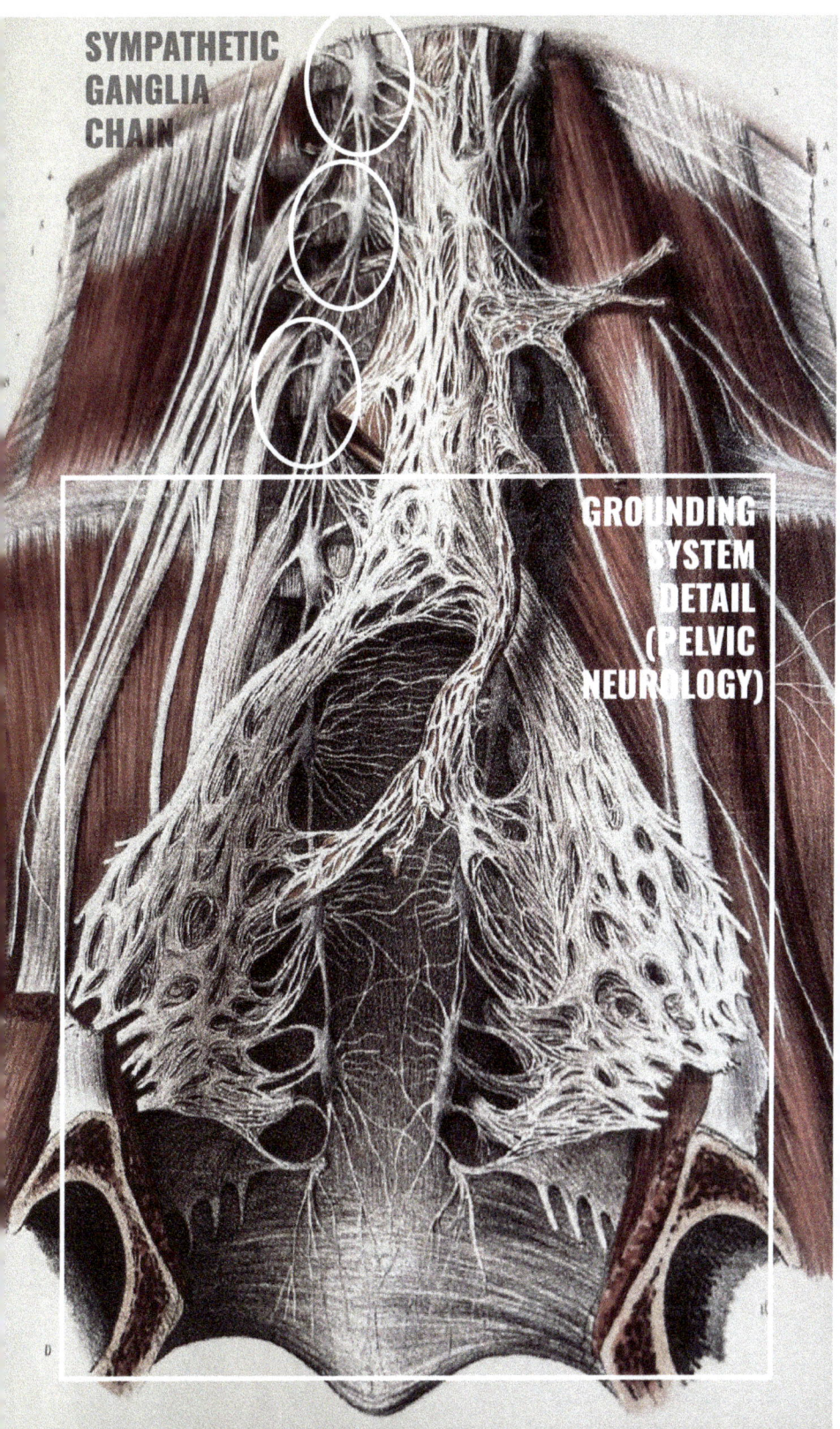

35 - I cannot bear it

An inquiry inward, and down, into what, if anything in my own story, in my own inward experience, might be getting in the way. An inquiry into what, if anything, in the story of my ancestors, in the story of my relatings, might be in the way. I want to know what is blocking the energy, what is preventing the flow; why I cannot feel my feet on the ground. And it begins not with something abstract, this inquiry, but a visceral awareness that there is a pocket of numbness in the joint of my right hip. A numbness that has come to the surface, edged into awareness. Has it been there all along? A numbness that seams the inward line of my psoas, on the right side, in a very particular anatomical location. A numbness that when I sense into it, deeply- for I have trained to do this- nearly takes my breath away. It is this numbness that is the occasion of this undertaking, this archeology. Numbness, a sharp vacancy, that is the telltale sign of a localized shutdown.

The trouble begins, it seems, when my paternal grandfather is 12 years old. This would have been about 1933. William is a bright and capable boy. He is deeply attached to his mother. I do not know what kills her. It has never been told to me, or I have not remembered it if it was. What I have been told, by my grandmother Beverly, his late wife, what I have been told sitting in the presence of my wife, who had the wherewithal to ask about this, was what happened afterwards. I hear this story sitting in the formal part of my paternal grandmother's living room, early in my courtship of my wife, at a time when we are already engaged to be married. I would have been twenty-three, my wife twenty-five.

In the wake of this devastation, the loss of his mother, William goes to live with an aunt. His mother's older sister. She will raise him, to the best of her ability, as if he was her son. Where the father was I do not recall. And yet, this is a time when a grief such as this was not metabolized well. I don't know anything about the funeral. I don't know anything specifically about what happened to my grandfather in the wake of this loss, beyond a knowing of what it is to be rendered homeless in one's own proper body. And a certitude that he never got over it.

I have the sense he was never the same. My grandfather shares a name with another William, a literary William. There is a moment, at the end of William Maxwell's aching autobiography, *So Long, See You Tomorrow*, when the protagonist, the author of the story, who is now in his late 60s, and living in New York, finds himself in the office of a psychoanalyst discussing the death of his own mother as a child. The occasion of this, in its particular circumstances, are different than those for my grandfather. Yet the two men are of nearly the same generation, and Maxwell, who became the fiction editor of *The New Yorker*, unarguably the premier literary destination of that generation, has an ability to articulate this loss in a way that my grandfather never was able. The end of the book hinges emotionally, a fulcrum, a pivot, on a single word that is spoken in the present-, and not the past-tense.

The author is speaking about an event that happened sixty years before, when he was ten years old. The book itself is a sort of archaeology of this time in his life: a moment before his early adolescence filled with events too large to be made sense of. For a good part of the book, we are following the story of another boy, not the narrator, but someone he knows. This narrative displacement seems to occur in part because bringing attention to his own direct experience was far too painful. Yet in the culminating and final chapter of the novel, we remember the death, with the narrator, as he tells the story to a psycho-analyst in a richly furnished office in midtown Manhattan, recalling the moments after the funeral of his mother, in a small farmhouse in Ohio, sixty years before. In Maxwell's own words:

After six months of lying on an analyst's couch—this, too, was a long time ago—I relived that night of pacing, with my arm around my father's waist. From the living room into the front hall, then, turning, past the grandfather's clock and on into the library, and from the library into the living room.

From the library into the dining room, where my mother lay in her coffin. Together we stood looking down at her. I meant to say to the fatherly man who was not my father, the elderly Viennese, another exile, with thick glasses and a Germanic accent, I meant to say I couldn't bear it, but what came out of my mouth was, "I can't bear it."

This statement was followed by a flood of tears such as I hadn't ever known before, not even in my childhood. I got up from the leather couch and, I somehow knew, with his permission left his office and the building and walked down Sixth Avenue to my office. New York City is a place where one can weep on the sidewalk in perfect privacy.

Other children could have borne it, have borne it. My older brother did, somehow. I couldn't.

I read the words of William Maxwell, but who I see is my own paternal grandfather, a vague etheric automaton walking in a slow loop around the first floor of the house, in the home in which the absence of his mother, her presence as thing (body), her absence as being (mother), is the predominant gravity architecture: a blackhole that has opened. Around and around the dining room table he goes, captive to a gravity whose presence is absence. Unable to parse spirit from matter he is fixed here, pinned, incapable of digesting the experience.

Maxwell, telling the story to his psychotherapist, tries to say, *I could not bear it*. And yet this is not the sentence that comes out of his mouth. What he says, nearly sixty years later, is in the present tense. *I cannot bear it.*

The sentence is a marvel: *I meant to say to the fatherly man who was not my father, the elderly Viennese, another exile, with thick glasses and a Germanic accent, I meant to say I couldn't bear it, but what came out of my mouth was, "I can't bear it."*

The fatherly man who is not my father...another exile. The Viennese psychoanalyst is a geographic exile, yet the Williams' exile, and here I am speaking of both Maxwell and my grandfather, is from themselves. The ground from which they have both been removed is not native soil, but their own inwardness. *I cannot bear it.*

The past is never dead, Faulkner reminds us. *It is not even past.*

What we know, and what we cannot know. What we cannot digest. In the presence of this absence, which neither William can bear, they absent themselves. But where to go if we are not at home in our own bodies? If we cannot bear to be inside them? And here is the synechdoche for modernity.

The other William's entire book, a heartbreaking and beautiful book, pivots on this moment of inability to place the event of his mother's death behind him. It remains present everywhen. And this is the nature of trauma. Something that cannot be contained by temporal structure, something that refuses to be digested, dissolved, placed into time, refuses to recede in the rearview mirror, refuses to take its place in the past. Something that we cannot get behind us. A crime scene that remains stuck in us. Frozen. Inaccessible. Everywhere. Everywhen. Unable to separate spirit from matter, allow each to return to its proper place, the grieving never happens, the flood of tears never comes, the ice never melts. We never recover the ground of being.

I know something about the writer's trajectory, not merely because of the public role he held as an editor of the premier literary magazine of the era, but because I know, well, how the architecture of a tragedy, such as that, takes a young boy, and moves him up into his head. Writing, for Maxwell, likely meant many things to him, yet among them it is a way to locate one's self in the flow of words, rather than in the flow of overwhelming and seemingly implacable emotions that we cannot bear. It is a way to create enough distance to hold an event- to grasp something too incandescent with loss, something that could burn you down, annihilate you- with the forceps of prose, so you can look at it without it setting yourself on fire.

It was not until later life that Maxwell published, *So Long, See You Tomorrow*, the crowning literary achievement of his career. It appeared in two editions of *The New Yorker* in 1979, when the author was seventy-one years old. It took him more than sixty years to be able to call forth the story: to temper the flame enough that it would not destroy him, and to cajole the language up from the depths.

My grandfather, William, does not seem to have been endowed with similar literary gifts, or an ability to surface the story. Instead, he pushes it down. This is why seeing the man in Brasil, the version of my grandfather who was possibly happy, was so startling to me. A version of my grandfather who was not an exile. A version of my grandfather at home in himself.

What I am told is that the gifts my grandfather had were mathematical. Brilliantly so. But the war came, as he moved into the later part of adolescence, and rather than going to school to pursue this ability, the heart-broken boy begs his uncles to let him stay in the family business: a fish business. What my grandmother told my wife and I, sitting on a couch in her home, years after his passing, was that his uncles had tried vigorously for quite some time to dissuade him.

I imagine that when she told us this she got a far-off look in her eyes, knowing as she did how the story would end forty years later. They knew he would not be happy. They knew that fish guts and a customer service counter would not satisfy him. They recognized in him an ability. A power. *Poder.* They wished that he would go and develop it.

But my grandfather, whose family had been stolen from him once, would hear nothing of it. To choose exile again after you have already been exiled?

He couldn't bear to leave them. He could not walk forward into his life. He was stuck circling the coffin. A blackhole opens inward and he could not put his feet back on the ground. And so he became a fishmonger. He worked with his uncles in a building on Biddle Street in downtown St. Louis. When he was young, he married my grandmother, Beverly. I have seen their wedding photographs. Both of them were beautiful. My grandfather looks more than a little bit like me. Perhaps a bit more Italian. A bit more Jewish. A beauty underlined by sadness that broods in his eyes. My grandmother, radiant in her wedding gown, has elegant curls that wrap her head and face. They look happy. The wedding cake is monumental. It is clearly an enormous celebration for both families.

Is it the mother-shaped hole in my grandfather's heart that causes him to treat my grandmother as though she is his mother? No one has ever told me that he did this. It is implied by my own wounding. I know he did this the same way I know I breathe. Unfinished business. It is implied also by my own excavation of my parent's relationship, where my father treated his wife as though he was her mother. Making her carry him, until it broke her back. And where I, in certain ways, have required that my wife carry me. When my wife first said this to me, it hit me like a slap across the face. I saw instantly that it was true. *How have I let this happen?*

None of this was conscious. Intended. Done on purpose. I doubt my grandfather realized he was doing it. My father would certainly be disgusted if I told him that I saw that in him. And I have been astonished when faced coldly with my own presumptions. Or, said better, my mechanically unconscious inertia.

A relational wound happens in 1933, and it is carried forward in the family for nearly 100 years, repeating. How does this happen? People want to say that it is epigenetic, but I don't think so. Part of my grandfather froze solid at 12 years old. He never thawed. My father, raised in the neurobiological imprint of a man partly frozen, *inherited* that freeze not genetically but *autonomically*. Not through DNA or environmental factors, but through felt resonance with something frozen. Something stuck in the cold, something dead, a place in his father that would not vibrate. Something from which all feeling had vanished, something numb. The bodies we are wearing are loomed relationally.

We feel ourselves because someone feels with us. This is the nature of attachment, and the wound of neglect. We can only feel ourselves, only develop boundaries, by being felt, and by having someone to push against. The way we feel to ourselves, the *feeling* of being in a body, is not inherited genetically, it is shaped by who we resonate with and who we push against. We merge and resist, merge and resist. This is how we come to feel ourselves. Indulge and fight. These are the rhythms. We co-regulate into interoceptive awareness, and those to whom we are attached provide the electro-magnetic templates for our embodiment or lack thereof.

My father raised by a father whose body was partly ice then raises me. And I, *not even knowing anything of the story until I was well into my adult life*, raised by my father, a man who had inherited a partly frozen body, inherited that freeze. In the imprint of its identical shape, with repetition. The multi-generational transmission of autonomic state. That is what we are talking about here. How the wound gets passed.

It is also why thawing my own body unearths the memories

of a hundred years. Why thawing our collective bodies unearths civilizational memories all the way back to the crime scene in the Original Garden at the origin of it all.

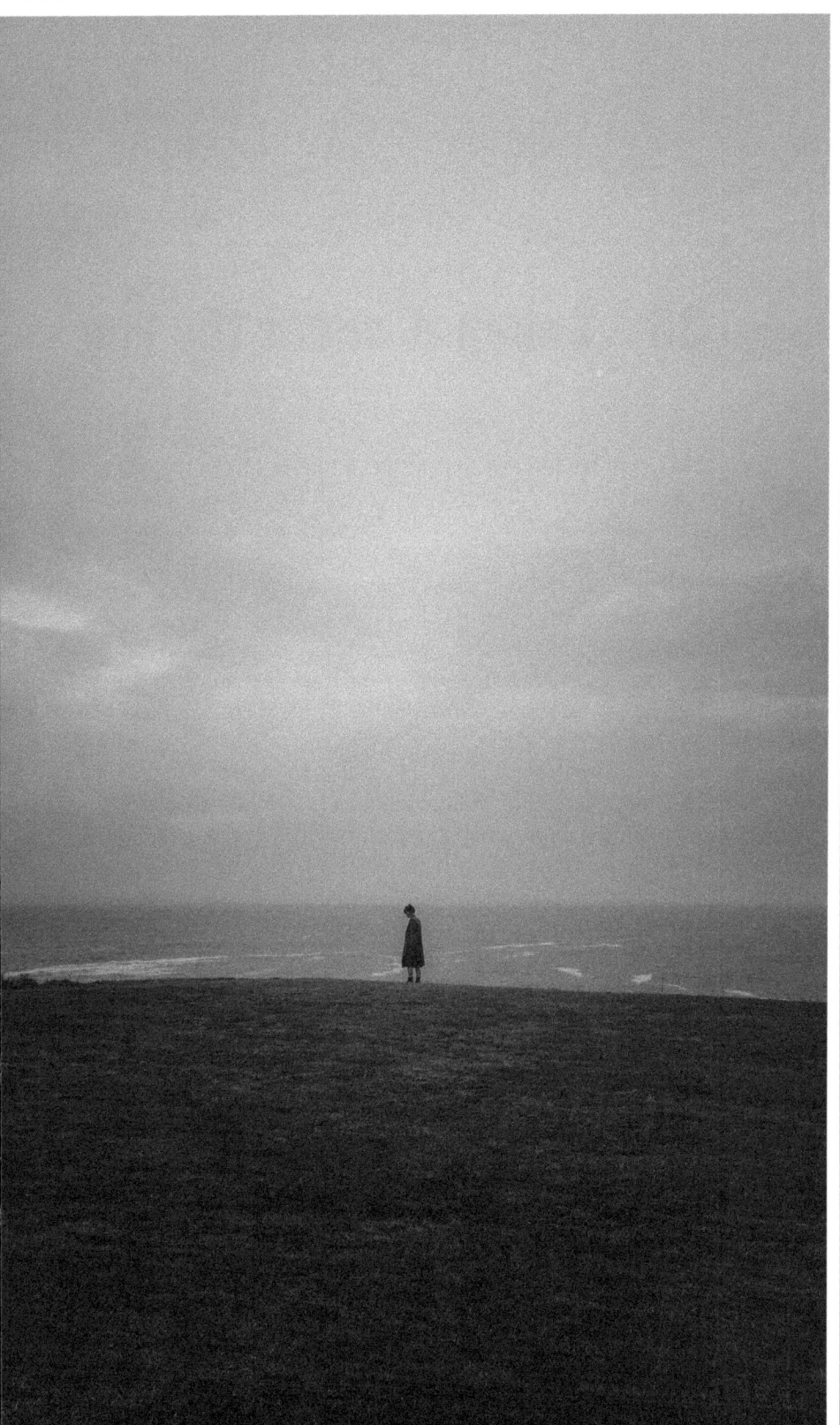

36 - Sweep it under the rug

There are technologies required to turn a corpse into an ancestor. It doesn't just happen on its own. Bodies, untended, unmourned, unwatered with the tears and lamentations of the living, putrify.

A mentor of mine recently told me that if you want to understand a culture, you look at their funerary practices. Culture, the real thing, has extensive spiritual technologies for alchemizing corpses into ancestors. Think about the rituals in Judaism, for example. Or Tibetan Buddhism. The grieving proceeds through distinct phases. Community is involved. The body is carefully and tenderly ritually washed. Grieving is allowed to happen, encouraged. Mourners arrive at the house and are nourished. People sit together, sometimes all night, sometimes for nights on end. The body of the departed is witnessed. Touched. Tears are spilled like wine from barrels, in great draughts. People cry themselves together, and tears pour over the corpse of the departed, great waves of veneration that tell the person and their spirit– *We love you, you are part of us, we claim you, we see you, we long for you, we miss you, we don't know how to go on without you, we....don't...know...how...to...go...on....* This loss must be alchemized. We have to reach the point of *we...don't...know...how...to...go...on.* Because only when we truly reach this point does the transformation– of us *and* the corpses–take place. Only when we cannot bear it, in the present tense, is there the possibility of spiritual alchemy. Only then do we see one another in our new relationship. Only then can we release one another. Only then can we be free.

A whole cycle of grief must unfold, and it must be metabolized by the community, and by the body of the departed. Is it not so?

But symmetrical to our lack of birth ritual, symmetrical to the way that we have forgotten the greeting customs required to welcome a new human into the world, we have forgotten, collectively, the way to release one from it. And so we end up in a world peopled with ghosts.

We are terrified of death because we don't know what life is. And in this unfamiliarity with it, with the mess of birth, with slicks of blood, baby poop black as squid ink, the squish of fluids, the nakedness of us all– this distance, this sense that it is something over there, something to be kept at bay– we don't teach our children either the customs of greeting or the customs of departing, and in this way we pass our ignorance forward in inadvertent generational transmission.

Corpses incompletely mourned because grief gets stuck in the breasts of the living, gets frozen, can't make its way out, because people do not know how to touch their hearts, open them, allow them to spill over–these corpses get swept under the rug. They pile up in the basement, in the root cellar, in the map of the ancient city beneath, where they tug on the living, haunt them, and the living, who if they allowed themselves to feel this would find it makes their skin crawl...the numb ones remaining, they tune this out, call it superstition.

We pour alcohol on the wounds to sterilize them, but we pour alcohol in the mouths to numb the pain, to release us, to ferry us away from all this loss. We turn the lungs into smokestacks, suck on deathsticks, the nicotine covering over the loss. We'd rather become drunks with emphysema than traffic with the dead we have improperly buried.

Outer darkness exists, but through our collective lack of attention to the ancestors here we have piled up quite a grand number of haunting agents no farther away than the basement of our own houses.

What is this mess, this catastrophe, this shame, this thing that we do not want people to see or know about? Uncle So-and-So has molested little Catherine, and we know this, but we can't talk about it, don't want to acknowledge it, don't know how and refuse to hold him accountable, nice people don't talk about these things, and so we'll just sweep it under the rug. So-and-So stopped taking his medication for manic depression, wandered off into the woods raving, has been gone for five days, they sent out search parties, his body was pulled from the river. We'll just open the door to the basement and throw the shameful things down there, into the darkness. Banish them from sight, speech.

But the basement is in the body, that's what I'm trying to tell you. The things we know and the things we can't know. The cellar, the body, the place where these things have been swept– it knows these things. All the way back and all the way down.

37 - Dreaming the Deepest Shutdown

When I awaken from the dream I lie there for a moment, stunned, not realizing I was asleep, my body slowly coming back to me, my hands numb, my face cold, my body inwardly frozen. Until I begin to realize I was dreaming, and then *what, what was I dreaming?*

It begins to come back, the dream, first its end, first the ending of the final scene, but within that only the feeling of it, what I remember. At the end of the dream they have all left, the ones who were in the house with me, the house that was the basement of something. They have all left or are leaving, and I am in a room with the last person, the last one there, and she is talking about a girl who has departed the room recently, who had a strange sex addiction, had some habits, she is saying, that were very difficult to change.

And then I am standing there, looking out the window, and I am looking far away, into the forest beyond, and I am thinking - *I want to be over there*. And what I mean by *over there* is not some other place exactly, but not here. What I'm meaning is that here I am shrinking. Here life is receding, it is harder and harder to get to, harder to feel.

What I am meaning is that I am longing, yearning, to climb up, to reach up and out of my body and span- fly- from this place, and this stretch, this impossible feeling of reaching, this helplessness to do it, my nose is numb as I say this, the cold is spiritually cold, of death, of permanence, of condemnation- this wanting to stretch and to reach up and out and away, this is the deepest aching feeling of the place and the last thing I feel in my body before I wake.

And then I wake and swim up to or back to myself.

There is more of the dream that I remember. But I want to sit here, for a moment, writing these words. I almost took a shower but I didn't want to warm myself, warm my core, feel like myself again until I had fingered the keys of this keyboard, gotten this down on the page. I didn't want to throw myself away from the feeling place of this, because what we always want to do is just get away from this feeling because this feeling - good God- it is the visceral feeling of alienation. It is the feeling of being unable to move, the feeling of being unable to escape the basement of this house where we are trapped with the mysteries of people unknown, cadaverous, strange, violent, unpredictable.

And what I start to remember of the dream is wandering through a house, and I believe houses in dreams are always a form of psyche, wandering through this house, remote, lost, unable to find anyone anymore, and the house is haunted but in ways to which I have become accustomed and so they do not frighten me in the dream anymore. I ramble through rooms daring almost the cupboard to open and rattle, talking and beckoning in a manner that furniture is not supposed to, knowing there is nothing in there except fear, fear that I cannot feel from this state, fear rendered somehow anemic.

The cavernous and haunted lurchings of the house I cannot escape make themselves known to me, but I know them without fright, they are emptied of menace, simply signals of entrapment, but the problem, the fucking problem is that I'm stuck here.

I cannot move forward, I am alone. There are people, others wandering these corridors here, but I am alone, I am elsewhere, this here is a non-place, outside of time, outside of forward movement, outside of the circadian rhythms of life herself– it is perpetually dusk or dawn in the house, but neither really, and all of this I know without knowing how I know it.

In the house, even in the dream, a sequence of strange things has happened. My nose is numb again, in real life, writing these words, it grows numb as if sniffing the strangeness of all of this, as if to acknowledge that in the dream I am bewitched, and as if to acknowledge that in the dream I am beguiled by being unable to breathe. I cannot feel my face.

For there is no oxygen there in that house, not really. There is no rhythm. No pulse. No life. There is the simulation of life, the apparent movements of it, people doing things, things happening, but without agency, without animacy. A simulation, a going-through-the-motions, and this is why, perhaps, at the end I am yearning, my heart nearly bursting though I cannot in the dream feel my heart, to get up and away and out of this place.

This is the deepest shutdown. This is what it means. This is who we are in this place, this version of ourselves. And you can see how here, in this place exiled from time, this place exiled from hope, we yearn for a savior. Yearn for someone to lift us up, yearn for a skygod. You can hear how people might cry out for Jesus if they had voices they could lift.

Earlier in the dream, and I know that I am working backwards, but this how it goes with trauma– we find a thread of something and we follow it back– earlier in the dream there were things that happened in the house. Let me see if I can remember, if I can re-assemble them.

There was a gathering of some kind, in fact an invasion. The house was over-run at some point by uninvited guests, this I remember. Uninvited guests making themselves at home. And I had a knowing that it wasn't really my house, so I couldn't remove them properly, and there were so many of them, and they acted with a sort of authority, or if not an authority an entitlement, and they seemed to know the place. One of them, a man on the back stairs, pointed out to me features of the back yard and distant ponds - *Is that a pond over there?* - I asked him. And he nodded, but why didn't I visit the pond? Only I know why: it is because we could not leave.

And so this house, which was also a psyche, which was also a prison, was at some point in the dream, earlier, over-run by a host of other people who were not invited or at least not by me, and yet who would not leave or at least I could not make them by force as I could not, in the dream, summon force.

And this is also what it means, the deepest shutdown, this helplessness. I awaken and my arms are buzzing in their roots as if they have been shut down at the trunk of my body, where they exit my torso. Like the electrical grid at the body has been powered off at the trunk. And of course, because I couldn't use them, couldn't summon them, these arms, I couldn't defend myself or throw those motherfuckers out, the group of them that came cavorting through the house, acting like they owned the place.

And this is shutdown also, because in this place, this place of dissociation, this place of being without a body, for this is what it is, the movement of the body, the central pattern generators taken offline, I could not act. Here, in shutdown, we are bereft of agency.

Action, acting, doing- it requires being able to move. And in this place, though the self-sense, the psyche, the identity, the 'I' or some version of it is there, it is not connected to the body. It is detached. The body is not available. And absent the body I cannot defend myself, cannot use force. Cannot boundary set.

Absent the body and its locomotive wherewithal we are open to the host of invaders trampling across the threshold, piling into the house. We are permeable to invasion. And this is true also, of course, because the chemistry of shutdown is dissociative. It is endogenous opioids required to release us from the body we are wearing, painkillers that ferry us up and out of the rhythms that organize our lives.

Startled into awareness, jolted by terror, and then disaffiliated from the organizing rhythmicity of the body we are wearing, the central pattern generators taken offline, breathing taken offline, the deep rhythms of the body offline, and so I am in an airless place where I cannot act, in a twilight ripe with invaders I cannot repel, but simply have to make room for, out of whose way I must stay.

This was earlier in the dream, but later most of them left. They came through in a stampede, and then most of them left.

⊕

I have paused here, writing this, the weight of it is enough. I got up, went upstairs, took a hot shower. I got dressed, said good morning to my daughter, came outside. When I stepped out of the house, encountered the morning air, I realized that I was not breathing. I had to recall to myself the rhythm of breathing. *This is how you do it*, I reminded my body. And I closed my eyes and listened to the rush of air hissing in, hissing out. I am now sitting in a coffee shop, it is 6:15 am, and there are people around, and I am still remembering how to breathe.

The smells of whatever they are warming, some sandwich with bacon, these drift through the café and I inhale them hungrily- not hungry for bacon- but for smell. For the facticity of life. In the dream there was no smell. There were no tactile sense qualities whatsoever, I am realizing now. No sense of temperature. No touch. No taste. No pain, no pleasure, no emotion. Because without access to a body, without any central pattern generators online, without access to motion, there is no *emotion*. No feeling. No color.

Without motion there is no emotion.

Unable to feel myself, I cannot feel.

And so I revel for a moment, in this archeology, this documentation, to taste the muffin I am eating, its warm sweet crumble. To really taste the coffee. Because every fragment of pleasure I derive from this is owing to having my body back online. You can't taste, smell, swallow, digest, pee, poop, make love, touch, be touched, or feel without a body.

And shutdown, if we are stranded in it, deprives us of all of this.

It is a place without rhythm: ecological circadian rhythm, the rhythm of relatedness, and the rhythms of the body, our inward physiological cadences.

And here then is the deepest antidote to this state. Rhythm is what creates the scaffolding to allow what we know in shutdown, know and cannot know, to be brought up from the depths where it is divorced from us in the murky waters of what the fathers of racist European psychology called the subconscious.

But they were wrong. There is no subconscious. Or, rather, the subconscious is that which we know and do not know. The subconscious is the aggregation of our collective shutdown. It is not psychological. It is the brain-based interpretation of a physiological experience, and what is held within its grip, unmetabolized. The frozen block beneath the surface, inaccessible directly, radiating strange emanations of loss. That is the subconscious. What is held in unmetabolized shutdown. No more, no less.

Learn to navigate down here, is what I am proposing, dredge it up to the surface, and it will help heal you. Remember though that this basement, permeable downward, contains not merely, not simply, your own history. It is collective also.

And here in the coffeeshop, sitting beside me, a group of men in earnest Bible study, and I want to get the fuck away from this shitty religion born of alienation. Let's get at the alienation directly, shall we not? Let us not seek some salvation to ferry us upward and away from all of this loss. Let us do the damn work to integrate, into the psyche, that which has become unmoored.

Let us do the work inward and downward, in the basement, in the dark, in the earthdamp of the cellar, with the bones. Let us stop escaping, cowardly, into the refuge of skygods, the upward, the fantasy of apotheosis. What if, instead of trying to become divine, we became human first? How would that be?

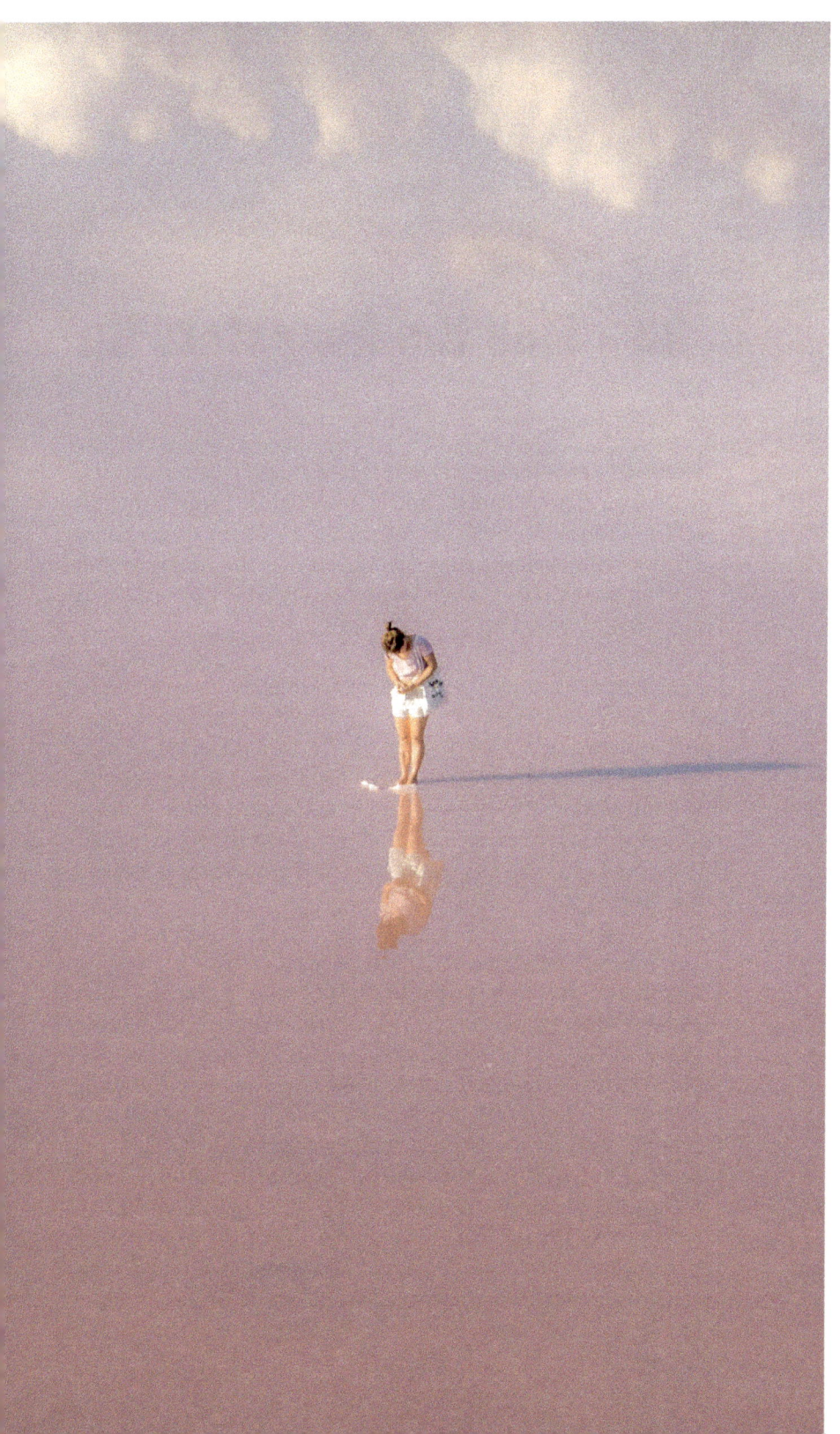

38 - Line the Ancestors Up

The call starts innocently enough. I haven't spoken to my mother in several weeks, and I finally clear enough mental space to be present with her. I am working about eighty hours a week, we complete a funding objective for the company, and I am able to exhale. I have a weekend: a Sunday fully off. I call her fairly early in the morning.

The conversation goes sideways pretty quickly. I am sitting in front of the coffeeshop, in my car. She asks me about work, and I answer her question, speak for about ninety seconds before she does this thing that she does. I hear it in a pause in her voice before it happens, and I know what is coming. There is a re-alignment in the center of gravity of the conversation. It moves from my side, the answer to the question she asked me, back to her.

There is an odd moment, a sort of grammatical scaffolding required so that the next move won't seem a complete non sequitor, won't seem crazy, as she takes whatever I am talking about, in the realm of autonomic physiology, and bridges the conversation to herself, and then she pours out a recitation, a lament, of all the things that are bothering her. She tells me about a new nerve treatment, a stellate ganglion block- *have I heard of it?* About her treatment team, about the functional medicine doctors she is working with (I know about this already, I was the one who referred her to them), about the series of challenges she is facing (I know, I've heard this dozens of times before), about what my brother said about this (I know), that she wants her life back (I know), that this is not really living, etc. This goes on for several minutes, a monologue, a soliloquy, a form of speech that could be mouthed into a mirror, doesn't really require an audience, is not a conversation.

At a certain point in this momentum, I feel myself taking a step back, a step away, energetically. I do it deliberately, the way you haul yourself out of a swimming pool with a lean on the edge and a quick and hard push up and away.

She feels this withdrawal of my presence, grows wistful. *It sounds*, she says, *like you don't want to talk about this*.

My mother and I are circling each other now, in a pattern that began in my adolescence.

At a certain point in a relationship, all arguments are the same. It doesn't matter what the argument seems to be about: its specific igniting. Once people know one another well, once the patterns of relating are grooved, all arguments are the same argument, energetically, until one person breaks, or cracks, or yields, or until an agreement is reached, a detente, a transformation, or a healing. Or until something simply changes. All arguments are dressed in the particular clothing of the particular circumstances they are wearing, but they are the same argument until it gets resolved, if ever. But how do we talk about this? And to her, in this moment, this is what I try to say.

By this point I'm driving. I've left the coffeeshop without getting coffee, because there is something about getting a coffee on a Sunday morning that feels like it is about setting your morning on the proper foundation, somehow espresso has a different taste, a different meaning on a day off, on vacation, on a weekend- and we have leapt sideways into something that is not the proper foundation for the morning I am wishing to have.

We talk about chronic pain, we talk about auto-immune issues, we talk about Mast Cell Activation Syndrome– all of these ways of medically describing things that are hard to get a hold of, things that are nebulous, things that describe the body turning on itself. But what happened? Someone broke someone else. That is what happened.

The received and felt architecture of our family of origin feels normal to us, no matter howsoever deviant it might be. This is how malleable humans are. We are trees that grow twisting and turning toward the light. We cannot control the soil we are born into, the exposure, how much rain comes. We simply survive the onslaught if we are able. What we survive seems normal to us, it cannot seem otherwise. It is just how things are. Our lives are just what happened. Shipwreck or victory.

My parents are not bad people: on the contrary. They loved me, love me, in the best way that they know how. I believe that they considered, deeply and methodically, what they believed would be of benefit to me. Yet this love, what they call love, is also shaped by a multi-generational contex of traumatic shutdowns and boundary violations. And so it is warped.

This story I am telling, this archeology, is particular, because I have to understand it in terms of the gravity of my own life: otherwise it is not useful to me; it cannot provoke liberation. The liberation that we are seeking is always particular: it is not abstract. And in this way it is specific, because there are particular events that occurred to particular people and require particular response. But it is not about my parents, or my grandparents, or even about me, really.

It is a story about *Us*. What happens to humans in families, absent the village, absent healed Elders, absent sovereignty, absent ancestral healing technologies that can touch the Source. It is a story about how wounds are passed. It is a story about how absence (loss of people, loss of contact, loss of safety, loss of access to interiority) structures the house of the psyche. And it is a story about how the generations born into these houses, which we all are, are shaped, energetically, by these gravitational forces, seen and unseen. By dead great grandparents under the floorboards who have not received proper burial, rememberance, or veneration. By encroaching parents. And how we, who grew up in houses with ghosts in the basement think this is normal.

This text is also a sustained question: how do we identify what is absent with enough precision to address it? How do we make visible the unseen such that we may heal it? Because what is missing has as great an impact upon us as what is here. This is the nature of cold stress. Of shutdown. It is defined by its absence. Black holes are not uniquely the province of astrophysics. They can be familial, cultural, and civilizational as well.

To do this, with my family of origin, I have attempted to direct attention not to the words we use, not to the surface ornaments of speech, but to the deeper dynamics. Down in the basement of my relating to my family of origin, the argument is very old.

It comes down to this: I have not trusted them since I was seven years old. My life has taught me, experientially, that I cannot rely upon their judgement. That were I to do so it might kill me. That it almost did.

I could choose to ignore what we call, for lack of a more physiological word, my deeper intuition. But this would be also to betray my own ground, and my own groundedness.

With my family of origin there is a boundary between us. Finally, an unambiguous clear embodied, *No*.

At last, I have put my foot down.

This knowing, when it comes, is not when I am on the phone with my mother. It comes when I am on the tennis court, in the middle of a match, my hands at work, my mind tracking something inward. The knowing, when it comes, is not in words. It is a feeling. Something in my body shifts, and it arrives whole, a gestalt, all at once. It is a vibration, a tension, a way that the leg changes how it is seated in the hip just a tiny bit.

Acknowledges the truth of the full body 'No' and finally accepts it.

A frozen place thaws suddenly like ice breaking up in a frozen river, comes back online, gives, releases back into flow. It is an adjustment of the nervous system, the autonomic, that then changes the muscular control and the sensory feeling of the right hip. I feel the joint awaken, come back to me. For a moment I feel like I will throw up, or fall over, stricken. Like a lightning bolt in the right leg, a sudden turning on. A strange taste comes into my mouth. Ozone?

I feel a new line of energy, of connection, run laterally from the socket of the hip into my genitals. Into the root chakra. And then I feel that line connect all the way down the inside of my leg, past my knee, my calf, my ankle, to the instep of my right foot. My entire right leg quivers and resets.

I take a tiny step, and the leg bears the weight differently. I feel like a newborn foal, for a long moment, moving gingerly as the organization of my weight changes. It feels deeply strange, and deeply reassuring. A reclamation and a novelty.

Testing the leg, feeling down through it tentatively and then with more certainty. Can I really feel in this place? Is this really ok? All of this happens within the span of about thirty seconds.

My breath hitches, and I breathe down through the right leg and into the earth. A neurogenic tremor passes up my right leg and through my whole body. My visual field trembles, wavers, time congeals and shifts on its axis. There is a buzzing in my head, I feel my vestibular system adjusting to a new sense of mass and balance in the right middle of my body.

I know, the hip itself tells me, *how to place a foot on the ground.*

I know how to stand upright on the earth. I learned this seven million years ago.

Some other part of me is talking now, and this is what it says to my ancestors: *Line up behind me.*

Just like that. It speaks with an unhurried and deliberate authority.

Get in formation. Find your places. For I have come to organize your ranks, move you into the places you need to stand to support this Now.

There is a certain silence after I say this. I don't quite know how to describe what happens. There is a slight wind, a sort of pause opens up in time. I am receiving serve, I am crouched down a bit, my opponent is serving, we are in the middle of a set, but time dilates, a few seconds expands into something deeper, something longer, something meta-real, anti-hallucinatory, and with the words still reverberating, *Line up behind me*, there is birthed, there is born, some new awareness.

I find myself crouching there, the serve comes, I swing, we play the point, I am moving across the court, I am striking a forehand, I am running in after the short ball, I am hitting an approach shot crosscourt, but there is some new awareness present, some new awareness that I can feel is very very old.

The point concludes, and I turn and walk back toward the baseline. This new, and very ancient awareness is arriving, and taking in the place. Landing, something vast touching down. And rising up, as if from the earth. As if mist. From in front of me, and from behind me. From the future, and from the past. It comes from all directions in space and in time at once, everywhere and everywhen, arriving. Settling. Organizing in.

When I called the ancestors, when I told them, with authority, to line up behind me, my gaze was trained on the last several generations of my family. That is who I thought I was talking to.

Yet who has showed up, and I don't know what part of me knows this, although it does, is much much older than what I was expecting. Than *who* I was expecting. This awareness, as it arrives, finds itself slighly bemused to be on a tennis court.

Finds itself slightly astonished by the material complexity of our modern world. The concrete walls, the right angles.

I am myself, and yet I am not myself, I am something deeper, something older, something taking in this moment, this environment for the first time, as if to say– *some things have changed since I was last here.*

As if the bones of the dead have been scoured clean, stripped of putrified sinew, emptied of fossilized grief, turned into rattles, alchemized by the Kalahari sun, the impurities eaten away, gnawed down by rodents to become the calcium they use to grow bones, distributed diffused and composted back into life, back into the animal realm, ten thousand creatures that have dined upon these remains, and spans of time have unspooled, all of them have died, melted back into the earth, dissolved into her, into humic matter, become soil, food for plants, the plants themselves, the energy cycle at their core, the chloroplasts, their cellular engines, become their respiration, their exhale, dissolved the energy patterns of dead families, broken them down into their atomic components, re-arranged the genetic lines, merged back into elements, water, carbon, calcium, nitrogen, phosphorus, distributed, taken up by clouds, rained back down, distributed around the world for aeons, dissolved into ether, and then lined up, ancestors as pure elementals...as if someone or something – *line up behind me* – has taken a vast rug outside into the sun, into the wind, to shake it out, all of the dirt fleeing, everything swept under smacked out by a broom, it snapping in the breeze, all of the particular filth...and then taken back up by my body in the form of ancient awareness.

As if I am no longer the son of a Jewish family with a dead great-grandmother, that particular history, as if all of that is in the past, behind me. As if my parents are not my parents. *Your parents are your parents, and not your parents.*

And I find myself sniffing at the wind, relaxedly stronger, my attention curious about the external world, my sense of smell more alert, my skin aware of the breeze in a new way, the racquet somehow lighter in my hands, carried on a current of peaceableness that expresses itself through an almost overwhelming affinity to simply marvel at the Living World around me and the profound uncanniness of it all.

I discover myself out there, on the court, swatting at a ball with a stick, but then this deeper older part begins to recognize, begins to remember – *a bird, a tree*– the elements, the elemental, and the pleasure it takes in this is so great, so broad and gentle and so loving, so deeply and profoundly peaceful, that I simply stop. My opponent on the other side of the net pulls up and looks at me rather strangely.

I stand, and stretch, and move this animal body, filled now with a peaceable and ancient awareness so primal, so oceanic, so vast– my skin drinks the light from the Sun, my nose quivers sniffing the melodies of spring deployed on the breeze: the faint exhale of sunwarmed soil, waft from some blooming tree, candy and violets buffered on gusts.

The blue of the sky elementally azure, depthless and profound, a transmission of blue, bluest blue: *sky*, I intone. The magnificent redwoods sentinel-like in their ascending verticality, endraped in leaf, needle, effortlessly being trees, not things, but beings. *Treeing*, I intone.

And everywhere there are verbs, patterns of energy swarming and constellating in mysterious expansion and contraction, breathing themselves awake, a scolding skittering Jay cavorting, a bumblebee humming like a tiny drunk bass amplifier thwacking its way unsteadily upbreeze.

My opponent is waiting, and it takes all of my focus to reel myself back in from all of this primal beauty, this original seeing, the call of it, its song to me, its song to us, its song to life– it takes all of my willpower to not simply set down the racquet and walk off the court into the forest.

39 - Sometimes God is a Blade

Mastery works with the material of the Real. The capital R suggests its objectivity. Reality is synonymous with Nature. Nature is both what we are made of, and what surrounds us, and yet most people will never come into contact with it, mired as they are within the labyrinth of the self.

Why are they mired within the labyrinth of the self?

Because parts of themselves have been left scattered along the way of their lives, fragments of two broad categories or kinds. Things that have happened that we would not have wished to happen, are overwhelmed by, and have not completely metabolized, and which have therefore left some part of us used up by the effort, some part of us left behind having incompletely apprehended and experienced the thing, whatever it was, such that it still lives in a part of us undigested, which is a way of speaking about the traumatic. To a lesser degree things that have frightened or angered us, raised our temperatures, and to which we have incompletely responded with motion, such that their incompleteness leaves an ache in the form of a gestural gap: some movement undone, in word or deed, that would signal to the deepest gateways inward (these are literally neurological gates in the brain) that we have set down this happening, again whatever it was, and the presence of which leaves the blood yet stirred in response to something that is no longer happening but that has not been released. These are the first category.

And things that we would wish to happen that have not happened, and into which we have therefore not been initiated, which is a way of speaking about neglect at one level, but more broadly is a way of speaking to the awareness that we have been marooned, we moderns, outside of a culture in any true sense of the word, which at its depths implies a wisdom capable of leading us to the throne, which is synonymous with leading us Home. Capital H.

The home to which you are really seeking to return is a psychographic location as much as it is a landscape, yet to call it inner misses the point, which is that if we actually contact the Real, actually find our way to the throne and can sit down upon it, the Sovereignty awakened thereby is nowhere *not* at home, because we have landed in the unutterable engine from which Being emanates, which some people call the Ground of Being, yet Ground here is a metaphor for something that is not gravitationally directional yet is rather omni-dimensionally in contact with the Real. From that place, experientially, Reality is not merely beneath our feet: we are surrounded: there is nowhere it is not touching us.

Let us call these two categories that restrict our contact with the unknown Real broadly *the traumatic*, and *the bereft*. One is things that have happened and that we have not completely recovered from, leaving parts of ourselves stuck behind or outside; the other are things that have not happened, and therefore yet unfolded upon the developmental origami of initiation, and about those we know nothing because we have not experienced them.

The first category of these, the traumatic, leads to automaticity, because choicefulness is the fruit of unity. To be in direct relation with Reality, capital R, requires all of us to be present, and the facticity of our fragmentation, the fact that we are cleaving off little parts of ourselves that have not made it through experiences that have happened to us, means that our bodies are woven and still carrying pockets of little localized death, places where the pliant flow of vitality has evaporated. I do not mean this metaphorically in the least. There is an autonomic science descriptive of these residual pockets (or more pervasively bodies) of mortification, parts of us stranded in winters of the body, frozen and unavailable to our greater unity.

Since apprehension of the unknown Real requires all of us to be united, these pockets of deadness in the body, which are trying to find their way to the surface and exhibit somber magnetism upon our trajectories, prevent such contact. Mired in our own stories of suffering, contracted into density, many retreat into chambers of cognition. Cognition does not touch the Real, for the Real is endlessly and eternally present, and never was a thought born that is not in the past or the future.

Dangers that arouse, things that have frightened us or angered us also pull. Their magnetism is not total, neither is it subterranean like the deadnesses, but active. We like, we dislike: we draw toward or away. This frightens us and so we avoid, this angers us and so we confront; yet here again our transit through space is marked by the compulsion to respond, preference this way or that, and so the present is marked by the past, pulling and pushing, we walk the path like drunks, staggering sometimes shadowboxing and sometimes fleeing the residue of ghosts from the past, the remnants of whose perturbations colors our present.

The labyrinth of self is the inertia created by these degradations of our limpidity and fluidity, into envelopes of steam and pockets of ice that live in the body and halo it, for there is no place else for them to live given their ties to our neurology and biochemistry.

The science of Autonomics was developed to address these aspects of neural automaticity as a result of deviations from our foundations in safety and connection, yet in the same way that the absence of danger is not safety, nor is the absence of illness vitality, it is not enough to merely clear the body of residual shutdown and activation: there is some affirmative relationship with Reality toward which we must direct ourselves.

In *The Neurobiology of Connection*, the first book in this trilogy, I wrote extensively about this pathway *towards*: a pathway in the direction of wellbeing that is ultimately a pathway in the direction of relating with *All That Is*. Through this movement from safety to connection to interoception to intuition to relating we can find ourselves back in horizontal relation with the Creation of which we are a part and from which we have become alienated. This is a movement into wellbeing that rebirths the body's latent potentialities for self-healing; moves us neurologically and metabolically into the burning of a more refined fuel in the body, takes off the jagged edges of activation, shakes off the deadened constriction of shutdown, and brings us humming into coordination of the fundamental autonomic systems is such a way that we become shimmeringly available to contact, inward and out. Again, this is not abstract in the least: when we move into this place we can feel is as limpidity in the body; its inner awakeness to vibration, its resonance with feeling. It is not necessarily emotional; though it is quite often tinged with feeling. In its vicinity we shiver awake.

Yet there is also a place in consciousness, an unmoving inward fulcrum, anchored immeasurably deep toward which we can orient, a center from which awareness can begin to emanate, and toward which we can train ourselves: I call this direction *sovereignty*. When I speak of this sovereignty, I am not merely talking about becoming the King or the Queen, I am not speaking of the external trappings of royalty at all, and we need to do some associative cleansing of these words because they are rife with obscuring associations.

The sovereignty toward which I am pointing has nothing to do with *authority* (*archon, auctoritas, potestas, imperium*) which is the Latinate derivation of most words for the Imperial (the Emperor). All of these words presence the notion of power over; of hierarchical structure.

What I am speaking toward is almost the opposite of this because it is under, or in service, to Everything. The sovereignty toward which I am pointing is accountability to the Real.

The more ancient Macedonian language, proto-Greek, from which this word derives, which was also translated as chief, king, or Emperor, is completely different. The word is *basileus*, and it means 'the Living Law'.

This sovereignty, innate and yet obscured, can arise as residual accumulations of autonomic defensive pattern are cleared, as we begin to come back into contact with the spontaneous throughput of our vitality, yet we are constantly shirking it because we do not recognize what liberation looks like and unless we have spent considerable time in its presence, or with texts or traditions that can point us to its visceral attributes, we have almost no idea what it means, how it feels, or what it looks like.

Liberation from the suffering of the contracted self is not vacation and it is not affluence: it is not a holiday, nor is it insulation from the vicissitudes of life: it is accountability to inhabit and occupy fully authentic the beingness gifted us. When this happens, the ordinary egoic self stops being the decision-maker. It dissolves because there is no contraction around which it can organize, and the ordinary sense of self most of us experience is in fact our inward gripping around a contraction to avoid relationship.

The radicality of what this actually looks like is alarming to those of us who have been socialized into a modern world, via factory schooling, into the utilitarian psychic economy of capitalism where we are existentially valid to the extent that we are useful to profit. To call it non-conforming would be an under-statement of the obvious. It doesn't give an actual fuck about conforming to anything other than the necessity of the Real. This makes it deeply inconvenient in a political economy consummately focused on trade, for it has little use for social niceties, no reason for accommodating, no use for being fawned over, no patience for being elevated. Like a still pool, it endlessly reflects; equally at home in stillness or in motion, receptive or directive. It has both complete optionality, and total allegiance to utility. It doesn't do anything, yet everything can be done through it.

The place in consciousness from which this happens is without friction. There is no apparent effort. When it is happening through us it draws on an inexhaustible supply of energy.

This is why, in the Tao te Ching (this is the Stephen Mitchell translation), it says

The ancient Masters were profound and subtle.

Their wisdom was unfathomable.

There is no way to describe it; all we can describe is their appearance.

They were careful as someone crossing an iced-over stream.

Alert as a warrior in enemy territory.

Courteous as a guest.

Fluid as melting ice.

Shapable as a block of wood.

Receptive as a valley.

Clear as a glass of water.

Do you have the patience to wait till your mud settles and the water is clear?

Can you remain unmoving till the right action arises by itself?

The Master doesn't seek fulfillment.

Not seeking, not expecting, she is present, and can welcome all things.

When we are in felt relational contact with someone who is operating from this place in consciousness, we can, if we are discerning, feel the degree to which what is arising from them, in word and action, is coming through them with authority (there is no equivocation, no apology in the place from which sovereignty emanates): yet an authority that does not belong to them; is not private; is not owned; is in fact no different than the wind in the trees or the crackle of the fire or the warning call of the dark-eyed junco or the deep silent animal communication of the head of a herd of horses whose band arrayed around it responds to its directive with motion and intent even though the old horse stands with eyes closed and unmoving.

A person standing in this sovereignty does not command through whimsy, or personal preference. Rather, like the horsetail growing in the middle of the stream, or the bamboo flexing in the wind, whose strength comes from the emptiness in its center, both plants a perfect cylinder, a radius in a flow, such sovereignty governs through its adherence to the currents of the Real: its total lack of resistance to what is required. Governs through the necessity of rendering the emergence of beauty, governs through service to what is asking to unfold. This is why, moving in the opposite direction of imperial authority, which is top-down, it can be described as moving bottom-up from the Ground.

For Reality is budding in each and every moment, a bloom taking shaping, waiting to unfurl into petal. And yet this emergence can, like a bud, in no way be forced. It must open from inside, of its own wilfullness to come into contact with the expressed. The yearning in the heart of the flower whose becoming arrives is the same yearning in the caterpillar dissolved in the cocoon yearning for wings is the same yearning in the heart of the person humble enough to realize they are not yet Home.

You can of course wait, as the millenary religions would have you do, for the coming of the Savior, your further reward in Heaven, the pearly gates and all of that et cetera et cetera. But what if that yearning for homecoming is ripening now? What if you could release the machinations of the clenched egoic self most us are dragging around, the husk of rumination and the reflex of cognition dragging around a corpse resident in your brain and relax into the limpidity of being governed by another geometry altogether.

At first it would feel like dying, a dying off, a cessation. A dissolution of all familiar points of reference. Yet because death is only the obverse side of being born, it would also feel like being born upon the next breath. A contraction, an expansion: the Zen Master points out that this is the fundamental pattern of the Universe anyway.

Beyond the death, another birth, on the other side of that gap a far shore, and on that far shore awaits the true groundedness of the sovereign.

Meleté Thanatou, says Socrates. *Practice to die.*

PHYSIOLOGY

40 - The Grounding System

So what has become of these bodies of ours? Cut off at the roots by millenia of domination, suffering the downstream impacts and neurobiological sequelae of multi-generational trauma? How are we doing, we hybrids of angels and apes? How has this uprootedness, this inability to know ourselves in relation to the ground, this untetheredness, this floating heads upon sticks, both impacted and shaped our wellbeing?

I don't have to answer this question, really. Look around. How many people do you know that are experiencing the shimmering vitality that is the hallmark of human flourishing? But setting aside, for a moment, the glaringly obvious fact that most modern humans are not well, let us look specifically at the forms of illness that are the neurobiological sequelae of humans who have been uprooted and are no longer in ontological and existential contact with the Ground, capital G.

For the neurophysiological system impacted most centrally by all this– our oldest, deepest, and most primal autonomic system– five hundred million years ancient, a system that has existed since the prevailingly available common body plans had radial symmetry, like a starfish, are the unmyelinated deep belly vagal systems in the guts.

These systems are centered around your umbilicus (belly button), and boxed at the upper end by the respiratory diaphragm that separates the belly from the chest, the organs of digestion from your lungs. At the lower end, they are enboxed by your pelvic floor. They extend forward and back to fill the inner volume of your viscera, your broad sense of your belly, your tummy, your ventral side. The part of you that a dog, when showing submission, turns up. These are your deepest soft parts, unguarded by the cage of ribs, unshielded from the world. Even porcupine, armored with quills even on parts of her face, has a soft furred belly.

And in this soft belly of yours are arrayed the neurophysiological autonomic systems that we know as the Grounding System. Their role is dual. In the Chinese and Japanese lineages these systems were understood as the elixir field, the place where the body makes the elixir of life. Known as the *dantien*, or the *tanden*, or the *hara*, this neurological field is understood to be a fulcrum of deep identity, a center of primary authentic movement, origin of deepest knowing of embodied self. It accords with the understanding of Ayurveda, which speaks of the *agni*, the digestive fire, as the primary hearth of the body. Many of the foundational recommendations of Ayurveda, the five thousand year-old mother medicine of India, center on the maintenance and tuning of this central digestive hearth. Because, as you may or may not be aware, this central location of digestion is not merely digesting your food: it is digesting your experiences. It is also the location of 80% of the immune cells in your body, and a seat of the endocrine system. So this field, what we are calling the Grounding System, in its health-creating aspect, is the intersection of a neurological, immunological, and endocrine center of intelligence responsible for metabolizing food into fuel, and metabolizing experience into wisdom. Or not.

From it, not from the cranial brain, not from anywhere else in the body, come our deepest gut feelings. While we do not have a compelling word, in English, for the embodied ways of knowing centered in the viscera, there are other cultures that do. In Japanese, a *hara o waru*, or split-belly person, i.e., one whose deep belly is open, is 'one who speaks the truth.' In Yiddish, *kishkes* means the specific knowings that arise from the deep belly. When it is available to us autonomically as our deepest center, this part of ourselves is an organ of deepest orientation: an inward compass. It helps us know ourselves at the deepest level, know what is ok and what is not. The knowing of the deep belly does not engage with surfaces. It has no use for chit-chat, gossip, pleasantries, matters of the mundane. But if and when something of real depth occurs, something that matters at an existential level, you will feel it in your guts. And then, we can hope that our deepest inwardness will be available to orient us; available for us to respond from. We can hope and pray that when the shit really hits the fan, we can find ourselves in this deepest center; that we are not exiled from this umbilical connection to deepest self.

Unless, of course, because we have become disemboweled by domination, frozen by multi-generational trauma, and shutdown by encounters with a hostile extractive transactional world being governed by elected and un-elected demons, this deepest autonomic system has shut down. In this latter case, the scene we moderns inherit, many people today are walking around with a deep belly system that has been pushed from being the center of the digestive fire, the deepest inward hearth, into a scene of winter. It has frozen over, become ice.

The fire has been extinguished. The body shifted into lifethreat. Again and again and again.

41 - Diseases of the Grounding System

It's a good idea to be careful what you wish for, because sometimes your wish might come true. In the summer of 2024, I received a longed-for professional wish, in that one of the world's leading mitochondrial researchers introduced me to a functional medicine doctor he asserted was the most brilliant physician that he knew. This man, whose name I will withhold out of courtesy, is an internationally sought-out functional medicine doctor who treats complex chronic illness. People fly in to see him from all over the world. He has patients who will rent apartments near his office so that they can be close enough to work with him for a period of time. They come from the US, Canada, Europe- as far away as the Middle East.

Over the past several decades, the incidence of complex chronic illness in the developed world has skyrocketed. There is an enormous proliferation of disorders that include entire classes of auto-immune disease and inflammatory bowel disease. The explosion of allergies, food allergies, gluten-sensitivity, Celiac Disease, Inflammatory Bowel Disease, Crohn's Disease, dysbiosis, SIBO, ulcerative colitis, infections like candida, Clostridium difficile, H Pylori, MCAS (Mast Cell Activation Syndrome), Myalgic Encephalomyelitis/Chronic Fatigue Syndrome (ME/CFS), auto-immune and inflammatory disorders ranging from arthritis to variations of rheumatoid arthritis (there are more than 500 different kinds), to fibromyalgia, migraines, etc.

This physician is one of the world's more sought-out specialists for dealing with complex chronic illness. He has a soft voice, fashionable spectacles, wears a bracelet gifted to him by an indigenous tribe from the Amazon, has the bearing of a patient detective, and an encylopedic understanding of bodily systems. He is accustomed to working on the most complex and intractable cases. The mitochrondrial researcher introduced us because he knows that there is a substantive autonomic component to all of these illnesses. He thought I could help the doctor achieve better results with patients.

Does he live in the United States? I asked the researcher.

In Northern California, the researcher told me, *a town called San Rafael.*

I also happen to live in San Rafael, California. So that is how it happened. The physician and I met, and hit it off. Turns out we have a number of connections, and interests, in common. And so he started sending patients over to me, twenty minutes up the road, two ridgelines and three valleys away.

⊕

The Autonomic Nervous System contains the deepest and most powerful levers that govern your moment-to-moment experience of wellbeing. When we have an overwhelming experience that pushes us into lifethreat, the three primary autonomic systems de-coordinate.

When you are experiencing enough safety, which is itself pulsative in nature, this brings all three of your primary autonomic systems into rhythmic alignment. Like an orchestra with a fine conductor, the bass, the cello, the violins all come into fruitful dialog: the full dynamic range of symphonic rhythms become coordinated and available. This synchrony is health-creating: the dynamic neurophysiology of wellbeing.

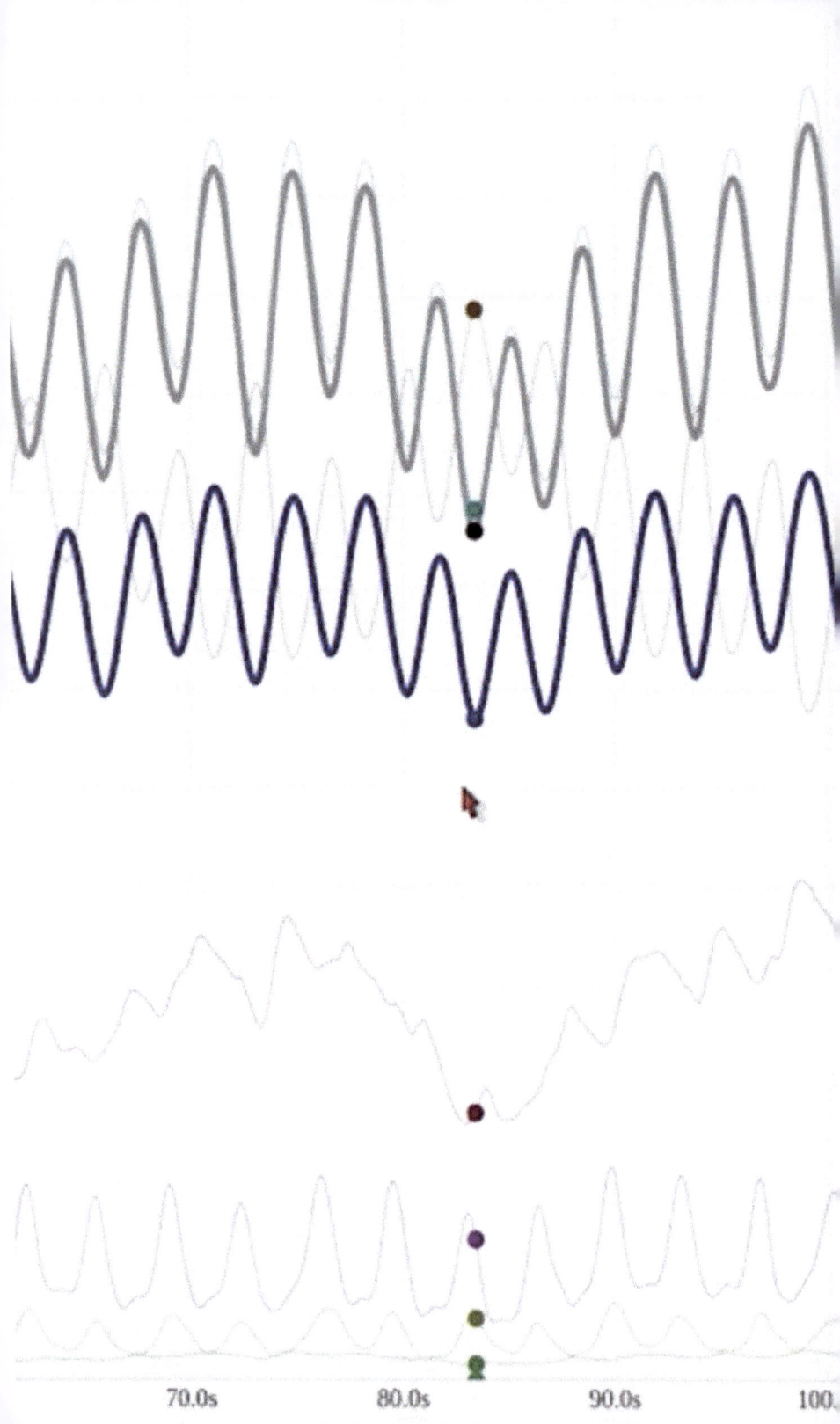

FACING PAGE: Sinusoidal coherence of autonomic waves stacking in a client whose autonomic systems are coordinated in a Connection state (©Heather MacDuffie, PhD & Samar Singh, PhD)

Absent the coordinating pulsation of safety and its affiliated neurochemistries of connection, the body moves into defensive responses, of which there are two primary categories. We have fight-or-flight responses, mediated by the spinal movement system (Movement System) – the movement architecture affiliated with the two hundred million year old vertebrate body plan, which coordinates Central Pattern Generators from the brainstem all the way down the spine, and organizes motor programs of attack and escape – in tandem with the activation chemistries of adrenaline and cortisol mediated by the HPA Axis. These are high-energy responses that have the twin characteristics of being mobilized (movement-based) and polarized (at a physiological level, our bodies discern who is with us and who is against us). The activation of this system is what most people think about when they think about stress.

Then we have the defensive response that is oldest, deepest, and most primal, and involves the most severe de-coordination of autonomic systems. This is the lifethreat response of the deep belly autonomic systems: what happens when every other autonomic system goes offline, and we are simply left with the oldest deepest immobilized sub-diaphragmatic gut architecture. This is the shutdown version of the Grounding System. Sudden winter in the body.

Usually, in my autonomics practice there is some detective work involved with discerning what specific defensive templates have been evoked in someone I am consulting with for complex dysfunction. There is a direct correlation between defensive autonomic templates and categories of illness. Certain classes of auto-immune disease, for example, arise from appeasing. Anxiety follows directly from chronicity of the flight response. The patients that the physician sent me?

All of them had the same fundamental autonomic profile: a decade or more in one of the three variants of the shutdown response. They were some of the sickest humans I have encountered. Nearly all of them had *extreme* digestive dysfunction, their digestive motility compromised so severely some of them had to have nourishment introduced into their bloodstreams directly through a port. All of them were dealing with various forms of mold toxicity, many of them had Lyme disease, nearly all of them had an entire host of immunological issues.

What I would like you to understand here is the following. Everyone on earth has mold exposure. Have you ever eaten peanut butter? Apple butter? Cherry Jam? Everyone is eating mold all of the time. Some people have more exposure, to be sure, or live in a home with it, but our environment is rife with pathogens. They are in the air, the water, the soil. Most people, whose Grounding Systems are functioning at least fractionally, whose digestive processes are intact, fight these things off routinely, as a matter of course. Your body does this so constantly that you do not realize it is happening. It is part of the everyday work of your immune system.

Yet if someone gets stuck in a prolonged or chronic state of shutdown; if their Grounding System truly shuts down, there are certain characteristic features of the way that wellbeing will be compromised. A sequence is set in motion: here is what happens–

Your body endures prolonged (or momentary) exposure to a lifethreat. The part of you that determines whether or not something is a lifethreat is not your ordinary sense of self, but rather your *autonomic self*, which is deeper, older, and more embodied. In the event of a lifethreat that puts you into a shutdown response,

1. Your autonomic systems de-coordinate.

2. The pulsation of safety is required to coordinate gut mo-

tility, because it is effectively a carrier wave that moves from the mouth southward to the anus, and must be passed from the evolutionarily newest autonomic system (Connection System) to the Movement System, to the Grounding System. In a lifethreat response, the Connection System and the Movement Systems go offline.

3. As gut motility decreases, the carrier wave pulsing food and experience southward slows. (Digestive motility decreases.)

4. The mechanism of the lifethreat response is connected to a 500-million-year-old diving reflex designed to radically conserve energy. This reflex inhibits breath.

5. Although the brain accounts for merely 2% of our body weight, the organ consumes nearly half our daily carbohydrate intake. Under acute stress it requires 12% more energy, and if the upstream hypothalamic gatekeeper (the nucleus arcuatus (ARH)) detects that the brain lacks glucose, it demands carbohydrates. In plain language, you crave sugar.

6. As digestive motility slows and breath is inhibited, the upper parts of the guts begin to de-oxygenate.

7. As the guts begin to de-oxygenate, their pH changes.

8. The gut microbiome is a garden. As any gardener knows, plants (in this case micro-organisms) are extremely sensitive to context. In a garden of plants, primary inputs include sun, water, nutrient flows, and soil composition. In the micro-biome, the equivalent is oxygen, pH, available food, motility (governs the speed at which material moves, or fails to move through as it is decomposing), and chemical context (e.g., what chemicals, endogenous or exogenous (i.e., produced by the micro-biome itself)) are present

9. As the gut motility drops, the pH changes, and you attempt to address the brain's need for more glucose by adding sugar, the microbiome is increasingly disrupted.

10. With changes in pH, the climate is less hospitable to beneficial bacteria (we digest our food in collaboration with trillions of specific micro-organisms). Some we absolutely need to even extract and synthesize classes of nutrients. As the Cleveland Clinic explains, "Bacteria in your gut help break down certain complex carbohydrates and dietary fibers that you can't break down on your own. They produce short-chain fatty acids — an important nutrient — as byproducts. They also provide the enzymes necessary to synthesize certain vitamins, including B1, B9, B12 and K."

11. Sugar eliminates certain types of bacteria that support classes of immune cells in the guts.[1]

12. As the bacteria we need diminish (think of this as the garden being filled with the plants you need) synthesis of required byproducts decreases, and the bacteria that we do not want to be there flourish (think of this as the garden filling up with weeds), there are increasingly systemic and predictable adverse effects.

Typically bacteria that we do not want, which are also breaking things down and excreting waste begin to cause digestive issues through several parallel and sometimes simultaneous pathways. Bacteria are eating and pooping, to put it bluntly. Beneficial bacteria poop things you eat (again, kind of gross but true, such as micro-nutrients). Harmful bacteria poop things that poison you. In tandem with this, they can disrupt the tight junctions between intestinal epithelial cells, creating larger gaps in the intestinal walls. The way that your intestines work is to selectively filter molecules from your food

[1] Microbiota imbalance induced by dietary sugar disrupts immune-mediated protection from metabolic syndrome, https://pubmed.ncbi.nlm.nih.gov/36041436/

and allow certain of them to pass into your blood stream as nutrition. You can imagine that having these molecules filtered correctly is both an extremely important, and an extremely chemically nuanced process.

Part of the reason that there is such an abundance of immune cells in the digestive system is because this is a primary place where things from outside of you (e.g., the food you have eaten passing through your inward pipes) are coming into contact with what is inside of you, and your immune system needs to monitor this filtration membrane closely. Disruption of the intestinal barrier, which is known as leaky gut, is the physical disruption of this fine filter of the epithelial cells in the intestinal wall. It can occur from bacterial excretion that irritates the epithelial cells, in tandem with reduction in the anti-inflammatory immune cells that need the proper balance of intestinal flora in order to flourish.

This negative feedback loop can lead to increased permeability of the intestinal lining, which can pass toxins and bacterial components into your blood stream. If this happens, it triggers an inflammatory immune response from the body that releases inflammatory cytokines systemically.

This entire process leads quickly to bloating, gas, diarrhea, constipation, and intestinal pain. But if the autonomic conditions undergirding this response do not shift, and the lifethreat state endures, the body enters an increasingly compromised feedback cycle.

It becomes internally cellularly compromised, in the form of an increasingly systemic cell danger response that Robert Naviaux, mitochondrial medicine researcher and Director of the Naviaux lab at UCSD has written about extensively. The metabolic climate of your cells becomes compromised. As this happens, they begin dumping ATP, which is their primary fuel, into the extra-cellular matrix, where it is highly toxic. This response causes local sites in the body to stop taking autonomic direction from the central nervous system, such that even if the CNS is sending signals of safety, the compromised cells cannot hear them.

It becomes immunologically compromised, as the immune system is forced to contend with molecular intrusion of magnitude, and a proliferation of toxic molecules incorrectly entering the bloodstream. The person become exponentially more likely to be adversely impacted by environmental contaminants, including mold, more prone to developing Lyme disease and other opportunistic infections.

The body becomes increasingly autonomically compromised, because the ANS is constantly scanning for both external and internal lifethreat cues. If the interior of the body is filling up with toxic byproducts of leaky digestion, as well as toxic bacterial metabolites, the ANS begins to re-inforce the lifethreat signals from within the body. This feedback loop, which puts people deeper into shutdown, is now running on internal (endogenous) momentum.

In parallel, the body becomes increasingly immunologically compromised, more and more likely to be unable to stop infections of all kinds. Things like mold and candida that are in the external and internal environment anyway are no longer kept in check.

It was in this state that most of the patients the physician sent me were residing. All of them had chronic fatigue, brain fog, movement limitations. All of them had extreme digestive issues, nearly all of them had extreme immunological issues. This is the neurobiological sequelae of having your Grounding System shut down for long timespans.

Once this process is in full swing, autonomic intervention is no longer effective in shifting autonomic baselines, because there are too many feedback loops engaged. And guess what? The prevalence of these types of responses, in the general population, is increasing exponentially.

42 - Eat More Dirt

In 2007 I took a trip to the Brazilian rainforest with about fifteen other Americans. We travelled to Manaus, in the state of Amazonas, where the Rio Negro and the Rio Solimoes unite to form the mighty Amazon. From there we boarded a rickety bus and drove several hours deep into rainforest, where we spent four days working with about fifty Brazilians preparing a tea commonly known as ayahuasca.

Before we took the bus into the forest, we drank the sacred tea in an outdoor temple on the outskirts of the city. Surrounded by a shrieking field of insect noise, about a hundred and fifty of us gathered in a metal-roofed structure in a relatively urban garden. At some point it rained, the water turning the tin roof into a mesmerizing drum. When the ceremony ended, at about two in the morning, I found myself wandering the lit pathways of the garden, studying the plants. God I love the plants in the Amazon. I love plants anyway, but the just absolutely wacky structural and architectural innovations of rainforest plants crater my mind. It was really late at night, and I was wandering around this garden, kneeling down periodically to look at flowers, studying leaves, an onrush of Portuguese all around, the smell of soup wafting: totally in my element. Underneath the arching canopy of a giant leaf I discovered a cluster of bats the size of your thumb.

The earth was an ochre color. It carries these hues, which look like the distillate form of oil paints: umbers, ochres, deep reddish hues, because of aluminum and iron oxide in the soil. I was kneeling down, studying it, looking at the lichen, the moss, the intricate micro-world of the soil and its tiny inhabitants when I started thinking about the micro-organisms. I was still feeling the rise and fall of waves of energy from the sacred tea, patterns of light swirled through my visual field eyes open, my perceptions were refined. It occurred to me that just about all of the micro-organisms in the soil here were alien to my body- I had never been in the Amazon before and that therefore my immune system was not going to be able to identify them. I had a vivid image of food poisoning then, and sat down on the ground. And with my butt on the earth, it suddenly occurred to me that it would be pretty easy to inoculate myself against this by introducing my body to them in a titrated fashion.

I'm not sure I would have done this in an ordinary state of consciousness; I'm not sure it would have seemed like a good idea. But what I did next was to move off the path into a part of the garden where it didn't look like any person (or any dogs) had been walking- I didn't wanna eat something off the bottom of someone's shoe or ingest a piece of dogshit- kneel down, pinch the earth to get the top layer off, grab a bit of soil between my fingers, and nibble at it. I let the dirt move around on my tongue, felt the particle size. There were some little rocks, some grains of sand, and some clay that shifted into a slurry as my spit moistened it. I sat there, closed my eyes, and swallowed this material.

I imagined my body meeting billions of tiny micro-organisms in this pristine particle of rainforest earth. Moss, lichen, and many tiny creatures. I imagined my immune cells arriving on the scene like so many tiny detectives with little magnifying glasses, beholding this strange array of diminutive creatures they had never seen before.

Eventually someone called me, and I found my wife and we drove home through the sodium lights in this old Amazonian cowboy town. When we got back to the place we were staying, maybe an hour and a half later, I chased the soil with a dose of colloidal silver (an anti-microbial) and went to sleep. By day five of the trip every single American had food poisoning except myself.

American children's immune systems are failing to fully develop because children are not eating enough dirt. To be of a place– to be grounded in a place, to be part of it– is to become one with it, and to become one with a place is to bring it into you, not simply metaphorically or emotionally or spiritually, but molecularly.

In Manaus I had done something immunologically courteous for my Grounding System– I had introduced it to a new place with intention.

Our immune systems develop through adequate challenge, and in a world where mothers are walking around with sanitizing wipes, where we are wiping down surfaces, our children's fingers, sterilizing play areas, and keeping kids indoors, they are not having enough molecular contact with the soil constituents of place to develop healthy immune systems. We don't feel comfortable acknowledging the degree to which we are animals. We are not comfortable with the biological facticity of this, with the reality that we ooze. We want a sort of sanitized world of right angles, napkins to absorb menstrual blood, corners with no dust, deodorant and anti-perspirant and no dirt behind anyone's ears. But we are animals, of the Living World, and we have to get more comfortable with blood and pus and mucus and bodily fluids and grime, because we come from them and we need them in order to survive.

When babies are born, they are slicked with vaginal mucus, and if they are born vaginally they are also coated with the mother's poop. Our first impulse is to wipe it all off without realizing it is all a brilliant immunological inoculation. The baby's first instinct is to climb up the mother's belly and attach to the breast, which would ideally happen wet and slimey if we could handle it, where the mother's body is going to produce colostrum, which is a close relative of pus or mucus, and contains enormous doses of the immunological material that the baby needs to keep it alive, having moved out of an inward ocean encased in velvet jelly into a world of blaring lights and honking horns and a blizzard of pathogens trying to kill you. The baby has no immune system at first- so the mother's immune system stands in for them. Mother's milk dynamically adjusts its immunological content based on pathogen exposure, so if there is flu going around, mommy's breastmilk is going to contain specific antibodies that baby needs.

Grounding means getting comfortable again (or for the first time) with the reality that we are animals, as dependent on the Living World as a baby is upon its mother.

Because it is our deepest inwardness, most people do not fully consider that our digestive system is in direct contact with the external world. What do you do all day long? You dump things from outside of you into it. You pour in liquids, and you chew up solids- things from the outer world- and these go into the deepest and most inward tube of you, where they slowly migrate southward through the wandering conduit of your intestines, as you extract what you can, pull the water out, and solidify the remainder into a turd.

People don't want dirt under their fingernails, but by law in the United States, the cherry jam that you just ate can contain up to 30% mold. If you ate it on a peanut butter sandwich, you've also just eaten at least one rodent hair and thirty fragments of insect, and peanut butter is one of the most controlled foods on the FDA list. You don't even want to know what is permissible in a hot dog. Let me just say that you've been dining on way more rodent feces than you'd care to know about for far longer than you would care to remember. Rat shit is part of what makes hotdogs great again. So the notion that you have mold exposure because there is mold in your house? Dude, you just ate a mold sandwich.

If your Grounding System is working properly, that's not a

problem. You've been eating mold sandwiches your entire life. (As a brief aside here, let me just note that if you do not want to eat mold sandwiches, you may specifically wish to refrain from eating cherry jam, and apple butter. And if you are not an enormous fan of eating insect parts, you probably don't want to eat cinnamon or black pepper again ever.) The point I'm making is that you find it disgusting to eat dirt, but you are eating dirt every single day of your life. The fact is that you get sick because you are not eating enough of it.

To be grounded means, in part, that we are eating the earth in the places we reside. Have a garden? Wash your vegetables a bit carelessly, that's what I'm saying.[1]

---

[1] Unless of course they have pesticides on them, or your garden soil is contaminated. But then you have other problems.

43 - Trinity

The primary purview of my work is autonomic physiology, and my most focused and longest running study is of the neurophysiology of the Autonomic Nervous System. Yet with the Grounding System specifically, although it is one of the three primary autonomic systems, we just cannot reasonably understand it without understanding its interaction with the immune and endocrine systems. I would go so far as to say that if we are looking at the body in terms of its functional organization, it makes more sense to think of the Grounding System as a sort of tri-system product (autonomic x immune x endrocrine) than it makes sense to think of them as three different systems sharing inputs. The integration is so tight, and so comprehensive, with such direct systemic effects on your overall experience that conceptualizing them as an integrated functional unit just makes more sense.

⊕

Digestion is an incredibly sophisticated gatekeeping function. Into the top of the tube you pour food and liquid, some of which your body will allow to enter your bloodstream, some of which is undigestible by the body (fiber, etc.), and some of which is straight-up toxic (mold, mouse droppings, insect parts, etc.). The dance of differentiation whereby your body determines what is nutrient, and should therefore be passed into the blood system as food or fuel, versus what is undigestible (excrete) or toxic (engulf and destroy) is an incredibly sophisticated act of filtration. In the digestive system, in addition to filtration based on particle size, roving immune cells pick through and pick off the things that could harm us. Add to the mix trillions of micro-organisms, some symbiotic, some irrelevant, some potentially damaging. The symbiotic organisms are breaking down food and creating nutritive products: these need to pass into the body. Irrelevant and toxic byproducts need to be protected from entering the body and either engulfed or excreted.

Part of what determines what passes from the digestive system into the blood is a question of mechanical filtration: the epithelial cells of the colon are tightly knit together, so large molecules cannot pass across for the same reason that the pasta doesn't fall through a colander: the holes are too small. Yet under sustained conditions of lifethreat, which predictably lead to various kinds of inflammatory bowel conditions, the tight junctions of the epithelial cells gap. When we look at the neurobiological sequelae of shifting into a prolonged lifethreat state, we find three factors coming together whose typical result is the perturbation of the mucosal layer and tight junctions of epithelial cells in the intestine that keep the filtration barrier intact and correctly differentiating what your body needs from what it cannot digest or what will harm it.

Safety is pulsative in nature, and the pulsation of safety literally coordinates our three autonomic systems: the Connection, Movement, and Grounding Systems, establishing the rhythmicity that draws foods from the mouth, through the digestive tract, and out the anus. If you watch the whole body of an infant sucking and swallowing, as Paula Garbourg, the Developer of the Paula Method did, you notice that the pulse of suck-and-swallow happens not merely at the top end of the baby's body, where you would expect, but all the way down at the bottom. The baby's anus is also pulsing, because we are observing a continuous rhythm passed all the way down the inner tube of the body.

Loss of safety disrupts this coordinated autonomic rhythmicity, and many other physiological rhythms. As these rhythms de-coordinate digestive motility drops. In the same way that a conveyer belt in a factory moves parts through it with a consistent velocity such that workers have a defined time period where the part they are responsible for passes by them, digestive motility is moving food through the intestines on a cadence. If the conveyor belt stops and starts, if it seizes and pauses, it is easy to imagine that work does not proceed as planned. Constipation is the cessation of digestive motility, while diarrhea is its explosive counterpoint. The quality of the product reaching the end of the tunnel tells us a good deal about its progress down the conveyor belt. When we have good digestive motility and the proper microbiome available to help us digest, the product is nicely formed and of uniform consistency. When there is poor digestive motility and we are having issues with the microbiome, we get rocks or splatter-paint.

Physicians will prescribe pepto-bismol, stimulant laxatives, and stool softeners for issues of digestive motility, but I've never heard of one prescribing safety. Yet if we go upstream far enough, to the source of the disruption of digestive motility, what we find every single time is that we have stopped neurocepting sufficient safety to coordinate all three autonomic systems.

There are two primary autonomic responses to threat, and while the simplified version of this includes a set of mobilized danger responses (fight-or-flight) and immobilized lifethreat responses (shutdown) the lived reality is more nuanced. Defensive patterns become grooved through use, and are also epi-autonomic, which means that we learn them in the context of family, community, and culture. They can also combine– the freeze response that has become popularly known since Peter Levine published *Waking the Tiger*, is technically called 'tonic immobility', which is a hybrid of fight-or-flight and shutdown states: imagine a deer in headlights, both rigid and immobilized. There are also many variants of the appease response, which overlays a defensive response (fight-flight, or shutdown) with elements of sociality to defuse the threat. My point is that there is a broad landscape of potential ways the body may respond to lack of safety, and for most people in the general population, who have not studied or thought about this very much, the particular ways the body responds are not well understood, either conceptually or experientially.

The shutdown response is a 500-million-year-old diving reflex that evolved at a time in our evolutionary history where the body plans of organisms were radially symmetric. Imagine a starfish. In the center of the body is the mouth and anus, where the organism ingests and excretes. At this point in our deep evolutionary history, predators did not have strong vision. They detected prey through movement and metabolic rate. The first and most ancient defensive response to lifethreat was this ancient diving reflex, which immobilizes the body and sends the metabolic rate plunging. Immobilized and with metabolism nearly shutdown organisms became undetectable to predators. Part of the mechanism of this shutdown response is a severe inhibition on breath.

Anybody who is in a shutdown response has neural inhibition on breathing. This is something you know anecdotally from your own experience. If you have every gone to see a really scary movie, you will notice, periodically, that when you are most afraid you are holding your breath. Breathing simply stops. We don't do it on purpose. It is a neurological cessation of breath; a prolonged apnea. The breathing central pattern generator is extremely sensitive to endogenous opioids.

If this has chronicity, it has very predictable effects on the digestive system. Our entire microbiome is conditioned on precise oxygen gradients within the human intestinal tract. Roughly, the deeper you get into the tube, the less oxygen is present. Although it was long thought to be a sterile organ, the stomach does in fact contain a core microbiome. There is more of the microbiome in your small intestine, yet most of it resides in the large intestine (colon). Oxygen requirements to maintain a healthy microbiome in the stomach are highest, they decrease along gradients as we move into the small intestine, and eventually the colon. Most of the microbial activity in the colon is actually anaerobic. Yet in addition to conditions inside the cavity itself, the entire digestive system is wrapped in a vascular and lymphatic network critical for nutrient transport and tissue oxygenation. And this system has high oxygen requirement.

During sustained conditions of stress, both fight-flight and shutdown, there are alterations to the oxygenation of the digestive system both within the cavity itself and in the surrounding vascular systems. Chronicity of stress responses also places metabolic demand on the body, leading us to alter our diets in characteristic ways.

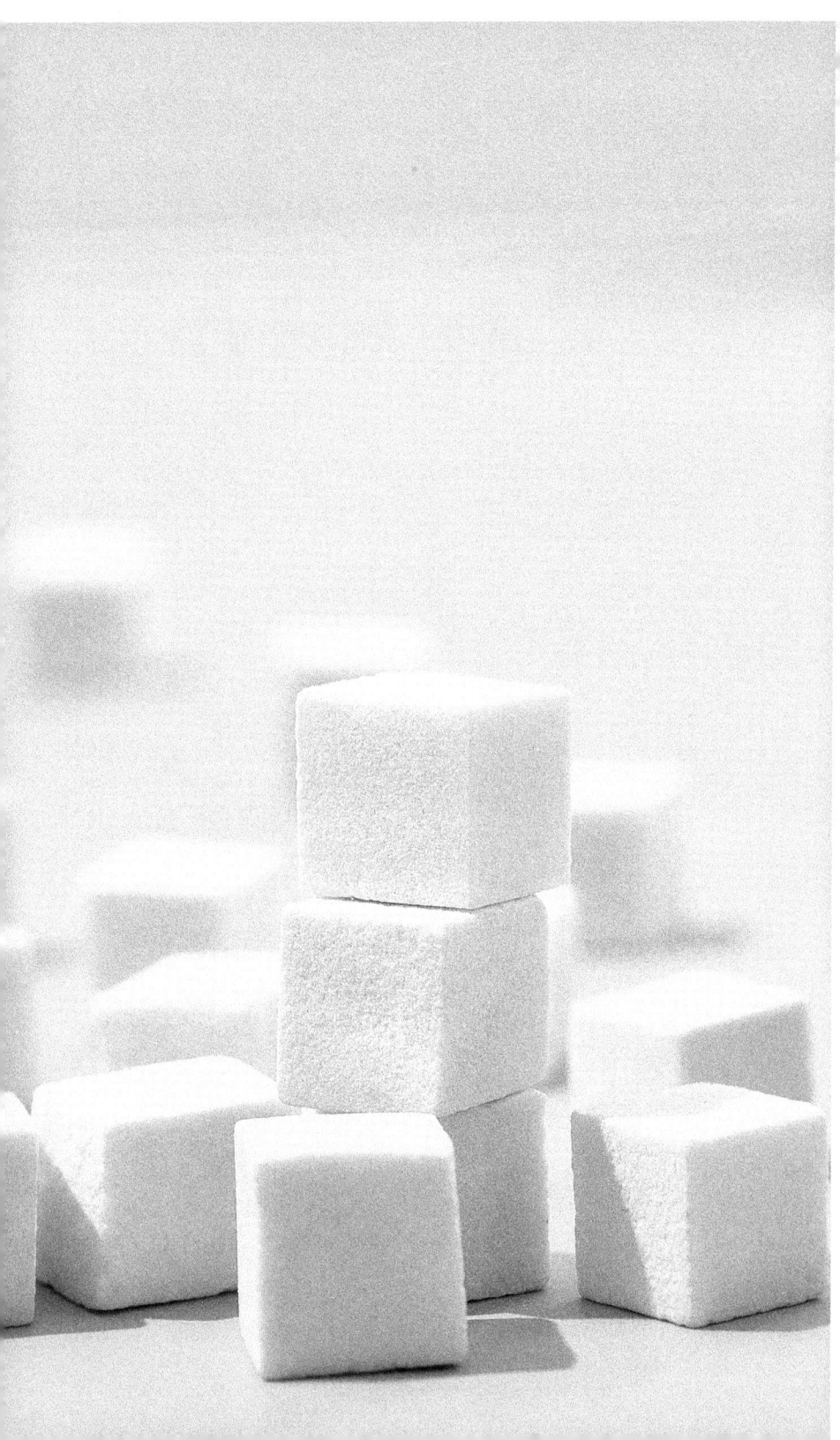

44 - Refined Sugar

Humans began extracting sugar from cane about six thousand years ago in India and Southeast Asia. By the first centuries AD, refinements of manufacture had led to a burgeoning sugar industry in India, where the crystalline granules were pressed into cakes and later cones, and considered for the next 1500 years to be an exotic spice. The plant – *Saccharum officinarum* – and the methods of sugar production eventually spread around the world. The expansion of the Islamic empire in the Middle Ages brought sugar to the Mediterranean, and then into Europe. In 1493, the second voyage of Christobol Colon introduced sugarcane seedlings to the 'New World'.

From the perspective of our deep evolutionary history, sugar is both an anomaly, and almost a perfect food. In our seven million year evolutionary history– if you count the origins of humanity in the moments we descended from the trees, moved onto the savannah, and shifted to a bipedal stance– for most of our lineage history we have struggled to obtain enough calories to survive. Of particular delight to our brains and Central Nervous Systems, and the degree to which they light up our reward centers is proof of this– are fats and carbohydrates. Fats are used to build brains and Central Nervous Systems. Most of what males are attracted to in females, at a biological level, turn out to be signals of fertility, and human fertility requires very specific kinds of fat.

Carbohydrates are what we burn metabolically to function, and so our bodies break down food into sugar (glucose). Refined sugar, which is made of– wait for it– refined sugar, mainlines cellular fuel into the body.

Accustomed as we are to its availability, we moderns take sugar for granted. But I want to invite you to see if you can remember the first time you ate a piece of chocolate cake? Or a candy bar? When I was about six years old, every Saturday morning, I would get an allowance of one quarter, and I would promptly march myself up to a corner store in Walpole, New Hampshire and buy a Mounds bar. If you've never had a Mounds bar, first of all I am very sorry, and second of all you should stop reading this book right now, go out into the world, and purchase one. I really don't know what you are waiting for.

Where I grew up in the Connecticut River valley, you could plant corn, and beans, and squash, but I understood innately that coconut was a sort of edible celestial sphere that only grew in tropical climes of bluest sky, in the presence of ultramarine waters, and that when shaved tasted like eating tiny bits of angel wings. A Mounds bar aggregated these heavenly shavings into a dense pillow held together by sweet nectar, and enrobed the mass in dark chocolate.

I experienced desire for Mounds bars that I can only properly call sexual. In late adolescence, when I really wanted a girl– the tenor of that yearning was the fuller expression of what my six-year old self awaited on Saturday mornings.

I do not remember the first time I ate a Mounds bar. I do, however, remember what happened the one time that my friend Galen convinced me to trade my precious allowance for Laffy Taffy. I was only fooled once. In a gesture of openness to novelty, I traded my quarter for something that was not a Mounds bar, and opened the package. I tried to take a bite. If Galen was not standing right there, happily chewing at his own taffy, I would have thought he was trying to pull a fast one on me. In a world where there were no consequences for your actions, the level of disgust and outrage that came over me as it dawned on me that I was going to have to go an entire week without eating a Mounds bar, that I had traded my precious once-a-week opportunity to chew at something that looked and tasted like a rubber tongue, I might have climbed onto the counter, grabbed the attendant by the shirt collar, and screamed, "GIMME MY MONEY BACK NOW! I NEED A MOUNDS BAR." This is, I think, a pretty clear sign of the addictive power of sugar, when a six-year old is thinking about threatening a grown-up store clerk because his supply has been cut off by his own folly.

The kind of sugar we buy by the kilo is not available in nature, for the same reason that the kind of heroine that we inject is not available in nature. They are both the highly refined condensate of something that occurs in nature in a much less potent form. To turn the sap of the opium poppy into heroine, you have to concentrate its chemical constituents. To arrive at the sugar we know, you have to take an incredible amount of sugarcane, crush it to get the juice, and boil down the juice, evaporating off the water. Sugarcane juice is already very sweet. On a visit to the Caribbean once I sucked on a section of cane, which just tastes like sugar water. But the stuff we grew up on, sold by the carton in the baking aisle at the grocery store, the stuff baked into cakes, and folded into chocolate, is pharmaceutical grade.

It is addictive at a level that we moderns do not understand, because we are already all addicted to it, and therefore desensitized. In order to understand the level at which it is addictive, you have to read stories about people encountering it for the first time. And these stories abound. Uncontacted Amazonian tribes that come into contact with sugar for the first time will trade nearly anything for it.

Part of its extraordinary efficacy, like most of the substances that we become easily addicted to, like opioids, is due to the way it locks into our bodily chemistry hand-in-glove. We get easily addicted to heroine, or oxycontin, or fentanyl, because the body manufactures fifty different varieties of opioids endogenously, and so our Central Nervous Systems are full of receptors for them. We get addicted to sugar so easily because our digestive systems turn our food into sugar so that we can fuel our cells. Refined sugar is the end product of this assimilation.

As I noted in an earlier chapter, the brain is incredibly hungry for fuel. Although it represents only two percent of our mass, the brain and CNS consume nearly 40% of our available carbohydrates. And when we are stressed out, its demand increases further. At an anecdotal level, you already know this. Most of us, when stressed out, start craving salt, fat, and sugar. This is the direct result of increased metabolic demand for these substances by our brains and bodies.

There is a bit of a biological paradox here. The stress response, in our long evolutionary history, was designed to come on rapidly and then resolve. Its resolution, broadly speaking, takes place in the context of community. Although our ancestors in deep time had incredible levels of physical stress, they had almost no social stress. For many modern people, however, this equation is inverted. Many of us spend long spans on the couch (no physical stress), but are incredibly isolated (profound social stress). Modern people endure chronic, toxic, and traumatic stress on the regular. And the long-term activation of stress pathways creates metabolic demand in the brain that sends it seeking SUGAR.

Refined sugar, which you would be well advised to think of as a narcotic, has specific impacts on the digestive system, in which the Grounding System we are talking about is housed. Its presence creates a novel source of easily convertible fuel for bacteria that you do not want to feed, while undermining the symbiotic bacteria that you need. A direct and fairly immediate result of this is the degradation of specific immune cells whose thriving is tied to beneficial bacteria. Sugar is essentially fuel for bad bacteria, and destructive to immune cells you need to fight off infection.

In this way, it ties in with the other two primary drivers of digestive degradation– decreased motility in the gut and de-oxygenation of the guts to create a sort of dark trinity of feedback loops that disrupt the tight contact between epithelial cells in the lining of the intestine, separating what is in the colon from what enters your bloodstream.

45 -The Body is the Sacrifice Site

If we are going to think in intelligent and accurate ways about autonomic physiology, it is crucial that we do not divorce these conversations, which are at some level neurobiological, from the discourse and context of culture, because in many cases our accommodations to culture, family, and society, literally necessary to survive, have co-opted our physiological responses.

It is for this reason that this book opens with such a long disquisition on the denaturing consequences of empire, and the domination paradigm writ large. As Nkem Ndefo, Developer of the Trauma Resource Toolkit notes, "Fight and flight are privileged responses to threat." If you don't understand what she is saying (because at a biological level these responses are not privileged: they are part of our basic repertoire of defensive responses) it is possibly because either you are not occupying a social location where appeasing is regularly required of you, or because you don't realize the degree to which appeasing is normalized and demanded in hierarchical social situations.

The small child dealing with an angry father learns to appease as if his life depends on it. The single mother feeding her family learns to appease her boss as if her life depends on it.

I am a straight, white, heterosexual man and I don't think of myself as someone who appeases other people regularly in my daily life, but a recent occurrence brought something home to me that I believe is instructive in this regard. I was recently introduced by a well-known mentor to the host of a podcast with a notably large audience (several million people). He asked me to appear on the show and talk about our work in Autonomics. When I first learned about the guy, and his show, I was intimidated by the size of the audience. It made me nervous, and I also sensed it as a large opportunity for our work. You can perhaps feel already the double-edgedness of this. Fear on the one hand (feeling intimidated is to feel afraid, and to want to get smaller), and excitement on the other hand, the sensing of opportunity. You can recognize that if we strip this impulse down to the most basic movements that might represent them, one is a movement of trying to get smaller (a movement away), the other is a movement towards. It feels also relevant to note where in the body each of these impulses came from, because they were not the same place. My guts, the deep belly (the Grounding System) was the place that felt overwhelmed. My head (thinking) sensed opportunity.

After the introduction, I went and listened to the show several times. I listened to the host get interviewed by another famous podcaster, and then I listened to the interview he did with my friend and mentor. A propos of nothing I said to my wife, "I'm not going on that show without training him first." It felt clear to me, as a teacher of autonomic physiology, that if I was going to go on a show to talk about autonomic physiology in front of several million people I wanted the person interviewing me to have experienced what I was talking about.

I was on the threshold of moving when we made contact, and told him I needed to get to the other side of the move before we scheduled anything. Once we had completed the move I emailed him and got no reply. Several weeks went by, with me thinking about the podcast daily. I finally emailed him again, with the name of my mentor, who he had already interviewed, in the subject line. The response came back five minutes later, in a single sentence. I had, in my email, explained again that our move was complete, that my new book was out, that I was excited about sharing our work, and had asked him if he wanted me to mail him a copy. His reply: *Love it. Production team cc'd; they'll find us a time to record.*

What happened next was that I did nothing. What happened after that was that I got increasingly stressed out. I got stressed out at a level that I do not generally get stressed out, stressed out in a profound deep belly manner. Stressed out in a– *this is the neurobiological sequelae of shutdown*– manner.

Days passed with no word from the production team. One night we had a neighbor over for dinner, which I prepared, and as a housewarming gift she brought us a jar of pistachio paste from the Greek island where she summers. At the end of dinner I opened the container and sniffed at it. It had the texture of any smooth nut butter, and was greenish brown, as pistachios are. There was only one single ingredient: pistachios. Foregoing dessert, I sat down with a small spoon, and took a single bite. The concentration of flavor was immense: pistachios ground down to a paste. Over the course of about twenty minutes I ate four or five small spoonfuls. Our guest left, and I started getting ready for bed.

I'm not saying that I got food poisoning. All I'm saying is that if someone brings you an unrefrigerated food product from the other side of the world, of unclear provenance, the temperature and conditions under which it travelled unclear to you, and you have just written a chapter about how nut butters contain mold, rat hairs, and insect parts, and the product is a nut butter, you might not want to sit down with a spoon and eat a heroic dose of it. *I* might not want to eat a great deal of it in one go. Particularly if I am extremely stressed. Note to self. After I had thrown up five or six times my wife, who was reading in bed, asked me if I was alright. This did not seem like a question that required an answer.

For the next several days, my digestion was, let me say with the word in airquotes, 'compromised'. Let me say that I could feel that my guts were leaking. If this has ever happened to you, you know when it is happening. Your entire abdomen is tender, you fart and burp like a monster, and your deep belly hurts. You have inflammation locally in the guts, some degree of brain fog. Generally, when the guts are leaking, my dreams are of invasion. I find myself in wars, situations of violence, houses entered by intruders.

For several days I did the kind of protocols that are standard in these responses. I took anti-candida tablets, I took extra digestive enzymes, I drank peppermint and turkey tail mushroom tea, I stopped drinking coffee, I cut sugar out completely. I made myself a large pot of kitcheree, which is a healing one-pot ayurvedic meal: an easily digestible complete protein. I ate oatmeal for breakfast.

For several days I coped with this level of inflammation and discomfort. And in several of these days I talked with friends and mentors about the podcast, without fully consciously connecting all the above.

The third night after the pistachio butter I awoke in the middle of the night with my stomach in knots, went to the living room, and began to meditate. In the meditation I became thirteen years old again, and I remembered, viscerally, what it had felt like when I had been accepted into seventh grade at the college prepatory school I attended, something I had, until that moment, not thought of for nearly forty years, and had no conscious memory of at all. If someone had asked me, "Gabriel, do you remember the pool party at the beginning of seventh grade?" I would have looked at them with a blank stare.

When my family moved from rural New Hampshire to St. Louis, when I was seven, I was enrolled in the local elementary school. This I graduated from in fifth grade, and then spent a year at the public junior highschool. My parents did not think I was being adequately academically challenged, and halfway through sixth grade I went to sit the enterance exam for a prestigious college preparatory school in Ladue.

Ladue, Missouri is the most affluent suburb in all of St. Louis County, and was not where we lived. The school had been there since 1924. It is called John Burroughs, named after the naturalist. Some fun trivia: recent graduates you might have heard of: Sam Altman (CEO, OpenAI), Ellie Kemper (actress, The Office, Unbreakable Kimmy Schmidt), Beau Willimon (Showrunner, House of Cards), Jon Hamm (actor, Madmen, etc.). I don't remember walking on campus for the first time, but I do remember sitting the exam. It was in an enormous gymnasium, called the Field House. In my junior year I visited several famous small liberal arts colleges in Massachusetts (Amherst, Williams college) and their field houses were shittier than the highschool's. I sat at the end of a folding table, took the exam, and got accepted.

I don't remember thinking much about the new school as I prepared for seventh grade, but a few days before the school year there was an orientation party. This took place on the field and at the pool behind the school. The kids I met, the kids who were going to be my classmates, came from social milieus that were alien to me. This was something I could feel the moment I stepped on the field. Many of them already knew one another: I knew one other boy who had gone to my middle school. Somehow he already knew many of them; it would turn out that this was because his family belonged to the same country club as a handful of them.

I remember details about the way they dressed: polo shirts, izod lacoste shorts, and these crocheted belts that appeared to be hand-stitched by mothers with time on their hands and included sets of initials - ESC or JAM - and little pictures of footballs, baseballs, baseball bats. They wore shoes I did not understand- why is there a slot in the top of your slip-on shoe for a penny? They had social rituals I could not make sense of. It was like being deposited in the middle of an uncontacted amazonian tribe, and being told, *Join right in!* I had no idea what to talk to anyone about. I didn't catch the references. I didn't know what Late Night with David Letterman was. I didn't know that colleges had football teams: I'd never thought about it. I had no idea that ABBA was a band.

After some games on the field, children forming into groups, some shy, some outgoing, we progressed to the pool, where both boys and girls went into the locker room to change, and then we met back up at the outdoor pool to display our two-thirds naked pre-pubescent bodies to one another. The upper classmen who chaperoned the gathering were so outrageously beautiful and adult-looking I could not even make sense of it.[1] Some of the guys had enough body hair that even without their shirts on it looked like they were still wearing sweaters. I didn't know how some of the seventh-graders knew them, or could manage to talk to them, or why some of them were getting picked up by these glamorous upperclassmen and tossed in the pool. I would not hit puberty fully for another couple of years, and starting seventh grade I was about five feet tall, probably about a hundred pounds sopping wet. I had no muscles to speak of, didn't even know what a weight room was.

I felt so embarrassed, so utterly out of my league that I'm not sure I said a single thing the whole day, other than *Thank you* to the seventh-grade principal when she handed me a plate in the line for lunch. All I wanted to do was become invisible.

Dr. Stephen Porges points out that we are social creatures, and that wellbeing is social in nature. He talks about the deep belly lifethreat responses as a kind of social death. The degree to which, in those moments, in that climate of luxurious affluence, casual beauty, and social ease I felt alien, ill-adjusted, and unprepared is an example of what he is talking about. Social death is, at some level, wanting to simply disappear. But that is not what happened, and instead I forced a smile onto the outside of my face, or at least some kind of a mask to hide what I was feeling inwardly.

---

1 Just to be fair here, and so you understand that I'm not exaggerating, one of them was the actor Jon Hamm, and other the actress Sarah Clarke (24, Twilight). So yeah, they were in fact unnaturally good-looking.

I became obsequious and overly polite. It would have been easier for me to feel at ease at that gathering if I was one of the staff serving lunch than I felt as one of the attendees at the party. Later on in life, after dropping out of Yale, I would start my working life as a busboy and then as a waiter, and I remember the feeling of serving rich people in that capacity, standing on the far side of the social gulf of service, wearing the uniform of the restaurant, and experiencing a sort of relief.

The world I had entered, of bar and bat mitzvahs, country club membership, kids going on spring break to Sanibel Island in Florida, which acquired a sort of mythical status for me, was filled with social codes and references I did not understand. My parents were useless in all of this, they were not socially adept themselves, didn't understand the shark tank they had thrown me into, and I didn't know how to explain anything about what I was experiencing to them without shame. They were focused on the academic side of this, and the opportunities it opened up for me, and although in one sense they were correct, as I would later go on to attend both Yale and Stanford universities, the social damage done to me attending that highschool was something I spent twenty years repairing.

That first gathering in seventh grade was not something I remembered at all until two o'clock in the morning several nights ago, when I found myself knotted up on our couch, my stomach growling, and I found myself, viscerally, there, at the opening of my prep school years, grappling with that 'opportunity'.

Some of the worst decisions I have made in my life have been the result of what appeared to be opportunities. I might go a bit further, and say that some of what appeared to be opportunities were in fact *very dangerous* opportunities. If we turn to Mandarin Chinese for a moment, we can discover that the characters for 'dangerous opportunity' comprise the english word 'crisis'. Most of these dangerous opportunities have been difficult to walk away from specifically because they were seductive. I do not necessarily mean this in a sexual sense, but I also don't refute its meaning in the sexual sense, because procreation and the attraction that accompanies it involves resonance with our most rooted frequencies; those closest to the ground.

John Burroughs was perhaps my first costly and dangerous opportunity. Some of these dangerous opportunities in my early twenties led to sexual trysts that did indeed turn out to be dangerous and costly, not to lead in the direction of wellbeing and happiness, but there is a deeper meta-pattern that I'm pointing at here. When we identify something as an opportunity- it might be a school opportunity or a work opportunity- we can feel that a door is opening in the direction of the destiny that is awaiting us, and this can create a certain amount of momentum and compulsion around seizing what presents. My highschool was like this, and I am thinking here also about a number of experiences that happened with my company over a period of several years as we stood on the threshold of making a major breakthrough in understanding autonomic physiology. Each of the opportunities- one financial, one related to disseminating our work, and one related to a partnership- presented as types of wish fulfillment scenarios, and appeared as though they would resolve some definitive issue in our favor.

And in each case, because of the internal momentum that I accumulated around seizing the opportunity, I found myself ignoring red flags that in hindsight were present from the beginning. Had I been more sober in my analysis of each opportunity, I would have realized each was a type of seduction. And had I been more sober in analyzing the costs of allowing myself to be thus seduced, more in tune with the hesitation I was feeling in my body, I would have terminated each of them earlier, possibly before they started.

Why am I bringing this up? I think that part of us *wants* to be seduced. We want to *be* more, *feel* more, *have* more. We want to be adored. We want to be needed. We want to feel important, and powerful, and beautiful. And while all of this is natural, none of these things are wrong to want, the reason that we want them in the first place– or the reason that we want them so much– is that we don't feel like we are enough as we are. Maybe that is obvious, but it bears repeating. Maybe this is the reason that we are not grounded. Maybe this is what it means. Because this dissatisfaction with things just as they are– the fact that this moment is not enough– is the reason that we are seducible.

Had I felt myself enough in 7th grade, possibly I would have said to my parents, "Look– I know you want me to have a universe of opportunities open up. I know you want me to be challenged. But being around these affluent entitled children makes me feel so insignificant, so deeply unimportant, and unsuccessful– so bad about myself– that I don't know if it is worth it. I don't know that I'll survive it." And that would have been true.

On the couch at two in the morning I asked my body then, *Ok, what if you felt enough? What would we do?*

And my thoughts went to the podcast, and the interview, this dangerous opportunity. And my deep belly said to me, very clearly, *If you are going to do an interview with someone that is likely to be heard by several million people, which you've never done before, don't you want to meet the person interviewing you first and make sure you trust him?*

The simplicity of which was undeniable.

And so I wrote an email at 3 am: *Hey, I'm not offering to go on your show yet. I'm just offering to have a conversation with you and see if we resonate.*

The literal moment I hit send, my entire body relaxed.

I had been appeasing him without even knowing I was doing

it, in the same way my 13 year old body began appeasing my classmates, without even realizing I was doing it. By the following morning my digestion had repaired itself. Two days later I was back to normal. My digestion was humming. My turds were snaking lincoln logs of uniform length and diameter, the settings back to factory specification.

From the moment I had solved the autonomic quandry I had not taken another supplement, or continued to alter my diet at all. I had gone back to drinking coffee, eating ordinarily, and my body had just figured it out, re-organized, and put everything back in order. No more sleep disruption, dreams of invasion, or gastric distress. I had found my way back to baseline: my feet were back on the ground.

Once I had resolved the autonomic problem (energy) the body repaired itself (matter). Repair the energy-processing template and the body re-organizes back into coherence.

Do you think the famous podcaster accepted my invitation to sit down and converse? He did not. Oddly, the last time I heard about him he had gone public about his own battle with a chronic stress-related disorder of the grounding system.

46 - Permeability

One of the features of permeability- and here I am speaking about it as a meta-pattern- is that when our guts are leaking, when our edges, our boundaries, our barriers are porous, they are porous not just to material but to experience.

If digestion is, in its essence, our ability to metabolize our experience- if food is a sub-set of what we are metabolizing but what we are metabolizing primarily is experience, it reframes a conversation about boundaries.

When our boundaries are not clear- and if our guts are leaking, our boundaries are not clear- it is not so obvious where we end and the world begins, where the world begins and we end.

The neurochemistries intimately associated with this boundary confusion are endogenous opioids, painkillers that immobilize, and provide the gateway for dissociation.

Endogenous opioids are the chemical gateways that provide us the grace of being able to leave a body under lifethreat. In our deep evolutionary history, where we were subject to the predation of apex predators, where we got killed in grisly and gruesome ways a lot, this chemistry provided the chemical portal whereby the spirit could exit the body. And make no mistake, this is a grace.

They recently found a trove of human skulls in the lair of a saber-tooth tiger from about 20,000 years ago. Apparently this tiger enjoyed featuring us at the center of its diet. The skulls all had giant holes in their rear base, because the tiger apparently liked to pounce on us from behind, as large cats like to attack their prey, and simply crunched right into the skull from the back, which probably killed us pretty good, given that their canines could be from 8 to 11 inches long. If you are being eaten by a saber-toothed tiger who has just pierced your skull all the way through, you do not want to be in your body feeling that. Endogenous opioids are the chemical gateway that releases us from the body.

Often, in situations of lifethreat this release happens under extreme states of arousal, the force of which provides the impetus for ejection. But there are other cases, where the arousal level is lower, or the level of opioids more moderate, and the chemistry simply makes us more porous to experience, less confident about where we end and the world begins.

If you start to add oxytocin to this mix, the chemistry of love and bonding, and you drop the fear factor to zero, this starts to look a lot like the chemistry of pure awareness. In many of the spiritual traditions that describe moments of awakening, you have a description of an experience of union with the cosmos. Neurophysiologically, if the chemical portals of permeability open (endogenous opioids) but instead of feeling in danger you feel safe, and the chemistry of love and bonding activates (oxytocin/ vasopressin), you don't displace but rather stay centered in the body and experience yourself connected to everything.

This is a state that can be fairly reliably induced by meditation, if you have the proper guidance.

It is also a state from which the world turns into a sort of massive portent, with signs and symbols everywhere: a shamanic state. The line here between the oracular and the psychotic can be pretty fine, and depends on underlying stability. We get uncomfortable in cases of insanity defense when someone says, "The birds told me to do it," because we are pretty clear that the birds said no such thing. But to someone in a high arousal state, running the chemistry of dissociation due to lifethreat, it could have sounded an awful lot like that is what they are saying. That same person, in a meditative state, with the same chemistry active, but who was actually stable, might have heard something very different, but it is quite possible that the birds were talking in an original language that they could understand because they were connected with them. In the same way that a neutral eye gaze means something different to a person in a connection state than a threat state, bird language means something different to a person in a connection state than in a lifethreat state.

47 - Open to Something that Hurts Us

The biological paradox that undergirded nearly all of the patients that the esteemed physician sent me can be summed up in the following sentence: his patients had internalized, and were operating from an energy-processing template (this is what an autonomic state is), where they were staying open to something that was hurting them.

The appease response, which co-opts our social circuitry in the presence of a threat, means that we continue to be available (open) to something that is causing us harm. We may or may not do this with conscious awareness. Hierarchy of all kinds requires this of us. It is a fundamental byproduct of empire. When Nkem says that fight and fight are privileged responses, I say only if you find yourself stuck in an empire. Because the imperial format, and make no mistake, we are all the unwitting orphans of Rome, will demand your submission if you are not at the very pinnacle of the power structure. The loyalty demanded by the heads of criminal syndicates, whether installed in officialized positions of power or wreaking havoc outside of them, requires this kind of sacrifice of self. Will you sacrifice yourself for the boss? For the dysfunctional family, company, mob, state, or religion- whatever the system of coercive oppression may be?

In the previous chapter, I explained to you how I realized I was doing this inadvertently with the podcaster, due to a perceived power differential. When I stopped doing it, which was a form of self-love, my digestion, which had become porous, repaired itself. My digestion had become porous- a physicalization of my boundaries becoming porous– because my energetic boundaries had become porous because I was staying open to something psychologically dangerous to me. When I fixed the energetic boundaries the physical boundaries repaired themselves. This is an important, and possibly axiomatic realization. While fixing the physical template (the porosity which expresses most typically in the chronicity of shutdown as ME/CFS, IBD, or SIBO[1]) does not repair the energetic (autonomic) template, fixing the autonomic template generally does repair the physical template. Energy organizes matter, not the other way around. This implies that if we change the manner in which we are relating, the physical body will follow.

I am saying staying open to some*thing* hurting us, but in actuality it is usually some*one*. It is usually a person. This is typically a habit of relating to other people, and it is a habit of relating to other people on whom we depend, which is another way of saying that it is a habit of relating to people whom we believe are more powerful than we are. This is a dynamic that is often learned by children in relation to unpredictable parents, or in family situations of violence, or substance abuse, or where there is parental or familial instability or mental illness. It is also, often, learned very early in life, and it is learned bodily and energetically, not cognitively.

Relationship is the exchange of patterns of energy and information. The relationships that offspring have with their parents are fundamentally asymmetrical until the offspring are capable of surviving on their own. Human offspring, in particular, who are born almost totally biologically helpless are utterly dependent on our caregivers. Consider this for a moment. A baby horse can walk within five minutes of being born, yet it takes a human baby over a year. If a baby horse is abandoned, it may (probably not but may) possibly survive. A baby human? No way.

1 ME/CFS - Myalgic Encephalomyelitis/ Chronic Fatigue Syndome, IBD- Inflammatory Bowel Disease, SIBO- Small Intestinal Bacterial Overgrowth

We are, to an extent that most people forget if they do not spend regular time around infants, totally incapable of meeting our own survival needs for at least the first 18 months of our lives, and in actuality much longer. We are unique among mammals with the complex kind of cortical enfolding our brains possess in being born after only nine months of gestation: other mammals with comparable brains spend two or more years in utero. This is impossible for us humans because our heads are so large that if we were to spend more time inside, we would not be able to be born because our heads would get stuck in the birth canal.

Nature solves this problem in an elegant yet paradoxical way. Human infants can be conceived as having a 27-month gestation period. The first nine months of this take place in utero. The next 18 months of it take place in two phases outside of the womb. Anthropologist Ashley Montagu calls this 18-month post-birth period the "womb with a view." It is the most developmentally sensitive period of human life (after our foetal stage), because it is the time in which our sensory and autonomic neurology is being completed and myelinated.

From a neuro-developmental perspective, a human baby isn't really born until the fontanelles close. Fontanelles are the sort of skylights in the skull that allows the cranium to slightly compress during the birth process, so the head can make its way out of the birth canal. There are two fontanelles. One is toward the front of the skull, one is toward the back. The first fontanelle typically knits closed at around three months of age, the second around 18 months of age. This closure of the fontanelles is contemporaneous with the completion of the infant's foundational neurological wiring. One of the insights of our research at Hearth Science is that the myelination of critical autonomic systems is not complete until this point, which means that our neuro-anatomical mapping of autonomic systems needs to include the neurology myelinated at this age. In indigenous and ancestral cultures around the world, for the first nine months of life the infant is typically carried on the body of a caregiver skin-to-skin. Often they are never placed on the ground. The baby is essentially given a womb with a view. They are in touch proximity with a regulated caregiver, and the cultures understood that this developmental period was so sensitive that keeping the baby in an optimal zone of arousal was a crucial part of building the baby's brain and nervous system in ways that were required for flourishing. For this reason, in intact ancestral cultures, many people will nurse the baby. The whole point is to keep the baby calm yet alert. This comes from a profound understanding that the baby is still being formed neurologically at nine months of age. There is typically a transition, around the time the baby begins crawling, and for the next nine months, through the development of walking, the baby is still kept close and monitored closely as they move through the final 9-month 'trimester'. Modern civilization has categorically and catastrophically failed to understand the significance of this 18-month post-birth developmental period.

Complex chronic illness is, to a degree that is not generally recognized, relational. And this is because the Autonomic Nervous System, which is the neural architecture of the mindbody connection, governs the energy-processing templates that shape the way that we relate to one another. What this means is that the roots of most complex chronic illness are laid down in early childhood, when we are learning non-verbally how to relate to those around us: our family, our siblings, the social systems in which we are enmeshed. This learning is not cognitive at all. It is, rather, deeply felt. It is primal: animal if you will.

When my daughter was born, she was so sensitive that I watched her startle awake at the click of a camera shutter. When a shift nurse in a bad mood entered our room, she would begin to wail inconsolably. From the moment she arrived, she could absolutely sense the energetic temperature of anyone around her. If their energy was clear, loving, and congruent, she would respond to this immediately. If a person approached her who was angry, irritated, frightened, sad, or upset, my daughter was immediately inconsolable. It became totally obvious that she was transparently feeling whatever energies were around her. She was picking up on the vibes.

Why is this happening? Because we are spiritual beings having a human experience, not the other way around. What does this mean? If I was going to rewrite this through an autonomic lens, I would say that we are not material beings having an energetic experience, we are energy beings having a material experience. I am fairly well aware that to someone who does not live in California, this sentence might sound a little bit New Age. But that's not what I mean at all. When I say energy, I'm talking about energy in the $E=MC2$ sense of it. In the Einsteinian interconversion between matter and energy sense of the word.

Your autonomic nervous system is the mechanism in the body that interconverts matter and energy: that translates the flows of energy that run through you into experiences that you can metabolize; or not. My daughter didn't have to learn to read people's energy because all of us are electro-magnetic towers broadcasting waves of energy out into the world detectable by a magnetometer at least eight feet away. When we are in a connection state: when we are congruent, when all of our autonomic systems are engaged, when they are coherent, when we are happy, the waveforms flowing off of our person are smooth, melodious, harmonized. And a baby simply feels that music, and it feels good.

When we are in a defensive state, there is no rhythmic pulse of safety, and our autonomic systems start to decouple. The Connection System comes offline, and in it is absence our bodies can no longer cohere their internal visceral synchrony. This too generates a wave pattern, but it is no longer harmonic, coherent, but chaotic, and confused. And this too we broadcast out into the world. These patterns of incoherence are not simply detectable by a baby, but by nature at large. Modern humans who walk into a forest, in a defensive state, broadcast their dysregulation in every direction.

When I began studying tracking with Indigenous traditions, this was one of the first things we learned. The reason that most people don't see animals in a forest is because their electro-magnetic signatures are so chaotic that the animals flee. And this is what my daughter was expressing when the dysregulated nurse walked into our room.

This was not something she had to learn. It had nothing to do with cognition at all. And she could not tune it out. She had no defenses against feeling the vibrations of any beings nearby.

I am bringing this up, because at one point you were that tiny being. And although I have met a lot of humans in my life, I've never met one who was born into a totally enlightened family. All of us come in with that level of sensitivity, then we are dropped into what my friend Shai Lavie calls 'the nightmare of the nuclear family'. The challenge we have as tiny, extremely sensitive beings, is that we are often being cared for by people who do not understand the degree to which we are permeable to their energies, and have likely themselves suffered lifetimes of under-care and stress.

So what happens for most of us is that we are taken home to houses with stressed-out parents and siblings. In order not to die in these environments, we have to learn pretty young how to defend ourselves against the onslaught of energies. And so this is where most of us begin to learn to contract: we learn, at an embodied level first, the defensive autonomic responses that will accompany us for most of our lives.

Children are indeed in a biological paradox, which can be distilled down to the following formula. We learn to appease when the people upon whom we depend to keep us alive are also trying to kill us. Usually killing us is not in the outright physical sense of trying to end our lives: usually they are only trying to kill part or parts of us off. Usually they are trying to kill the parts of us that have been killed off in themselves, or were killed off by their own parents, which tend to be the parts of self that are sovereign. It is again, a multi-generational transmission of woundedness, and it typically happens outside of conscious awareness, by which I mean that most parents are not doing this to their children on purpose. Parents who have been beat down (by their own parents, by the world, by what or whomever) generally cannot tolerate sovereignty in their children. Often, if we get right down to it, they believe that it is better for them to beat their own children down than to the let the world do it: they describe it as adaptational.

The structure of empire is organized around power over (vertically) rather than power with (horizontally). Sovereignty, in the sense I'm using the word, the antique sense of direct unmediated contact with Source, is not about having power *over*, but about having power *with*. It is about animist and vital and imaginal power. It is about full expression of authenticity, about creating kinship relations with the universe entire. Many of the peoples and cultures who do this most naturally and inculcate it in their children most effortlessly are indigenous, and they would not recognize or relate to this word, which has the effect of invoking images of kings and queens in our modern minds. We cannot think of kings and queens without imagining pomp and circumstance, but what I'm talking about has nothing to do with tiaras and courtly dress. I'm talking about knowing at a fundamental level who you are, that you are intrinsically valuable, and about being unwilling to sacrifice yourself to stay in the good graces of a tyrant, be they father, boss, or president.

When we are six years old, and our father is enraged, and we weigh fifty pounds and he weighs two hundred, exhibiting sovereignty is likely to get us killed. And so we learn, most of us, to appease him. This comes at a tremendous cost, and if we don't unlearn the habit, and we don't figure out how to excavate the rage and terror that we have been shoveling down into our own guts– *because where else do you think we store these unmetabolized emotions?*– we are going to have a real problem down the road.

Furthermore, we will have a problem of two distinct kinds. One of them is a problem of excavation, of learning to exit the allostatic load and neurochemistry archived deep within from stuffing our anger and our fear. And the other of them is a problem in that unless we become conscious of how, at a primal feeling level we are working with the onslaught of these forces (threats from others), we are likely to internalize the pattern of staying open to threat.

I remember the moment, at age sixteen, that I grew taller than my father. I remember this not because I remember making a line on the bedroom doorframe where I kept a record of my height from year to year, but because when I surpassed his height my father made me sit down when he wanted to punish me. From the time I was sixteen until I left my parent's house, at age eighteen, to go to college, if my father was going to punish me he made me sit. I remember the living room chair where this happened, its shape and the way the base rocked (it was a kind of easy chair) and the pattern of the fabric, which was green with tiny flecks of red and orange. Just remembering this puts me in the body and mindset of appeasing.

As a grown man, fifty years old, I can feel the way that my body rises up in resistance to this. In classical chivalric paintings from the Middle Ages, you can see that everyone drops to a knee when the King enters the room, to recognize his authority. And in his own way, this is what my father was asking. *Recognize my authority. Make yourself smaller. Be diminished before me.*

I'm not singling him out here, and he was not a violent man. And I would not have wanted to father my own teenage self. I'm talking about the pattern. And because I depended on them, financially, and at that point also emotionally, because I was living under his roof, eating food they bought me, wearing clothes they bought me– I did it. I sat down. And inwardly, I shovelled this down into my guts. I swallowed down the rage: I forced myself to eat it.

Numberless generations ago, my ancestors in deeptime stopped moving over the face of the earth in deep rhythmicity with the seasonal migration routes of animals. They became shepherds perhaps, permanized their relationship with the flock, eventually settled down in a village that became a town that became a city. They demarcated land boundaries, began to pass 'property' from one generation to the next. Their primary cosmovision shifted from being horizontal- moving across the land- to being vertical: arranging in social heirarchies. The lineage encountered the Romans, was more deeply contaminated by empire. My peacable and sovereign ancestors in deeptime, who were not concerned with coercion, gradually turned into people who felt the need to circumscribe the liberty of others, because they had their own liberty circumscribed. Thousands and thousands of years pass, parents non-verbally teaching childen how to be in their bodies through the relational contact of co-regulation, how to survive the onslaught of domination, and because these ancestors lose the technologies of healing that would restore them to sovereignty, over the millenia they begin to freeze inwardly.

I'm not talking about being cold, I'm not talking about the weather outside of us: freezing winters. I'm talking about inner weather. I'm talking about the way that we lose contact with the ground. I'm talking about the way that trauma, repeated, ground into us, generationally- all of the insults of overwhelm- accumulate within us as allostatic load. Only this is cold stress. The stress of shutdown. Stress that makes its way into the psoas muscles, the junctions between the legs and the back: the muscles that join the parts of us designed to move across the landscape to our feeding centers.

Millenia of being told what to do; of being coerced, forced to conform. Of having our instinctual responses domesticated. Having them tempered by religion, by political necessity: *You may not weep like this, unrestrainedly, for the dead!* (Solon, 6th century, Greece) I'm talking about seeing people beaten, and beaten down. I'm talking about a thousand times a thousand times a thousand moments of being suppressed, of being uprooted, of being ripped from the arms of our caregivers, of being ripped from the land to which we belong.

I'm talking about the long, epi-autonomic, multi-generational experience of loss, of terror, of rage, and the not-knowing how to clear these autonomic wounds from our bodies. I'm talking about the way that we come into the knowing of our own embodied sense of self by resonating with our caregivers, and what happens when these traumas of shutdown have come to reside within their bodies as pockets of deadness.

I'm talking about how losing a great grandmother well over a hundred years ago has shaped the very immediate contours of my life, not in some abstract way, but in the very foundations of how I feel myself in the body that I am wearing.

I'm talking about how, over hundreds of thousands of years, we went from animals with radar in our feet, sensitive to the minutest vibrations emanating from the deep belly of the earth, to heads on sticks, modern people floating untethered, who can barely feel the ground, have forgotten they are earth-based creatures.

This is the pattern I am describing: the *how* of it. I am talking about civilization, and lineage. I am talking about culture. I am talking about how the millenias-long acculturation to domination has led us to the precipice we stand on.

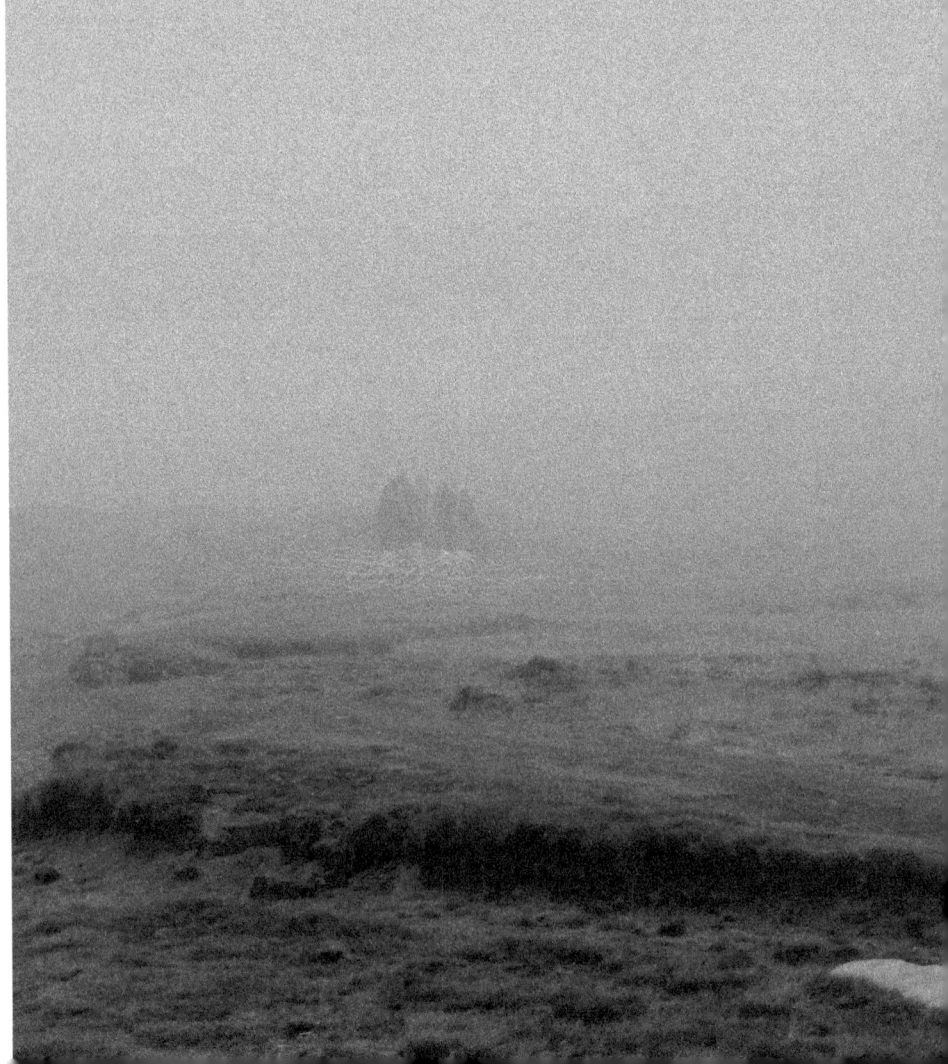

48 - Audacity

There is something astonishingly arrogant about me offering a formula here for fixing all of the aforementioned issues, twelve thousand years of uprooting, multi-generational histories of complex trauma, and profound physiological dysfunction. So take all of this with a grain of salt: it is all just my humble opinion. It is, however, a humble opinion informed by an extraordinary amount of suffering research I conducted through the catastrophe of my own life and its transformation, as well as a thirty year study of autonomic physiology.

At some level, what we have been talking about in this entire book is the manner in which modern people have become de-indigenized. The myriad ways in which the origin of modern civilization so-called, what used to be called 'Western Civ', is the reification of embodied alienation. What I have attempted to do thus far in the book is sketch this out for you, first at the level of the origin stories (Adam & Eve, Cain & Abel), and then at the level of the activities (the schizophrenia of supremacy, the creation of right angles to denote property boundaries, the enclosure of the Commons, etc.) that scaffolded the project of modern civilization, then through a representative example (my own) of the multi-generational epi-autonomic transmission of trauma, then through understanding the ways in which the physiology is compromised by lifethreat responses, their neurobiological sequelae, and their characteristic arcs of illness.

These layers are, I believe, fractal: self-similar at varying levels of scale. All of them, if viewed from a sufficient remove, are about humans becoming uprooted. Losing anchoring in place, losing their cosmological moorings in relatedness, losing the sovereignty of their bodies, their sovereign grief, access to the full range of their innate stress responses, and the transformation of those in community and healing ritual. A long arc of the way that our original knowings have been corrupted by imperial domination, and then the ways that we have subsequently internalized this domination paradigm, so that even if the outer empire were to crumble, we have instantiated it deep in our own psyches and modes of relating.

In transparency, understanding all of this took on a certain urgency for me several years ago when I realized that a spiritual group I had belonged to for nearly fifteen years had, somewhere along that pathway, devolved from a culture into a cult. As I tried to assess, soberly, just how this had happened– how an organization with an extraordinarily beautiful mandate had transformed from being something spontaneous and liberatory into being something profoundly hierarchical, reactionary, and bureaucratic, I was confronted by how deeply we have internalized domination. This particular organization had taken a plant medicine referred to in indigenous communities as the Grandmother, and transformed it into a global organization whose formal leadership structure is comprised entirely of men. From a feminine spiritual medicine, the organization had created an entirely patriarchal system.

I saw, in the organization, a synechoche for modernity, a part standing in for the whole. A fractal to the entire arc whereby modernity had blamed the falling out of relationship with All that Is on a woman (our feminine nature) and on a snake (our indigeneity).

Over the duration of my career, I have consulted with probably eighty organizations. And again, despite the fact that many of them are doing profoundly egalitarian work, are profoundly concerned with social justice, I watch them continuing to replicate the modes of domination that undermine and contradict their visions of the world our hearts know is possible. Again, this paradox.

It is very difficult to address these problems in their complexity outside of the context of communities of relationship. But because we modern humans are so wounded in our relating, whenever we come together in groups, we create cults. We have no idea how to create a culture.

I offer this section therefore not as an invervention, as a protocol, or as a formula, but as a series of inquiries: provocations designed to confront our inheritance from Rome.

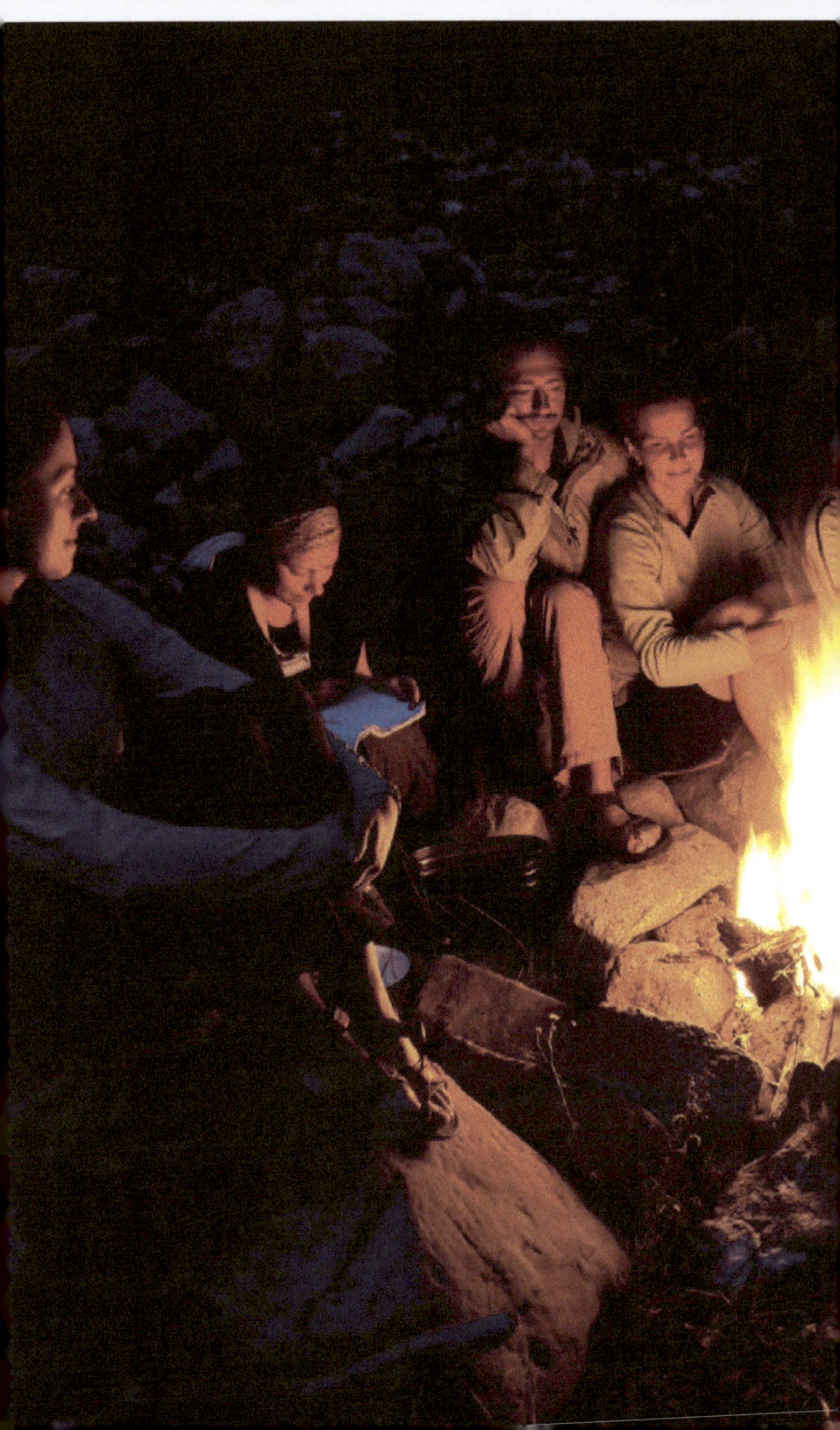

49 - Ancestral Fireplace

My favorite word for the Sacred in any language comes from Aramaic, and is a word that Jesus used frequently. It is transliterated as *Qadash*, and is comprised of two roots. QD, and ASH. QD can be translated as the centerpoint. ASH is the circle of light and heat around it.

When I say the word, the image that comes to mind immediately, almost unbidden, is a circular fireplace in the middle of the savannah. In the image, it is a time before time. Around the fire, there is a circle of us, a small band, sitting on the ground.

The image for me is so profound, so archetypal, so deep in the lineage history of our humanity, that it is what I named our work after (Hearth Science). The original fire, the sacred fire, with its centerpoint, and us, the people, the humans, the village arrayed around it in a circle. I want to begin the provocation of redressing our imperial injuries with this image. I ask you to hold it close. It is an image of our lineage history in deep time. If I was a doctor, in the deepest sense of the word, and you came to me and told me that you have been uprooted by empire, and I could prescribe for you one thing, one remedy, it would be this.

I would prescribe a campfire in the middle of an aboriginal forest.

I would prescribe that you sit with others in a circle around it. I would prescribe that you humble yourself to the awareness that the fire itself, not a person, not a leader, but the elemental center, is your portal to contact with the Source.

I sincerely doubt that reading about this will do you any good. It is like seeing a picture of chocolate, and listening to me describe its taste.

What you need to do is eat the chocolate. If you would be fully provoked, go *do* this. Gather a group and go make a campfire in some aboriginal context of the wild.

Set time down altogether: spend hours there. Stay deep into the night: the genuine depths of its darkness. Stay beyond the front edge of night, into its depthless center. Stay through the hours of darkness that seem as though they will never end, when all light has been gathered, when the only beacon is the embers of your small fire. Do not let the fire die.

If you ask the fire with enough sincerity, and enough recognition that it is sacred fire, it will begin to teach you, and then I would advise that you discard this book and simply listen to the fire. If you were to run out of fuel, once the fire starts talking to you, you can feed it this book, page by page, from the end backwards. The book won't mind. The book was sourced from this fireplace; you are feeding the fire to itself.

At the peak of the darkness, the fire will teach you about the difference between life and death, the difference between lifeways and deathways. These teachings are reserved such that they can only be called forth by the depth of the darkness. Only then are they truly necessary.

It will teach you about sovereignty, if you allow it. It will teach you relating. It is capable of teaching you everything, in a language original.

Soften your eyes. Forget what you have been told the fire is. Recognize that you are in dialog with a being. The fire is not a thing. Trees are not things. Rocks are not things. They are all verbs. All beings. All animate. Entelechies awaiting your noticing of their sentience.

Regard the fire recognizing that you do not yet know who you are looking at, nor the language in which its awareness will reach you. Regard the fire with the awareness that it is sensing you as well–that the direction of observation is not one way only. Listen through your ears, but from your interoception, the Mother of your Senses, your deep inwardness. Move into the liminality between sleep and wakefulness, but do not fall asleep. Listen through your body entire.

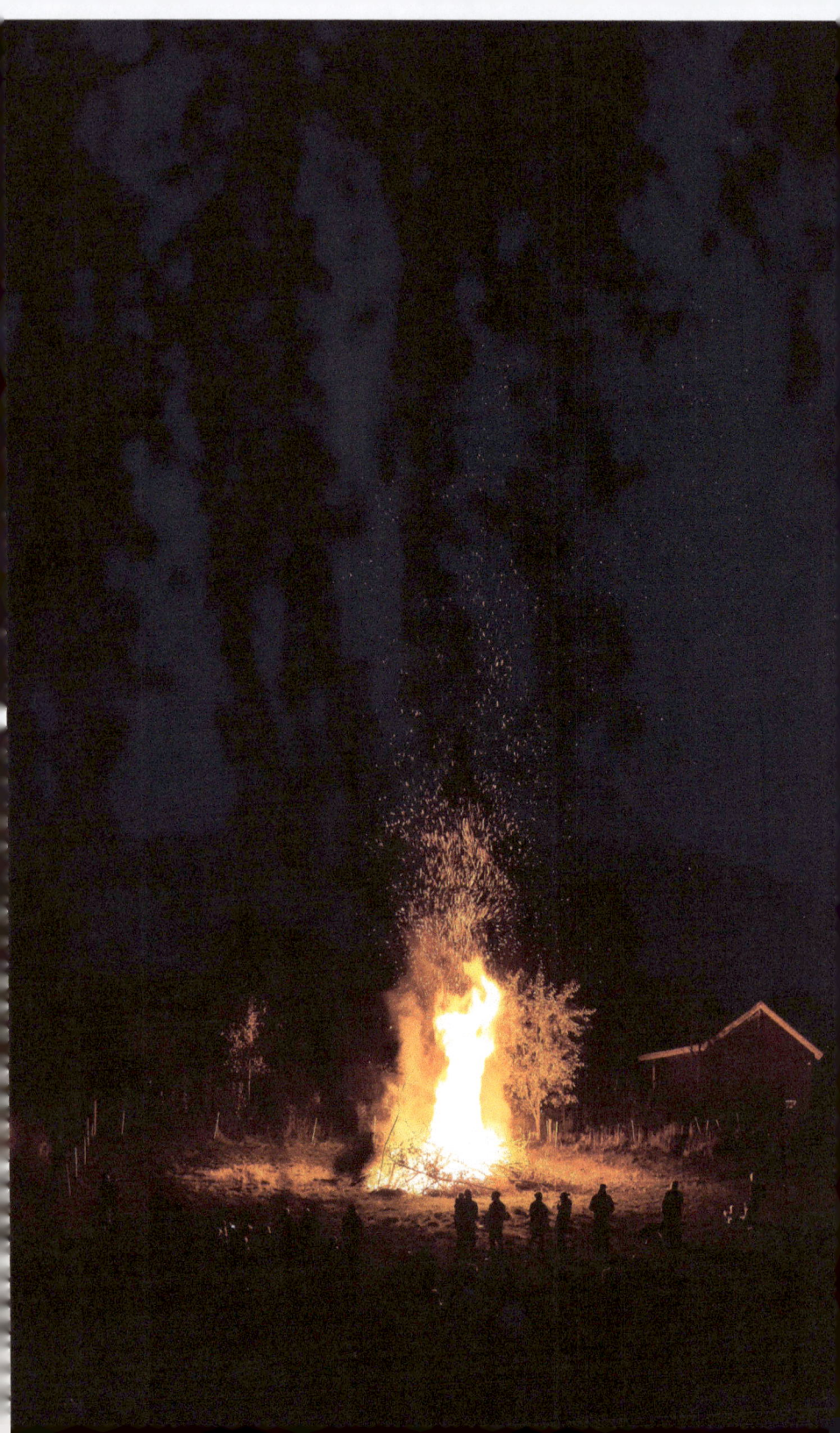

50 - Observations Derivative Thereto

Sitting in the circle, a couple of things become obvious.

First, there is no privileged position in a circle. It has no head. It has no location of greater subjective importance. It has no place from which the view is privileged, although from each seat the view is singular: unique.

Another way of saying this is that everyone sitting around the perimeter of the circle is equidistant from the Source.

Second (and not because it is second in importance, but simply because it flows in this manner), if we are sitting around the fireplace, at night on the savannah, and we are sharing the savannah with apex predators, it is the small band that helps confer our sense of safety.

Safety is, clearly here, not an individual affair. It is a collective enterprise: keeping one another safe. In modernity we have drifted, entrusting our safety to institutions. Bureaucracies of one sort or another. Losing the image of wholeness of ourselves, we have differentiated all the functions of the small band and apportioned them to varying governmental entities beholden to other interests. Yet safety, to the degree it exists, is here with the small band.

Furthermore– the person who is most likely to keep you safe, the person whose default view is to see what is behind you, which is exactly what you cannot see, is the person sitting opposite from you on the other side of the fireplace.

Another way of saying this, sociologically, is that the person who is most different than you are, structurally, is the person most easily able to see your blindspots. They are structurally located in such a place that what you cannot see is easily visible to them.

This is a teaching about diversity.

If you would survive, it is imperative that you place people all around the circle. Which is to say that the resilience of the circle is a function of its diversity. Put too many people on one side, facing the same direction, and you are vulnerable to being snuck up on. You are vulnerable to confirmation of your own bias.

Put people at all points around the circle, and, without effort, you (the small band) can see in every direction. Fill the circle and seeing becomes omnidirectional. Of course, I am not speaking about seeing in an optical sense merely: I am speaking about sense-making. I am speaking about tracking the flows of the felt such that we can maneuver our shared boat through the rushing rapids and over the crashing waves.

A hypothesis: the number of people that can fit around a fire, in the savannah, of the size that it is possible to create and sustain in that ecology, where wood is not so abundant, soles of their feet toward the fire, without burning themselves, dictates the size of our small band hunter gatherer bands: 25-35 people.

Assertion: the proper unit of human flourishing is the small band. It is not the nuclear family. It is not the individual.

Human wellbeing is social in nature because the proper unit of humanity is not an individual: it is this band, with its collective sense-making, its holism of collective vision, in the interoceptive sense of that word.

This social structure is innate; intrinsic; hard-wired.

Our deepest evolutionary biology is designed to unfold, elaborate, inflate, become fully aware in the context of a small band kin group of this size. Your body knows, and is innately hungry to be witnessed in this manner.

The subdivision of the tribe into the marriage dyad is a fulcrum of alienation. You belong to a nuclear family, yes, but the body wants to enfold along the oragami lines of the small band. Assemble the band and you will find the scope of your true capabilities. And not simply *the* band, *your* band.

51 - Furthermore

Consider please, the sound of the fire, and what it is. Consider the whispering voices of tongues of flame: consider the combustion itself.

The fire is made from wood: the wood is the dried-out bodies of trees. You are burning kin, replete with its own endogenous knowings of interbeing. Consider the trees themselves: all around you, their intelligence and animacy. The husk of their bodies is the material the fire makes itself known to you through. And all around you, exchanging air with the village, are the trees.

Your neurology is dendritic, which is to say, in Greek, arboreal. Your nerves are an inward forest. The forest your outward nerves.

Beneath the forest, the underground network sharing resources to enrich the collective: mycelium. This too has an inward analogue in your myofascia.

So to look outward into the forest and to look inward into your body: these are not all that different. Around the fireplace, this becomes obvious at dusk.

So the fire will tell you, if you ask.

Down at the cellular level, a fire is burning as well. It is not wood that is combusting, but glucose; yet your mitochondria, the cellular engines that power life, are combusting as well.

How does this sugar arrive to them to be combusted?

It is conveyed on inward waterways, known to you as arteries, blood vessels, capillaries, not that different than the river, stream, and creeks coursing past.

It moves through an inward ocean, not that different than the outward ocean.

To be divorced from Nature, outwardly, is to be divorced from your Nature inwardly, because there is one pattern language of Nature.

And one slight substitution in the associative matrix of who you've been told you are makes it obvious.

We have been told, "Humans are made in the image of the Divine." What we have forgotten is that it is the image of Divine Nature, which is to say Nature, with a capital N.

So you are made in the image of Nature. Which means that staring into the greengold forest, the shimmering sea, the lucid desert– the jewelled night sky, the motion of celestial bodies, the pattern of the raptor catching thermals, the otter with his babe on his chest, the kelp undulating in the swell: you are looking at yourself.

That tremor in your body just now, as you read this? It is recognition. It is Nature becoming known to itself.

To be divorced from your Nature inwardly, is to be divorced from Nature outwardly.

As above, so below.

It is not enough to know it, you need to feel it.

It is not enought to feel it, you need to be saturated with it.

It is not enought to be saturated with it, you need to dissolve into it.

Like sugar in water, surrender to the shaking. Identify with the shaking, not your resistance to it. Dissolve into who you actually are. An I in the whole body.

If you would know who you are, dissolve into the mirror of Nature. Your church cannot be indoors if you would become who you are.

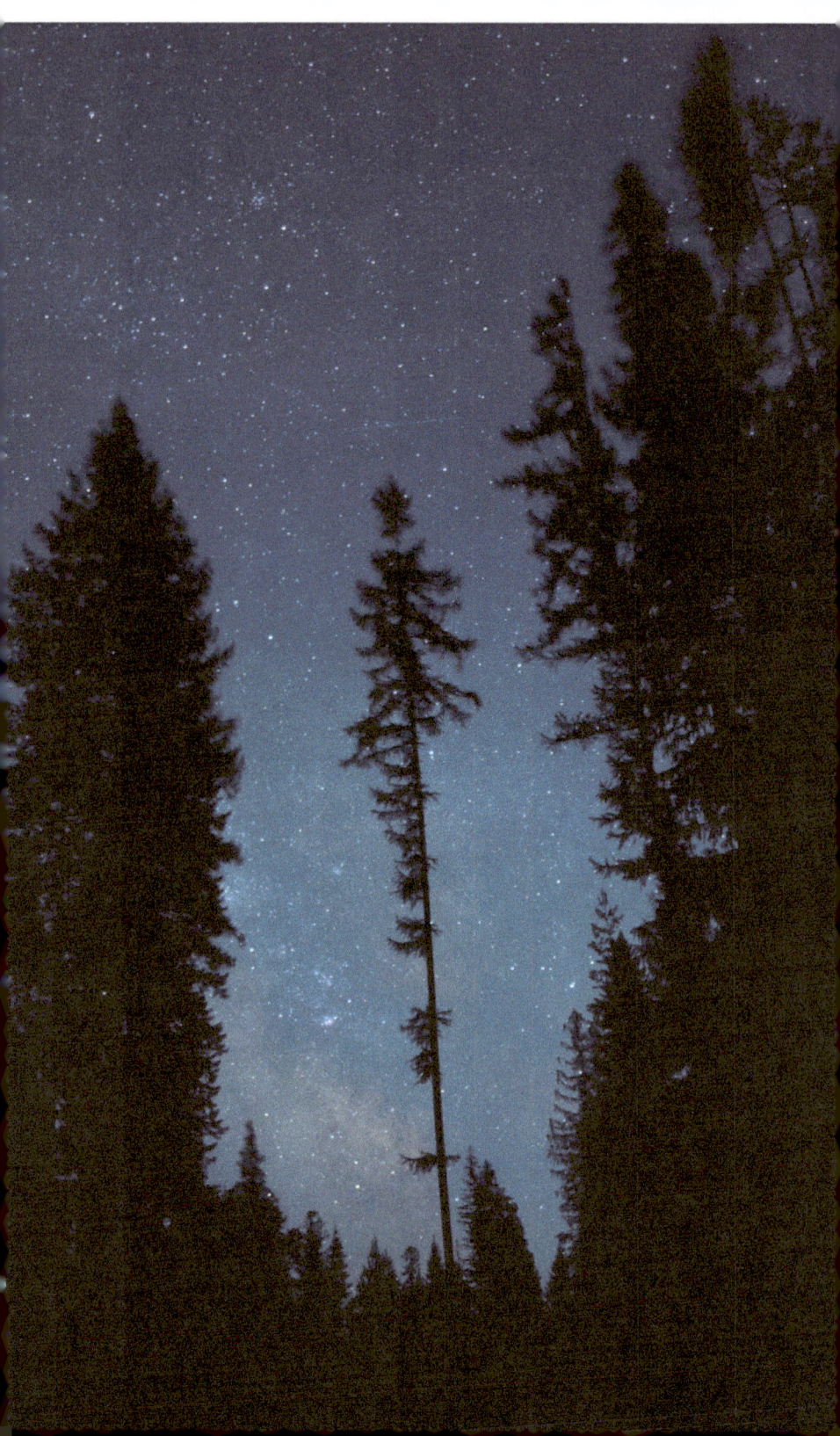

52 - Breathe

Are you really, do you think, breathing? Because if you were, you would smell the woodsmoke. You would watch the embers fly up, and the smoke curl, but you would inhale draughts of it when the wind changed, and if you were paying attention, you would know by its smell whether we are burning alder or ash, bay laurel or Douglas Fir. The smoke of each, tinted by its proper resin, you would know.

And you would know the smells of dirt exhaling under the moonlight, the fecundity of it, soil-smell, the scent of the aromatic herb that gets crushed underfoot, its aerosol of mint.

You would open your nostrils, and the air would spiral into them (this is how it works), and because the air is aromatic with campfire, with mint, because the trees are literally an oxygen factory, you would want to draw all of this deep deep deep into the recesses of your body.

You would want your breath to move and oxygenate your blood, you would want the oxygen to enter into everywhere you are wearing a body.

And when you exhaled, out of generosity, because you recognized that you were feeding the trees, you would make sure to empty yourself of carbon dioxide. You would hold nothing back.

You would see that you and the trees were holding one another, breath to breath, in a perfectly circular exchange. And empty of all concern, you would give yourself over to the breathing itself, you would let it breathe you.

And under the moon and the stars, in the safety of the band, you might close your eyes and allow your breath to re-organize, to find its way back into coherence, to become fluid as the tidal exchange, unperturbed as water slipping up and sliding back down the beach.

53 - Allowing

And if all of this happened, which is to say, if you allowed it to, because you cannot *do* any of this, *doing* is useless...

you might find a spaciousness, somewhere between the sound of the fire and the wailing wall of insect noise, in which your ordinary sense of self loosened a bit, the way it feels to loosen a necktie after a formal evening, the way it feels to step out of heels that are too tight, unhook garments that are restrictive in a way that you are accustomed to, and that is yet constraining. Your ordinary sense of self might, for a moment, dilate. It might, for a moment, grow less solid, less certain, less heavy. Chatter in the mind might cease. Rumination, recrimination, commentary.

You might simply become receptive; open to listening.

While this occurrence would be context-dependent, neurochemically it might also be a function of the release of endogenous opioids, yet they would be releasing into the flow of oxytocin (we are here together with our peoples) listening at the cadence of safety. You might perceive that the harmonic of frogsong is happening at this same cadence. That Nature herself is pulsing, breathing, oscillating. Rising and falling like the sleeping baby's chest.

And in the spaciousness created by the winding down of the machinations of self– *Good God, running this program takes so much energy!*– you might experience contact with that which moves through you.

From this place beneath

behind

below

your daily sense of self, you might notice that you do not feel *separate*.

And the poetics of this viscerality- an experience of being part of- are not linguistic but deep-bellied. Not cognitive but existential.

Were this to happen, I would invite (no, even recommend) that you bow down. For you have come to a holy grove; a place the bards and mystics have been writing about since things could be written down.

A place people have journeyed far to reach, thousands of miles to reach the Oracle, fasting for days, ingesting various indole alkaloids, enduring various ordeals to catch a glimpse of.

You have arrived in the vicinity of the wellspring. How interesting and necessary that you cannot arrive here with your ordinary sense of self.

The accretion of deadness, allostatic load, the reification of believing yourself to be a thing, something solid- the whole mass of it sinks to the bottom of the pitcher under its own weight- none of that can come with you to this place.

In this place the only thing you can bring is your originality; your essence.

And in truth, most modern people are afraid of it, this gate to actual life. Most modern people arrive here trembling, terrified, stand at the gates convinced that to step across is to die.

But what dies?

It is true that to kneel down here, in the grove, in moonlight is to let go of the self you cling to. You will have to release your storied and deeply cherished attachment to your own victimization, yes that is true.

But the thing that dies? It is an accretion, a residue, a husk.

I cannot encourage you here. You must dwell here in the encounter yourself. The terror is real. It cannot be reasoned with, or walked around. I won't invite you further. I have the duty to lead you to the throne, but I can't make you sit down on it. That work is yours, and yours alone. You will have to face your deepest fears: that's how it works. Dying will present to you in the image of what you are most afraid of.

Forty days and forty nights
we are told
Jonah in the belly of the whale
Jesus in the desert

this is how long it takes us to face ourselves;
to become what we were meant to be:
a biblical span.

Was a story in *The New York Times* recently
about a teenage kayaker got swallowed by a whale
and spit back up

Long long moments down there in the close dark.

But 40 days?
How long will it take you to face yourself?

Do you think you can do it by reading a book?
At the pace of flipping pages?

Do you really think this is a book?
I grip you in a transformation engine.

This is not a book.
This is an ancient technology
a ceremony

an initiation

I have a sword drawn at your neck
trained on the carotid pulse.
The flat of the blade rests against you now, can you not feel it?
The steel is cold.

But why would I do that?
You thought I was your friend.

The friend I am has no allegiance to your delusion.
No allegiance to your contracted self.
I am here to help you out of the slip knot of your alienation.

I have the practiced hands of a neurosurgeon.
I have done this thousands of times.
My hands are steady.

We separate what is alive from what is dead.
Cell by cell.
Molecule by molecule.
Adam by adam.

What is dead may not pass through this filter.

You must strip your self naked as a babe.

I would pray, if I were you.

Not to something up there.

It won't help you.

This is chthonic work.

Deep belly work.

Pray downward, to the Ground.

To Our Mother that art the Earth.

Like this:

Dear Mother,
which art the Earth

Forgive me,
I knew not that you were sentient.

To the Father I have prayed
in lines practiced and rote
nightly even

As I desecrate you daily.
As I, complicit in normalized destruction
consume

like a virus
pollute
like a virus

assured in my entitlement
to convenience
the luxuries of the modern world

burn carbon
eat endlessly of your bounty

bottomlessly hungry for
more

and more
and more

And yet it occurs to me
all this time I have relied upon you
I did not realize there was a *you*.

As I have relied upon you
as a babe relies upon its mother,
I have been utterly ignorant

never considered the relationship
from your perspective

that in poisoning your air
I am poisoning my breath

that in poisoning your water
I am poisoning my blood

That in poisoning your soil
I am poisoning my belly

Forgive me.
Now I see that you are me,
I have been poisoning all of this time
and I do not know what to say.

How must you, Dear Mother
which art the Earth, regard me
destroyer of worlds
?

and you say nothing, Mother?

54 - Full Spiral

I am once again sitting at the circular wooden table with the sunburst pattern long before dawn. I have a different beverage than that with which I began this project, this time it is espresso-based, but my feet are bare. Outside, I can hear the wind and a smattering of rain, but it is a different season.

In a way I have come full circle, back to the starting point, its elemental configuration, but the arrow of time has progressed, so perhaps I shall say I've come full spiral. I began to organize this book in autumn, now it is spring, not of the same year.

Each book, I find, has its own innate logic, if I can trust it deeply enough to reveal itself. Writing this concluding chapter reminds me, for some reason, of staking down a teepee. I have moved in a wide circle outside the structure, and now I am close to where I began staking it down, yet on the opposite side of the doorflap. This is the final peg to nail, but somehow I also know that the interior of the space is not finished with its work yet, or its work on me: I am merely tapping down the stakes at its perimeter. I am confident that although this will be the final chapter you read, it will not be the final thing that I write in making the book as complete as I can make it.

The first book that I wrote front to back, the first one that had the kindness and simplicity to unfold in linear fashion, was my tenth book. The first several I wrote backwards, and I am aware that this is because all of them were trauma narratives. I think that the only honest kind of book a traumatized person can write is a trauma narrative, and since trauma definitionally interrupts the progression of linear time, the coherent forward moving of beingness, it makes sense to me that my first several books, which were assemblies designed to put me back together, were written backwards.

The first novel I successfully completed, which has not been published, was completed at an artist's residency in Rabun Gap, Georgia, where I was staying in a house reputed to be haunted, although no one told me that when I moved in. If this was true, the spirit there had a playful side and a sewing kit, because I was constantly coming in the front door and finding tiny things on the windowsills that had not been there before. Old buttons, pins, once a thimble, things like this.

I had been working on the novel, by this point, for almost a decade. I still didn't fully realize that I was re-writing the story of my life, using structures of narrative to transform it back into something I felt that I was steering. The book, though interesting, was a map of fragments, and what I had done was commandeer the dining room table, which was large enough to seat twelve people, turn it into a sort of war room, and lay the manuscript sections out on the table in piles. In the center of this was a large folio sheet that contained a map, my intricate notes on how it all fit together. A scrawl of lines and arrows and circled chapter titles and intricate glyphs meaningless to anyone other than myself. It was on a single piece of paper, maybe 16 x 20 inches, that I had quartered for easy transport and then unfolded. It looked kind of like the map of a city's sewer system; intricate and convoluted at that level.

This was about halfway into a six-week residency. I had been there for three weeks working, and I had re-read everything twice. The book swam in my head in fragments, sections bobbing loosely in the water like bits of flotsam in the same eddy, yet unconnected. The map at the center of the table was my understanding of how everything fit together, the thread I would string it all with, and it cohered a set of timelines that jumped forward and back, through present tense narration, back into the past, and back to the present again many looping times.

I remember leaving the house for dinner and locking the door. I had been working most of the day. We took dinners communally, all of the artists of that particular cohort, in a more formal dining room near the entrance to the Arts Center. I don't remember what we ate. I remember trudging back up to the cabin, up the dirt road, in the close dark. It was late October of 2005. I unlocked the door, and went back into the dining room, turned on the light, which pooled, an island in the old dark wooden-walled house. I reached toward the map at the center of the table, and realized belatedly– as I was attempting to pick it up– that there was nothing in the middle of the table, that I was reaching for air. Time stopped for just a moment as I recognized I was trying to pick up a mirage.

I had been using the map an hour prior.

There were screened windows open on a sleeping porch behind the dining room, and the first logical thing that occurred to me was that while I was at dinner a breeze had blown in, and carried that single piece of paper like an oragami bird up off the dining room table. And so I looked for it on the floor first on one side of the table and then the other. Then in the kitchen that abutted the dining room. Then in the front room. My heart rate began to pick up. Fifteen minutes later, I had scoured the house top to bottom, and was shaking. My heart was racing. I could not catch my breath.

The map had vanished.

I never found it.

As I attempted to go to sleep that night, continually reassuring myself that I would find it, I had a sinking feeling. Over the next several days, as it became apparent, somehow, that a single piece of paper sitting in the middle of the dining room table had been removed, a piece of paper containing the entire map of the underground city of the world of my book, useful to no one but me, nothing else in the house touched, no other papers ruffled, I bottomed out, and entered a sort of depression in which I dwelled several days as though it were a pit I had fallen into deep within a sunless forest. Eventually I was forced to come face-to-face with the reality that I could either pack it in and give up, or that I had to carry on. I was running out of time, and I needed to finish the book before I concluded the residency. Too much depended on this. I had been working on it for a decade. I needed to buck up and get it done. I had to move on with my life.

And so I made myself release the map. I pried my fingers off it, mentally, because I could not get them to let go. They held onto it out of habit: the cartography of that story, what I could remember of what it said, how I thought it all fit together.

I did not try to recreate it. I made myself drop it, pried it out of my mind the way you force a dog to drop a stick. *Drop it!*

Then I spent several days confronting the fragments of the text and I allowed the sense of order to melt off of them. I stopped fighting. I surrendered. I let it collapse. This terrified me. I thought I might go crazy, become totally overwhelmed by chaos.

In the cocoon the Monarch caterpillar simply dissolves. Cut one open and the incipient butterfly drips out as goo. The caterpillar is gone, dissolved down to cellular soup. The butterfly has not yet organized.

I passed through a liminal state. The temperature plunged, I had to close the windows, I couldn't get warm no matter how many blankets I piled on and foxes screamed at night. There came into the air a sort of yearning melancholy I cannot explain. A sadness that seemed to condense hundreds of years of pain aboriginal to that place and its tortured history rose up in the night, and I sincerely feared my heart would break. I convulsed on the bed, broke out in a cold sweat. There were several nights where a kind of formless grief stalked its way through the hills, reverberating, and I curled tight into a ball, dangerously lonely, vibrating with the feeling of being forsaken. The sun would rise and burn off the mist, a sort of relief and benediction. I would blow on my hands and yearn for someone to share my bed. I was newly married: my wife thousands of miles away in California.

This continued for several days as I shivered and then the wife of the caretaker of the property died. I did not know her, and I did not know her story, but I felt the seduction of the grief emanating immanent and I could easily imagine how it could catch you if you gave it a surface to attach to. I had curled into a ball at night like an armadillo, presenting the bony back to the world, no soft ventral side available. With her passing, which swept the community around me, of which I was peripherally a part, into a coherent form of mourning, gave this formless grief a focus, an outlet, a shape, the energy consolidated and passed through.

And this gauntlet pulling us down and inward run, what happened next was that I started to be able to feel tiny islands of coherence. The edges of the chapters became, for lack of a better word, slightly magnetic. I started to be able to feel where one scene wanted to stick to another. Where a scene wanted to be preceded, or followed by another. And little by little a sequence emerged that was totally different– I mean utterly and completely and unrecognizably different– than what had been on the map that disappeared.

Is it possible that because I had a map I thought I knew the territory and had therefore stopped really listening to the text itself? I am convinced, to this day, that if the map had not disappeared I would not have succeeded in completing the book. And since what I was really re-writing, despite the fact that I did not know this, was a story of self, I am not sure that my story of self would have come into coherence.

I was tempted to say 'come back into coherence' but it did not come *back*. It did not revert to some previous form. It came forward into coherence. A new story, a new constellation, a new organization, nudged forward by a prodding from the unseen.

Through a provocation, the minor chord of its unresolve, my bringing myself to the collapse (a pit in a forest) and then through and out the other side of the grief, avoiding the temptations and distractions along the way, I had passed through something alchemical, and eventually out the other side.

Two days before the end of the residency I sat with my laptop in the front room where the buttons and thimble had appeared and typed out the ending scene of the novel. Then I cried my eyes out, wept with abandon, unable to stop, moved to my core for reasons I did not understand fully at the time.

When I finally stopped shaking, and my hands were once again steady, I rolled a cigarette, smoked it, and came back into time.

THE END

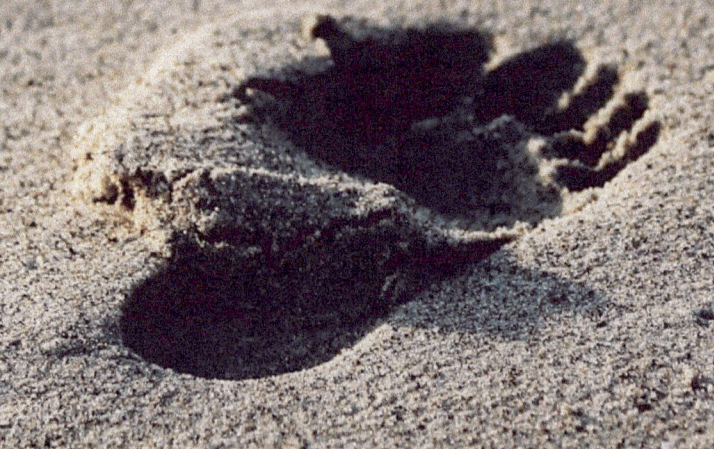
RESOURCES

Grounding Practices

In this section, I am going to shy away from standard issue practices and invite you to think more holistically about the notion of creating more physiological opportunities for the autonomic Grounding System to function as it was meant to:

-**Get (or make) a Standing Desk**. If you must to spend long periods of time working in a stationary position, get (or make) a desk that you can stand in. While you can buy a fancy motorized standing desk, and for many people this is a worthwhile investment, if affordability is a primary consideration, figure out what desk height is required for you to work comfortably standing, and then change the legs on a traditional desk to make it taller. I work at a standing desk most of the time, and there are really only two high positions I work at. One fully standing, the other leaning back against a stool. I built a standing desk for our office at the height required to stand, which was much less expensive and does most of the job.

-**Instead of an office chair, get a stool that swivels**. The modern chair, and I'm talking about office chairs, sitting chairs, dining room table chairs: all of them, with the knee-bend at ninety degrees and the thighs parallel to the ground is totally alien to the natural motion contours of the human body. Humans ancestrally would squat, low to the ground.[1] Never in

---

1 Squatting is ancestrally the birthing position. Modern gynecology, with tables that position a woman on her back with legs splayed, are the idiosyncratic preferences of the French monarch Louis XIV, who wanted to watch his babies being born. The notion that this position

our evolutionary history did we sit as we do in modern chairs. The modern chair makes it very hard for us to keep the core engaged and the proper curvature in the spine. Sitting in a chair it is very easy to lose contact with the ground.

-Barefoot Shoes are an extraordinary simple and powerful way to deepen your proprioceptive contact with the ground in an effortless daily way. Without exaggeration, I can say that switching my primary footwear to barefoot shoes five years ago was one of the most powerfully transformative and nearly effortless healing technologies I have encountered. In addition to immediately decreasing anxiety (anxiety accelerates when we have an impulse to flee and lose contact with the ground), the proprioceptive inputs totally change the way it feels to be standing. Barefoot shoes are a modern adaptation of the deeply ancestral practice of

-Going barefoot. For many modern people, living in cities, walking on sidewalks, moving across surfaces that are jagged, going barefoot out in the world is not really practical. That said, dramatically increasing the time you spend barefoot, with intention, as a wellness practice, is something I recommend to everyone. It is unlikely you will step on a nail indoors. If you do go barefoot, take the time to

-Feel the Ground beneath your feet. It sounds simple, right, but one of the proprioceptive sequelae of walking around with a slice of rubber under our feet for most of our lives is that we cannot feel the ground in a granular way, and so most of us stop paying attention to these felt sensory inputs. Simply increasing our attention to the felt contact with the ground, and becoming more aware of the way our weight can rest into gravity is the awareness foundation from which the utility of barefoot shoes and going barefoot spring. The soles of your feet (and the palms of your hands[2]) are radar.

---

is the result of evidence-based medical practice is horseshit. Like much of the modern medical canon around birth, it is done for the convenience of the doctor, who was, until recently, usually a man.

2 I've written about the hands as radar at length in *The Neurobiology*

-**Lie on the ground.** If you want to, you can spend several hundred dollars on grounding sheets, which have a thin copper wire extending from them that plugs into the ground of your electrical. Alternatively, you could spend more time lying on the ground. If you are worried about insects, put a blanket down. Be advised that the earth is infinitely specific in the energies that radiate from place. Some places radiate benificent energies and some places, in part because of things that may have happened in or on them, do not. If you are going to spend time lying on the ground it is a good idea to check and see how it makes you feel. If it makes you feel good, chances are that you are lying on a place with beneficent energies. If it makes you feel bad, you might want to move.

-**Rest into Gravity.** One of the principles here, of lying on the ground, is this notion of resting into gravity. Alot of the time we are in motion, and we are making a lot of effort to hold ourselves up, and we are moving quickly. Letting ourselves lie down, letting ourselves feel the pull of gravity, letting ourselves allow the body to be heavy: this is a way of harmonizing with the Earth herself.

-**Slow Down.** Study the pace of natural cycles, and you will notice that nature is not in a hurry. She is not rushing around, hectic, crossing things off her list, feeling frazzled. No, that's only us. One of the simplest and most profound ways that we can GROUND is by slowing down. Moving at an earth-based pace. What is *not* moving at an earth-based place? The internet. Your iPhone. Tiktok. Snapchat. The news cycle. Celebrity gossip. The stock market. Politics. War.

What *is* moving at an earth-based pace? Building a fire. Letting the house get dark when the sun sets. Lighting a candle. Watching wind move through the trees. Listening to the sound of water. Or insects. Or watching raptors catch thermals. Or watching sunlight filter through leaves. Analog things tend to exist at an earth-based pace.

-**The Analog.** Record players. A dedicated camera. Newspaper.

---

of Connection.

Clocks. Maps. Calculators. Landlines. Compasses. Protractors. Hammer and nails. Mallet and chisels. You will notice, perhaps, that many of these tools, with their own form factor, their own uses, have been co-opted by modern digital bricks. Your iPhone can do all of the above except pound a nail and chisel a block of wood. Yet what gets lost? What happens to our sense of grounding, our sense of visceral contact with our surroundings, when all of our tools get digitized, and no longer require the use of the hands?

–**Hammocks are good.** In an autonomically-informed version of the healing arts, every medical and therapy room would have a hammock in it. I'm talking about the Brazilian variety, a *rede*, or net, not the kind with the cross-piece, but the kind that can wrap fully around you. A hammock can give you touch compression across the entire body, while rocking. The restorative autonomic inputs from being rocked while under touch compression track all the way back to the oceanic context of the womb.

–**Inhale earthsmells**: compost, rainwet leaves, new-mown grass. Do you remember the moist and particular exhalation of ferns in rain? Most of us have less traffic with the sense of smell as we grow older because the modern world is so heavily indexed on visuality. But smells, particularly smells from the living world, anchor us to the body, to the senses, to place, to earth. Become purposeful about your use of scent, and smell, to help yourself feel more grounded. (There is nothing that makes my body relax faster than the smell of a campfire. Right?)

–**Get your feet in mud.** Foot-based sensory slickness. When was the last time you let yourself wander outside, barefoot, in a rainstorm?

–**Bidet.** Dare I point out that having a waterjet tickling your anus is proprioceptively useful to maintain contact with the far end of your tailpipe? We recently rented a house with a bidet, and I'm not going back. Again, I know talking about this can make people uncomfortable because we are a culture that is coprophobic. We don't want to think about, look at, or focus on feces. We under-appreciate the degree to which that part of the body is rife with sensory neurology. All you have to do to know this is watch how much fun a baby will have squishing around in a dirty diaper.

-**Understand Systems.** One of the most subtle and insidious ways that Empire, and modernity at large decouple us from our birthright of experiencing ourselves as earth-based creatures is by obscuring the cyclic and systemic nature of our interactions with the Earth. When we can walk into a grocery store, approach the deli counter, and order thin slices of an animal that has been raised by someone else, slaughtered by someone else, cooked by someone else, and prepared by someone else, it is pretty easy to lose touch with both our sense of gratitude, and an understanding of what is required to present this animal as food. I have both experienced, and been regaled by many parents with stories of the shock their 5, or 6, or 7-year-old experiences learning that hamburger comes from a cow. The children are uniformly disgusted by this; many of them feel betrayed. As adults, we can ask how this happens, but the answer is right in front of our faces. If we walk into the grocery store with our kids and order hamburger from the Meat Case, they think that is where it comes from. Our failure to understand complex systems is part of why we get into our gas-powered cars everyday. These decouplings preserve the status quo of alienation. It is possible to disrupt this; here are a few simple ways:

-**Pee outside:** One of the peculiarly malignant ways in which capitalism operates is to teach us that our biological outputs are disgusting, and must be vacated and swept away. I actually got suspended in highschool for peeing through the fence of a tennis court during a match at an opposing school when I couldn't find my coach to authorize a bathroom break. *Disgusting! How rude! An insult to our opponents!* Here's the thing though: we are the only animals that don't pee outside. We've been socialized to pee into a little basin of water in our bathrooms, which then flushes, whisking our turds and urine away into an underground labyrinth of sewers, or a septic system. So you flush your urine and feces down the drain every day. These biological outputs though, intriguingly, are actually the building blocks of fertilizer. Think about it. When you fertilize plants, what do you do it with? Ammonia-based fertilizers, and manure-based fertilizers. Manure is the linguistically non-defiled word for animal feces. We are taught to throw away our foodscraps, our eggshells, our urine, and our poop, yet every one of these things is actually required as inputs to create soil and to nourish plants. We then have to go out and pay money to buy fertilizer, when we have just discarded, as though it has no value, all the things that our bodies naturally produce that we could make fertilizer with. Do you see how ironic this is? To be clear, I am not advocating for farming with your own feces.[3] I'm just pointing out how the systematization of this disconnection is self-reinforcing to create deeper dependency on capitalistic systems, which are fragile, rather than self-sufficiency, which is anti-fragile. When we understand the systems, we can make different choices.

-Stop burning carbon. What would be ideal is if we could walk, and bicycle, and use mass forms of transportation. What would be ideal is if our homes were solar-powered, and harvested sunlight to run them. No one ever mentioned this as a selling point for EVs, but from the moment I started driving one I felt more connected to the earth, because I didn't have to dissociate from my awareness that I was damaging her every day.

-There is no such thing as away. Ecologist/ activist Julia Butterfly Hill pointed this out a long time ago. We say, "We are throwing it away." But there is no *away*. If, like nature, we were required to use all of our inputs as outputs, if, like nature, we could waste nothing– what would we do? How would we build? The primary reason we are not in touch with this is because nothing in the modern economic world is correctly priced. We externalize all of the ecological costs of our harm

---

3   This is actually called humanure if you'd want to dig deeper into this shit ;)

back to the earth herself. If things were priced accurately, that petroleum-derived single-use plastic fork would cost forty dollars, not two cents, because it will not degrade for thousands of years, and it is therefore a problem that we are passing forward for dozens of generations. If we, instead of the earth, had to pay the price for this indulgence, it would be prohibitively expensive. So too would be oil, air travel, takeout food, fast-food, fast fashion...

Thanks to Lu Hanessian, Molly Weingrod, Vera Love, Garrett Whitney, Tosca DeVito for contributing to this list

Illnesses of the Grounding System

While out of deference to the global scientific community and the peer-review research process this list must be considered anecdotal, as it is not yet validated by empirical peer-review research (that is on the way...), our research team at Hearth Science has, for the past decade, been rigorously studying the relationship between autonomic states, autonomic injury, and pathogenesis: the etiology of disease. The following is a list of diseases and conditions whose development, in our experience, cannot take place without truamatic stress injury specifically resulting in chronicity of the shutdown response (and its variants of Placate and Tonic Immobility), which is what happens to our Grounding System under lifethreat.

You will note, as well, that some of these issues are 'physical' and some of them are 'mental health'. From the lens of autonomics, this distinction becomes antique, because all stress-related issues are mindbody issues given that the Autonomic Nervous System is the neural architecture of the mindbody connection.

⊕

Addiction, certain types (as I've pointed out in the book, most of us are self-medicating to a degree we do not recognize, in the moment-to-moment modulation of autonomic state throughout the day. This has varying degrees of adverse consequence for us, depending on what we are self-medicating with, but often the root of addiction is our unwillingness to be present with an internal visceral experience or feeling.)

Categories of Inflammatory Bowel Disease, including:

Crohn's Disease, SIBO, Ulcerative Colitis, Mast Cell Activation Syndrome, etc.

Auto-Immune Illness broadly construed

Billionaires

Cancer

Complex Chronic Illness broadly construed, including co-infections such as Lyme Disease, mold toxicity, etc.

Complex Regional Pain Syndrome

Depersonalization, De-Realization

Developmental Trauma

Digestive Difficulties (anytime the body moves into shutdown digestion is compromised)

Dissociation, and Dissociative Disorders

Eco-Detachment (pervasive in modernity, not diagnosed as a disease or disorder, unquestionably a disease and disorder)

Major Depression and **Bipolar Disorder**

Myalgic Encephalomyelitis/ Chronic Fatigue Syndrome

Parkinson's Disease

Personality Disorders

Post Traumatic Stress Injuries (this is typically referred to as PTSD, and conceptualized as a Disorder, but this class of disease is the neurobiological sequelae of an autonomic injury, not a disorder)

Psychosis (shutdown and extreme pressure)

Risk-taking behaviors of various kinds (if we feel dead inside, we may engage in risky behaviors to feel more alive.)

Shock trauma (usually what we mean by shock trauma is that someone got shifted into a shutdown response: either pure shutdown or tonic immobility)

AUTONOMIC MANDALA

12 COMPETE

11 PLAY

10 CONNECT

9 ENJOY

8 RESTORE

7 UNION

1 ACCOMMODATE

2 APPEASE

3 FIGHT / FLIGHT

4 FREEZE

5 PLACATE

6 SHUTDOWN

© HEARTH SCIENCE, INC.

An Interview with Natureza Gabriel about GROUND

Q: *The book has a quality of existing in what I'm going to call a 'suspended present'. Can you talk about this quality?*

A: When I'm working on a project like this, by which I mean a book that I'm going to fully invest in, as compared to a guide, or a coursebook, or a summary, I am really surrendering to it, and allowing it to take me where it wants to go. I have this sense, which is probably common among fiction writers and maybe less common among non-fiction writers, that I don't really know where the book is trying to take me, what I will learn along the way, or where we will end up. If you are writing fiction, you learn to expose yourself to the possibility that your characters will surprise you. This is part of what makes it interesting to read. Fiction that is fully plotted in advance feels formulaic. You get drawn into a story when your readerly revelation is happening in tandem with writerly revelation because the writer didn't know their character was going to say that, or do that, either. This attitude in fiction writing is a kind of tracking. You put yourself in the presence of characters, in situations, and you permit your characters to spontaneously respond, and you document this.

What I'm doing has more in common with this methodology than what is usually happening in a book about neuroscience. In the Autonomics Trilogy, what I've been trying to do is allow the neurological systems themselves, in what I'll call their manifest or archetypal wisdom, to speak through me. The books are, I hope, transmissional. I'm making myself available to something coming through me. And my method in this book, of taking off my shoes and putting my feet on the ground when I wrote, was part of this invitation to the Grounding System, and the earth with which it is in contact, to speak through me.

William Faulkner says this thing in *Requiem for a Nun: The past is never dead. It's not even past.* And one of the strange things about working on the book, strange in a way that I hope is useful, is that when I allowed the grounding system to speak through me, this had nothing to do with time. I found myself in this temporality, or a-temporality, that is what you are referring to as a 'suspended' or sustained present.

Part of what I'm proposing in the book that is radical- I don't know if I say it outright, but I want you to feel it- is that that the story of Adam and Eve is not in the past. It's right here, because it is an embedded fulcrum of culture. It purports to be speaking about something at the origin of things, but let's be honest: humans have been here somewhere between several hundred thousand and seven million years. No one writing the story of Genesis was there when humans originated. The story is an explanation of something that the writers did not witness.

And this explanatory power- what it means- is baked into modernity in the west the way that yeast is baked into bread. It is part of what made the bread rise the way that it did. Because this story of Adam and Eve, and orginal sin, is baked into the Catholic church, and the Catholic faith, and this sense of antecedent guilt (alienation) gives rise to Supremacy, and this Supremacy, among other things, creates the legal and cultural foundations for colonialism, and colonialism births the modern incarnation of capitalism, which is the water we are swimming in. So all of us, modern people, are embedded in a culture that is structured by all of these things. I've taken a handful of what I think are the most potent structuring ingredients- these Biblical stories, the origin of right angles, the origin of enclosure, and I'm asking how these foundational expressions of alienation have gotten baked into us. Not at some time in the past: how are they alive in us now? How do they operate within us, as a structuring of our inner worlds, and how it feels to live in our bodies, and how might we transform this.

Because the alienation, which is part of our ungrounding, is very old culturally. It didn't start with us. Those of us alive now were born into at least 12,000 years of this. I'm wanting to shed light on this cartography of alienation.

Q: The book begins with a dedication that reads: This is not a book. This is an initiation. Prepare accordingly. And it sort of ends with a question. The second to last chapter contains pages and pages of empty space. What are you up to here?

When we listen to a piece of classical music, let's say a symphony, there is a way that a composer will typically organize embedded motifs such that they elaborate during the piece, and then come together and resolve. When you are listening to the concluding movement of a piece of music like this, there is a bodily registration of the whole orchestration coming together, and we tend to experience this moment cathartically. It releases the tension that was built up during the movement.

But what about when you are interacting with art that asks something of you? If that resolution happens in the artwork itself, it doesn't require anything from you. No critical engagement. So self-examination. No internal friction. It doesn't make you work.

There is a moment in the history of theatre where playwrights and theatre companies started breaking the fourth wall. The fourth wall is a term that began to be used in 19th century theater, and it refers to this kind of imaginary wall between the stage and the audience. This is the traditional theatrical conceit where a play takes place before you, as if you are looking into the rooms where action is happening. This is obviously an artifice, but it is the artifice that theater depends upon.

When the fourth wall is broken, it might be that a character turns to the audience and addresses them directly. Or that we can see the ropes and lighting of a prop on the stage, making it harder to accept the simple veracity of the object. In a way this shatters the illusion of the imaginary world. It is a rupture in the framing of representation. But once that fourth wall is broken, the audience is implicated. The audience is now part of the play. And this changes our understanding of who we, as an audience are, related to the theatrical work that is happening.

This was done as far back as classical Greek plays, it happens sometimes in Shakespeare's soliloquies, but it wasn't really used as fundamental technique until Berthold Brecht, the German playwright, elaborated this theory of *Verfremdungseffekt*, or the 'alienation effect' that was designed to keep reminding the audience that they were watching a play, such that they would engage with it critically.

Part of my objective in GROUND is that the reader experience themselves as being implicated in the text. I'm talking about a modern sense of self, so I'm talking about *us*. I'm not just talking about me. I'm talking about the conditions of the collective: the cultural milieus in which we find ourselves.

And so the book is turning to the reader and reminding you that it requests and even demands some sort of transformation in order to complete itself. For this reason the text resolves on a minor chord, but I hope that completing the reading of the text is not where the work of the book ends. To paraphrase a Zen teaching, *It is a finger pointing at the ground, not the ground itself.* I don't want the reader to get caught up on the finger, I want them to find the ground.

Q: You have written a lot elsewhere about Artificial Intelligence, and the dangers of endstage capitalism, but you are pretty restrained in talking about this in the book, aside from throwing shade on some of the more egregious examples of hoarding, apocalypse merchantry, and ultra-rich white men trying to get off-planet. Why didn't you spend more time in the book talking about the contemporary intersections of psychedelics and AI that seem like very extreme examples of present-day ungroundedness and expressions of domination mind?

I live about fifty miles north of Silicon Valley, which is close enough to experience its emanations pervasively configuring how people where I live think, and far enough away to live in a forest backstage of many of its day-to-day impacts. I deeply appreciate California as a place where when people meet you, they ask you what you do, not where you went to highschool, or what your last name is.

Part of the reason California is a such a hotbed of innovation is because it is not fixated on the past: people here want to know where you are headed, not where you came from. But there is also a danger in this disregard for prior norms and what has come before. Because people in Silicon Valley have succeeded in generating such ungodly sums of money, truly staggering coin, the place has this ethos of thinking it is correct about everything. This creates a hyperbolic narcissism. I have nowhere on earth encountered the density of arrogance you find strolling down almost any street in Palo Alto.

My friend Tiokasin Ghosthorse, of the Lakota, says progress is another word for domination. And Silicon Valley is deeply - DEEPLY - under the sway of domination mind. It has taken domination mind to scale.

People out here are also doing a lot of hallucinogens. Whether it is attending ayahuasca retreats in Costa Rica, or micro-dosing to improve business outcomes, psychedelics are part of the culture. They have been since hippies in Haight Ashbury were tripping LSD in the 1960s.

Psychedelics are non-specific amplifiers. When people take them, the strangeness and intensity of the experience makes them believe that they are experiencing some fundamental aspect of reality. But some of the most delusional people I have ever met regularly use psychedelics.

TESCREAL is an acronym that was proposed by computer scientist Timnit Gebru and philosopher Émile P. Torres. It stands for Transhumanism, Extropianism, Singularitarianism, (modern) Cosmism, Rationalists, Effective Altruism, and Longtermism. Gebru and Torres propose that these ideologies should be treated as a sort of cultural framework that formats much Silicon Valley thinking, and allows the threat of human extinction to justify extremely asset intensive or detrimental projects (transhumanism is essentially eugenics dressed up in new clothes). This ideological stew provides the framework required to justify Artificial General Intelligence, work on life extension, and work on space colonization: three areas with which Silicon Valley is totally obsessed.

This tech elite rhetoric– and the attitudes that it creates– have become foundational justification for much of the global capital flows over the past several years. In the United States, without the AI trade the country would likely already be in a recession. The scholar Nese Devenot, in her illuminating 2023 paper *TESCREAL hallucinations: Psychedelic and AI hype as inequality engines*[1], focalizes the many ways in which the TESCREAL worldview is an accelerator of inequality.

Emil Torres explains: *The key idea at the very heart of the TESCREAL worldview is this techno-utopian vision of the future whereby we develop advanced technologies that enable us to radically reengineer the human organism to create a new post-human species — so-called transhumanism. We will spread beyond Earth, colonize Mars and then the rest of the galaxy, and ultimately create vast computer simulations full of trillions and trillions of digital people.*

It would be interesting if this constellation of ideas were original. It is not. It is simply the latest, psychedelically-addled, AI-infused, digitally-inflected format of the domination paradigm uprooted humans have been refining since Rome.

Since my goal in this book is to speak to something fundamental in human nature, more deeply than its specific formulation at this moment, I have opted not to dwell on it in the text itself.

---

1 Devenot, Nese, 2023, *TESCREAL hallucinations: Psychedelic and AI hype as inequality engines*, Journal of Psychedelic Studies, Volume 7: Issue S1, pages 22-39
https://doi.org/10.1556/2054.2023.00292

What I would point out categorically, is that the most vocal exponents of this worldview, people like Peter Thiel, Elon Musk, and Sam Altman, in addition to being billionaires, share incredible asymmetry in their brain functioning. These are men who have organized their sense of self profoundly in the left, literal, linear, 'rational' side of the cranial brain. All of them were *severely* traumatized as young people. The legacy of this early childhood adversity cannot be overstated. These are people who have not healed.

Everything we are talking about in GROUND has to do with embodiment. Embodied experience flows up from the body into the right hemisphere of the brain. People who do not have access to their embodied experience because they are inwardly frozen, whose grounding systems are not available, do not have access to the right hemisphere of the brain, and therefore live exclusively on the left side of it, become mentally unbalanced in specific and predictable ways.

If you add to that asymmetry copious quantities of ketamine, for example, which is dissociative, you end up with someone so deep in a reality distortion field of their own creation there is no exit from it. If that person has functionally endless resources at their disposal, you end up with Kings of Delusion doing everything in their power to build a future for us all, little different than what the Emperors of Antiquity were up to in their day.

My invitation to all of us who don't want to live immobile in pods pluggeed into a digital simulation is to find the GROUND beneath our own feet, so that we can create a different set of futures. For all their bluster, certainty, and grand rhetoric about super-intelligence, humanoid robots, the Anti-Christ, and life on Mars, you will notice that none of these people appear, in the least, to be happy.

To the Emperors of the Ancient World, and the present World: you are merely Masters of Outer Darkness.

About the Author

Natureza Gabriel (aka Gabriel Kram) is the principal neural architect of Autonomics, a cutting-edge & ancestral re-imagining of living autonomic physiology, which he has developed over 30 years of trans-disciplinary study and research with input from well over 5,000 wellness professionals, and 100 mentors and advisors from 25 lineages of healing in 24 cultures. His mind was trained at Yale and Stanford Universities, his heart has been educated in ceremonies and circles. He has spent 30 years studying connection through the lenses of neuroscience, mindful awareness, social justice, deep nature connection, non-cognitive ways of knowing, Indigenous Lifeways, and cultural linguistics.

Gabriel is Founder of Hearth Science: a translation research firm pioneering the union of neurophysiology and ancestral awareness to turn on the deepest drivers of human wellbeing. He leads the Autonomics Clinic, develops autonomic neurotechnologies, and teaches internationally. He has been asked to teach Autonomics to people in 50 countries, executives in Fortune 500 companies, the faculty of medical schools, governments, international NGOs, and tribal leaders. GROUND is the second book of the Autonomics Trilogy, which begins with *The Neurobiology of Connection*, and concludes with *Body as Verb*. You can find more of his work, as well as that of the extraordinary faculty of Hearth Science at

HTTP://www.hearthscience.io

HTTP://www.naturezagabriel.com

www.ingramcontent.com/pod-product-compliance
Lightning Source LLC
Chambersburg PA
CBHW052126030426
42337CB00028B/5048